21.00

D1329495

SAUNDERS MONOGRAPHS IN PHYSIOLOGY

CLINICAL RESPIRATORY PHYSIOLOGY

AUBREY E. TAYLOR, Ph.D.

Professor and Chairman
Department of Physiology
University of South Alabama
College of Medicine
Mobile, Alabama

KAI REHDER, M.D.

Professor, Department of Anesthesiology
Mayo Clinic
Rochester, Minnesota

ROBERT E. HYATT, M.D.

Professor of Physiology and Medicine
Mayo Clinic
Rochester, Minnesota

JAMES C. PARKER, Ph.D.

Professor, Department of Physiology
University of South Alabama
College of Medicine
Mobile, Alabama

A SAUNDERS MONOGRAPH IN PHYSIOLOGY

1989
W. B. SAUNDERS COMPANY
Harcourt Brace Jovanovich, Inc.
Philadelphia/London/Toronto/Montreal/Sydney/Tokyo

W. B. SAUNDERS COMPANY
Harcourt Brace Jovanovich, Inc.

The Curtis Center
Independence Square West
Philadelphia, PA 19106

Library of Congress Cataloging-in-Publication Data

Clinical respiratory physiology / Aubrey E. Taylor . . . [et al.].
   p.   cm.—(A Saunders monograph in physiology)
   ISBN 0-7216-2484-7
   1. Respiration. 2. Lungs—Physiology. I. Taylor, Aubrey E.
II. Series.
   [DNLM: 1. Respiration. 2. Respiratory System—physiology. WF
102 C641]
QP121.C55 1989
612'.2—dc19
DNLM/DLC
                            88-6717

Editor: Martin Wonsiewicz
Designer: Maureen Sweeney
Production Manager: Carolyn Naylor
Manuscript Editor: Amy Eckenthal
Illustration Coordinator: Brett MacNaughton
Indexer: Nancy Newman

Clinical Respiratory Physiology   ISBN 0-7216-2484-7

Last digit is the print number: 9   8   7   6   5   4   3   2   1

PREFACE

As we began this book, we defined only one major objective and that was to produce a textbook that *not only* contained the basic physiological principles to provide an understanding of respiratory physiology to medical and graduate students, but also a text that contained logical explanations of the many mechanisms responsible for the functional aspects of respiration in all areas of lung physiology. The final goal of each chapter was to expand these concepts and ideas to integrative problem solving.

To accomplish this specific objective, we set several goals: The first was to combine our individual expertises in such a fashion as to produce a "single-authored text." Although each author obviously imparted his own expertise into his respective area of interest in some chapters, each author also provided equal input into all chapters, so this approach has truly produced a "single, four-authored text." Second, the classic areas of respiratory physiology are carefully presented in chapters dealing with lung structure, cell function, lung mechanics, ventilation, gas exchange, ventilation/perfusion, acid-base balance, and respiratory control, and in each area precise explanations for all phenomena are carefully developed. Third, we boldly included chapters usually not fully developed in basic respiratory physiology texts, such as pulmonary and bronchial circulations; lung fluid balance, which includes epithelial transport and pleural fluid formation; clinical pulmonary tests, including the most comprehensive table of clinical tests now available; therapeutic ventilation, including high frequency ventilation arguments; and altitude adaption and diving physiology, including a discussion of gas exchange in exercise. These chapters present the student with state-of-the-art knowledge in several areas of respiratory physiology by providing an integrative approach to learning lung physiology. Fourth, we provide questions and answers for each chapter that are designed to acquaint the student with a working knowledge of the basic equations and theories that are necessary tools to understand respiratory physiology. In addition, these problems and examples introduce the student to clinical situations in a problem-solving mode that requires the knowledge contained in each chapter, as well as previous chapters, in order to incorporate an integrative approach to respiratory physiology in every step of the learning process. Fifth, we have provided a few general references for the readers who wish to gain additional information in any specific area. Sixth, we redrew and simplified many familiar respiratory function curves in an attempt to make them more readily understandable to the student. We have also developed many new figures that describe less generally known lung phenomena, such as airway and alveolar transport, pleural fluid dynamics, and respiratory function in exercise.

Finally, we strove to produce a text that would allow the respiratory community and its future practitioners to experience the joys and pleasures of learning respiratory physiology that we have experienced with our peers over the years. Few other workers in medicine or science consider each other's areas of expertise with the same excitement and helpful criticism as occurs among the various disciplines in respiratory physiology and respiratory medicine. We tried to make this book reflect this attitude of our peers and colleagues, and we hope this book will be useful to them and their students.

We have worked hard at this pleasant task, but there will be errors, misstatements, and omissions for which we apologize in advance. We encourage the readers to make us aware of these problems when using this text.

No text is put together without a tremendous amount of help from many friends and coworkers. In Mobile, Sandy Worley retyped the chapters until her trusty IBM Displaywriter had to be replaced with a new IBM-PC. Penny Cook conveyed ideas for design and redesign of the figures to Wendy Hill and excellent figures resulted. At the Mayo Clinic in Rochester, Kathy Street provided expert proofreading of various developmental stages of the text, while in Mobile Drs. Morgan Smith and William Womack undertook daily proofreading with lively discussions of chapters. The book would not be possible without the inputs from these individuals, as well as the input from many other colleagues and students at the Mayo Clinic and the University of South Alabama College of Medicine. We also thank our respective universities for allowing us the time to develop and produce this book. We wish to thank you for reading our book; we hope you like the end product as much as we have enjoyed writing this text.

AUBREY E. TAYLOR
KAI REHDER
ROBERT E. HYATT
JAMES C. PARKER

CONTENTS

CLINICAL
RESPIRATORY
PHYSIOLOGY

1

ANATOMY AND FUNCTION OF THE LUNG

HISTORY OF PULMONARY PHYSIOLOGY

From the beginning of recorded time, man wondered why he breathed and what constituent of air was necessary for his survival. The basic idea that air and blood meet within the lung dates back to the earliest cradle of Greek science, located in Ionia. In the 6th century BC, Anaximenes postulated that *Pneuma* (or air) was related to breathing, and Diogenes later proposed that *Pneuma* was necessary to maintain life in both man and animals. The term "artery" was first used to describe the trachea and bronchi, which were thought to carry *Pneuma* to the heart. In the 5th century BC, the Hippocratic Corpus defined how arteries left the heart to distribute blood to all the body and "supplied the human body with life." Plato commented on the lung's ability to cool the blood, which was believed to be heated by the heart. Praxagoras,

3

in the 3rd century BC, made the distinction between arteries and veins and felt that the left ventricle and arteries were filled only with air, whereas the right ventricle and veins were filled only with blood.

It remained for one of the distinguished scientists working at Ptolemy's Library in Alexandria to first define lung function. Herophylos, who had studied in Cos with Praxagoras, defined pulmonary function as "absorption of fresh air, distribution of this air to the body, collection of air returning from the body and evacuation of vitiated air to the exterior." Galen, the most famous of all physicians, postulated that blood flowing through the lungs gathered its nourishment from *Pneuma* and, in turn, nourished the body. Thus, Galen was the first to realize that *Pneuma* was the source of energy. In addition, he defined the pulmonary circulation as a unidirectional flow of blood into the lung but also speculated that air entered the left ventricle. Ibn Nafis, an Arab physician living in the 13th century, ascribed the mixing of venous blood with air to the pulmonary circulation (which "purified" the blood) and described the return of the oxygenated blood to the left chamber of the heart. Servantes was burned at the stake when he further developed this theory to explain the change in the color of blood after it passed through the lungs. William Harvey demonstrated that the right heart pumped blood into the pulmonary artery and returned it to the left ventricle, but he still felt that the major function of the lungs was to cool the hot blood from the heart. Malpighi described the pulmonary capillaries and the alveoli, finally providing a complete anatomical understanding of the blood vessels in the lung.

Robert Boyle, in the late 17th century, studied the properties of air and recognized that it was necessary for life. Richard Lower performed several ingenious experiments that demonstrated that venous blood exposed to air turned red and that this process was not due to heat transferred from the heart. After Lower's experiments, research in the area of vital gases rapidly expanded. Hales actually tried to measure air exchange in 1731, and Joseph Black discovered CO_2 in 1757. The existence of CO_2, however, was not well accepted until 1774 when Priestley rediscovered it. More importantly, Priestley also discovered a gas (oxygen) that caused a candle to burn brighter. In 1775, Priestley showed that mice lived for longer periods of time in the presence of oxygen than in its absence. In the 1780s, Lavoisier showed explicitly that air entered the lung where oxygen was exchanged for CO_2, causing the blood to turn red. From this time on, pulmonary physiology blossomed as a discipline, and the amount of information in the field mushroomed. No discussion of the numerous studies or the great respiratory scientists of the 20th century will be made here, but this book relies quite heavily on their experimental data and ideas.

ANATOMY OF THE RESPIRATORY SYSTEM

The upper respiratory tract, as shown in Figure 1–1, includes the nose, nasopharynx, larynx, and trachea. The nasal turbinates provide a large surface

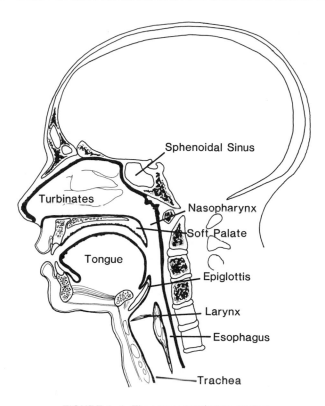

FIGURE 1–1. The upper respiratory system.

area for heat and water exchange. The volume of gas that fills the upper respiratory tract, down to and including the larynx, constitutes about one-half of the volume of inhaled gas that does not exchange with blood.

The trachea, with its cartilaginous rings, extends from the lower part of the larynx (at the level of the sixth cervical vertebra) to the upper border of the fifth thoracic vertebra. Here it divides into two mainstem bronchi. The right mainstem bronchus is wider and shorter than the left. Since it deviates less from the axis of the trachea than the left, foreign bodies enter the right mainstem bronchus more easily than the left. The right mainstem bronchus gives rise to (1) the lobar bronchus of the right upper lobe and (2) the intermediate bronchus, which then divides into bronchi supplying the middle and lower lobes. The left mainstem bronchus gives rise to the left upper and lower lobar bronchi, since the left lung has only two lobes. The conducting airways include the trachea, the mainstem bronchi, the lobar and segmental bronchi, and additional branches down to and including the terminal bronchioles.

The visceral pleura covers the surface of each lung and dips into the fissures that separate the lobes. This pleura is continuous at the hilus with the parietal pleura that covers the inner surface of the chest wall, diaphragm, and mediastinum. In man, each lung has its own separate pleural sac. The intrapleural space is located between the visceral and parietal pleural membranes. It is a true space in healthy individuals, averaging some 20 μm in thickness. The intrapleural space contains a small amount of fluid, which is thought to arise from the parietal pleural and visceral pleural surfaces of the lungs; this fluid is transported downward and removed by lymphatic-like structures located in the parietal pleura and diaphragm. The pleural fluid pressure is subatmospheric and in an upright lung is more subatmospheric at the top of the lung relative to the bottom of the lung.

The lung is served by two sets of blood vessels. One set of vessels is derived from the low pressure pulmonary arteries and is responsible for supplying the blood involved in gas exchange. The other group of vessels arises from the high pressure bronchial arteries and supplies blood to meet the metabolic needs of the larger airways, visceral pleura, and large pulmonary vessels. The pulmonary arterial system accompanies the bronchial tree down to the level of the alveolar ducts, where it terminates in a dense network of capillaries in the alveolar walls. The surface area of the alveolar capillaries is tremendous and facilitates gas exchange in the lung. The pulmonary venules arise primarily from the pulmonary capillaries of the alveoli. They coalesce into the pulmonary veins, which do not accompany the corresponding bronchial and arterial trees. Instead, the pulmonary veins course in the intralobar septa to the hilus.

The bronchial arteries generally arise from the thoracic aorta but can originate from the intercostal, internal mammary, and subclavian arteries. The bronchial arteries accompany the airways down to the level of the terminal bronchioles, where they merge with the pulmonary capillaries and venules. There are extensive postcapillary anastomoses between the pulmonary and bronchial circulations, but venous blood from the large bronchi drains into the bronchial veins, which empty into the azygous and hemiazygous veins.

Pulmonary lymphatics, which remove fluid from the pulmonary interstitium, are found superficially in the visceral pleura as well as deep within the lung in the peribronchial and perivascular spaces. These lymphatics surround the blood vessels and bronchi and extend down to the respiratory bronchioles. No lymphatics have been found within the alveolar walls. The visceral pleural lymphatics course over the surface of the lung toward the hilus where they anastomose with deep lymphatics. The larger lymphatics contain one-way valves, which prevent reflux of lymph from the superficial back to the deep lymphatics. Pulmonary lymph flows to the hilar lymph nodes and eventually reaches the blood stream through the thoracic and right and left lymphatic ducts. The lymphatics have an intrinsic pumping action that provides the pressure necessary to propel lymph through these valvular structures. In humans, most lung lymph enters the right lymphatic duct, and only the left upper lobe drains into the thoracic duct. In contrast to pulmonary interstitial fluid, the pleural fluid is cleared via the extensive lymphatic system in the chest wall through structures called lacunae, which are most abundant in the lower region of the chest wall.

FUNCTIONS OF THE RESPIRATORY SYSTEM

Gas Exchange

Gas exchange is the major function of the lung. The normal human usually breathes 15 times per minute; each breath contains approximately 500 ml of air. Thus, the lungs ventilate at least 10,800 l/day. In addition, approximately 5,700 l/day of blood flow through the lungs. About 600 l/day of oxygen are transferred from the inspired gas into the pulmonary blood, whereas 460 l/day of CO_2 are removed. The remaining oxygen (140 l/day) is combined with H_2 as water. The lung also functions as an impressive regulator of acid-base balance by excreting 12,000 mEq of carbonic acid per day. This is a tremendous amount of H^+ exchange as compared with the kidney, which can only excrete 80 mEq of fixed acid per day.

Speech

The thoracic cage can be thought of as a respiratory bellows that supplies expiratory gas flow to the vocal apparatus for speech. This gas flow is generated by the elastic recoil of the lungs and chest wall and by contraction of the expiratory muscles. The inspiratory muscles can modify the expiratory forces in order to fine tune the driving pressure that forces gas through the vocal cords. Experienced speakers and trained singers exert precise control over the size of the glottis and supravocal tracts. Pitch, loudness, and quality of the voice depend upon an exact interaction of the functions of the chest cage with those of the glottis and supravocal tract. This precise control of speech requires that carefully programmed sets of nerve impulses be relayed to the speech apparatus. Feedback control from various auditory, proprioreceptor, and tactile receptors helps to develop these patterns during learning. Muscle spindles indicate the relative state of muscle contraction, and this information is integrated in the spinal cord in relation to impulses arising from higher centers. There are many muscle spindles in the intercostal muscles and in the muscles of the pharynx that are responsible for control of subglottic pressure. In contrast, the diaphragm, which plays no active role during speech or singing, has few muscle spindles.

It has been suggested that human speech developed when man began to assume an upright position. It is thought that this postural change led to structural alterations in the supravocal tract that caused the descent of the larynx and the development of a long, mobile pharynx, a necessary component of speech. An interesting example illustrating the nature of normal speech is seen when an individual switches from breathing air to breathing a less dense gas mixture such as 20% oxygen and 80% helium. Initially, the voice becomes high-pitched and squeaky; however, if the subject breathes this gas over a long period of time, the speech pattern changes to accommodate the gas density, such that the voice returns toward normal pitch.

Cardiovascular Effects

The state of lung inflation alters the pleural pressure and directly affects the heart. Decreases in pleural pressure lead to an increase in the transmural pressure of the heart, which improves filling of the ventricles and increases cardiac output; conversely, increases in pleural pressure, such as those associated with positive pressure ventilation, cause filling of the ventricles to decrease, and cardiac output falls. Venous return is also compromised by high pleural pressure, resulting in a decrease in cardiac output. A complete discussion of the cardiopulmonary interactions is beyond the scope of this book, but the student should remember that the cardiovascular and respiratory systems are linked mechanically, and ventilation can greatly affect cardiac pumping effectiveness.

Metabolic Functions

Since the entire cardiac output passes through the extensive pulmonary capillary bed, the lung is ideally suited to perform certain metabolic tasks. Figure 1–2A is an electron micrograph of the pulmonary capillary. Figure 1–2B shows the luminal surface in detail. The pulmonary capillaries are lined with a continuous type of endothelium, with junctions of about 20 to 50 Å in radius between the endothelial cells. Small molecules and water can easily move into and out of the pulmonary capillaries through these junctions, but large plasma proteins cannot easily cross the endothelium. The apical surfaces of the endothelial cells form caveolae, where a number of physiologically important enzymes are located. Angiotensin-converting enzyme, which converts angiotensin I to angiotensin II, is located in these caveolae. This same enzyme also degrades bradykinin. The lung can also degrade several other compounds, including norepinephrine and epinephrine. In addition, large vesicles are seen in the endothelium. In some instances, these vesicles appear to coalesce to form a continuous channel (radius of 200 Å) between the capillary and interstitium.

Conditioning of the Inspired Gas

Inspired gas must be warmed to body temperature and fully saturated with water before it reaches the alveoli. By the time it reaches the posterior pharynx, gas is warmed to 33°C, and warming continues until a temperature

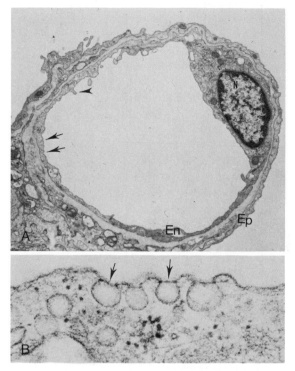

FIGURE 1–2. Electron micrograph of a pulmonary capillary. A, This micrograph shows the alveolar epithelium *(Ep)* and endothelium *(En),* and the endothelium nucleus *(N).* B, The luminal surface is lined with small pits called caveolae (arrows). (Reproduced courtesy of U. Ryan.)

of 37°C is attained in the distal airways. Moderate amounts of water are required to humidify and fully saturate this inspired gas. For example, 12 mg of water per liter of gas, or about 120 ml per day, is required to achieve 100 per cent saturation as the gas is warmed from 30 to 37°C.

Another function of the upper airways is to remove noxious particles and gases from the inhaled gas. The turbulence that develops as gas passes over the nasal turbinates causes deposition of particles on the nasal mucous membranes and dissolution of noxious gases in the liquid lining of the turbinates. For example, concentrations of sulfur dioxide as high as 25 parts per million are almost completely removed as gas passes through the nose. The high ventilation rates seen during exercise cause breathing to occur mainly through the mouth, bypassing the turbinates, and the SO_2 trapping efficiency decreases by 65 per cent.

The morphology of the airway epithelium changes greatly between the large bronchi and the respiratory region. As seen in Figure 1–3, a ciliated columnar epithelium, goblet cells, basement membrane, small glands, and a rather large interstitial space, with smooth muscle cells and cartilage, are found

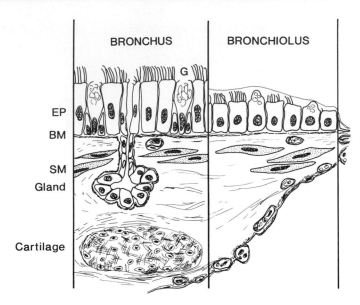

FIGURE 1–3. Schematic representation of airway epithelium. Note ciliated columnar epithelium *(EP),* goblet cells *(G),* basement membrane *(BM),* glands, smooth muscle *(SM),* and cartilage in the bronchus. In the bronchiolus (or terminal bronchiole), epithelial cells become cuboidal and there are no glands. (Modified from Weibel, E.R.: *The Pathway for Oxygen.* Cambridge: Harvard University Press, 1984, p. 236.)

in the large airways. In the terminal bronchioles, the epithelial cells become smaller and cuboidal. This region also contains Clara cells and goblet cells, but submucosal glands are absent. In the alveoli, the epithelial cells are classified either as thin type I pneumocytes or as type II pneumocytes that contain lamellar bodies.

The epithelial cells of the airways are covered with a thin layer of fluid. The fluid is formed by an active Cl⁻ secretory process that causes Na⁺ to passively follow. The accumulation of these ions on the outside of the epithelial cells creates an osmotic pressure that pulls water across the epithelial layer, producing the isotonic fluid layer that surrounds the epithelium. The mucous glands and goblet cells secrete a mucous coat, which floats on top of this fluid layer. The cilia have small claw-like structures on their tips that actually dig into the mucus, moving it toward the pharynx with a rapid, whip-like action. The result is propulsion of the mucous layer, along with any trapped particles, up and out of the terminal airways until it is finally either expelled by the cough mechanism or swallowed. Cilia are found from the nose down to the terminal bronchioles and beat as frequently as 1,000 times per min, moving mucus out of the airways at a velocity of about 10 to 15 mm/min. It is now thought that mucus contains antioxidants that may reduce oxidant-induced injury. So mucus is protective because (1) it coats the epithelial structures with a relatively impermeant, viscous lining; (2) it entraps large particles and aids in their expulsion from the lung; and (3) it acts as an antioxidant medium. The isotonic fluid layer that supports the mucous layer provides water for humidification of the gas and serves as a low resistance pathway so that the cilia can beat more easily than they would in a viscous mucous layer.

The alveolar epithelial membrane is relatively impermeable to small molecules. The alveolar epithelial cells do, however, have the ability to actively transport Na^+ and Cl^- out of the alveoli into the interstitial space, creating an osmotic pressure that pulls water out of the alveoli into the interstitium. This process is necessary to prevent excess accumulation of water in the alveoli, since there is normally a tendency for water to enter the alveoli because of surface tension effects (see hereafter). Under normal conditions, the tendency for water to move into the alveoli is balanced by the tendency for water to be removed; the final result is a thin fluid layer lining the alveoli.

Defense of the Lung Against Infection

The lung normally remains sterile. This is remarkable in view of its continual exposure to an unsterile environment. Although the mucous layer and cilia aid in protecting the lung, the main line of defense against noxious agents, large particles, and bacteria is provided by the macrophages of the distal airways and alveoli. These alveolar macrophages contain lysosomes that digest ingested bacteria and foreign particles. Lymphatics also remove particulate matter, either in its free form or in macrophages contained in lymph. In addition, tissue macrophages can attack any substance that crosses the epithelial membrane. Finally, the blood polymorphonuclear cells act as a last line of defense, since they migrate to the lungs and attack organisms that escape the alveolar macrophage system.

Maintenance of Airway Patency

For normal gas exchange to occur, the airways must remain patent and offer little resistance to gas flow. The respiratory system has several means of maintaining airway patency. For example, neural impulses originating in the respiratory center stimulate the genioglossus and superior pharyngeal constrictor muscles and dilate the pharyngeal airway during inspiration. Contraction of these muscles counteracts the subatmospheric intra-airway pressures generated during inspiration. When this system fails (e.g., in obstructive sleep apnea), a marked narrowing of the airway can occur during inspiration.

The pharynx and the larger airways have considerable amounts of cartilaginous support. The extent of cartilaginous support decreases progressively as the airways become smaller. The smaller airways are composed mostly of elastic tissue and collapse when they are dissected free of the lung. In the intact lung, these small airways are held open by the elastic recoil of the lung parenchyma.

Maintenance of Alveolar Ventilation

The conducting airways of the lung form an enormously complicated branching system in which the terminal airways are surrounded by thousands of alveoli and alveolar ducts. This arrangement of branching airways is illustrated in Figure 1–4. In this figure, the human bronchial tree is considered to be symmetric, with each parent branch giving off two smaller daughter branches of equivalent size. Gas moves through the conducting airways to the respiratory bronchioles, alveolar ducts, and, finally, the alveolar sacs. The primary purpose of this system is to properly ventilate the primary lobule or acinus, which is served by a first-order respiratory bronchiole. There are approximately 600,000 such acini in the human lung, each accommodating approximately 0.01 ml. Figure 1–5 shows an acinar unit receiving gas via the terminal bronchiole (TB), which branches into the respiratory bronchioles (RB), their resulting alveolar ducts (AD), and alveoli (A). The blood enters *via* a small pulmonary artery and exits *via* the pulmonary vein. Note the absence of lymphatics in the alveolar walls. Because of airway branching, a remarkable increase in total airway cross-sectional area occurs distally from the trachea (Fig. 1–6).

Maintenance of a Large Alveolar Surface Area

For adequate gas exchange, a very large contact area between alveolar gas and pulmonary capillary blood is necessary. In man this is provided by 3 million alveoli, each with an extremely thin wall, producing a total surface area in the neighborhood of 140 m², the size of a tennis court. An electron micrograph of an alveolar wall is shown in Figure 1–7. An erythrocyte (RBC) occupies most of the capillary. The tissue barrier that gas must pass through is composed of

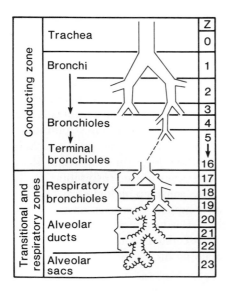

FIGURE 1–4. Schematic representation of airway branching showing the division of the airways into functional zones *(Z)*. (Modified from Weibel, E.R.: *The Pathway for Oxygen.* Cambridge: Harvard University Press, 1984, p. 275.)

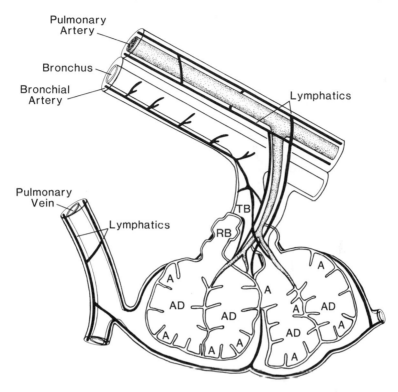

FIGURE 1–5. A primary acinus showing its blood supply and lymphatic drainage. *TB* = terminal bronchiole, *RB* = respiratory bronchiole, *AD* = alveolar duct, *A* = alveoli. (Modified from Comroe, J.H.: *Physiology of Respiration.* Chicago: Year Book Medical Publishers, 1970.)

the alveolar epithelial cell (EP), two basement membranes (BM) separated by a small interstitial space (IS), and the endothelial cell (E). The total alveolar-capillary thickness is approximately 0.35 μm, which is about 1/50 the thickness of a piece of thin airmail stationery.

The lung has developed several adaptations to maintain a thin alveolar membrane and a large total alveolar surface area. Connective tissue fibers weave in and out of the capillaries in the alveolar septum. This crisscrossing network of connective tissue fibers provides support to the alveolar septum but adds little thickness, thus minimizing the distance between capillary blood and alveolar gas. These connective tissue fibers are anchored at both ends to support the alveolar septum. At one end, the fibers are contiguous with the connective tissue fibers that dip into the lung parenchyma from the pleura, whereas at the other end they are anchored to fibers that accompany the pulmonary artery and bronchus. Therefore, alveolar walls are under tension as the lung expands, so that they lengthen and flatten, producing a large surface area.

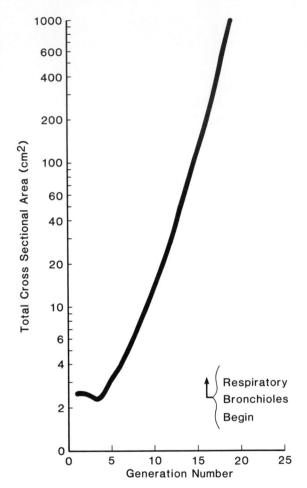

FIGURE 1–6. Total airway cross-sectional area as a function of the number of generations from trachea to alveolar ducts. Note that the scale is logarithmic and that the total cross-sectional area increases dramatically in the small airways.

Prevention of Lung Collapse at Low Volumes—Surfactant

The alveoli are lined by two different types of cells as shown in Figure 1–8A and represented schematically in Figure 1–8B. The epithelial type I pneumocytes (EP1) are extremely thin squamous cells that are similar to the endothelial cells of the capillary walls. The type II pneumocytes (EP2) are characterized by microvilli (MV), a large number of mitochondria, and large lamellar bodies (LB). These lamellar bodies are related to the production of surfactant, which lines the alveoli and reduces their surface tension. The number of type I pneumocytes is only about one-half that of the type II pneumocytes, but their apical area is 25 times that of the type II pneumocytes. This phenomenon is due to the flattened morphology of these type I cells as shown schematically in Figure 1–8B. In fact, the total area of the type I pneumocytes is at least four times that of the pulmonary capillary endothelium. This flattened

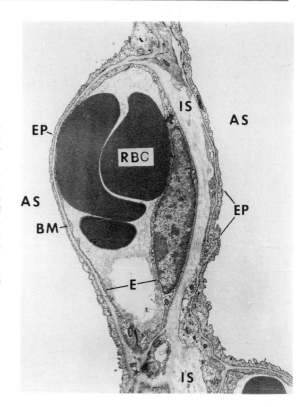

FIGURE 1–7. Electron micrograph of an alveolar capillary in a human lung showing the alveolar space *(AS)*, interstitial space *(IS)*, basement membrane *(BM)*, endothelium *(E)*, continuous epithelium *(EP)*, and an erythrocyte *(RBC)*. Note that the thickness of the alveolar-capillary barrier is extremely small (0.35 μm). (Reprinted with permission from Murray, J.F.: *The Normal Lung.* Philadelphia: W.B. Saunders Co., 1976, p. 47.) (Original provided by E.R. Weibel.)

morphology of the type I cells results in a thin alveolar barrier to gas exchange but also creates a problem since these thin cells are fragile. Type I cells do not replicate; instead, the type II pneumocytes divide and differentiate into type I pneumocytes.

There is an additional challenge in the maintenance of a large uniform alveolar surface area. Since the alveoli are covered by a very thin layer of fluid, a force (called surface tension) is generated at the gas-fluid interface that tends to collapse the alveoli. This tendency to collapse is counteracted to some extent by the connective tissue network described previously, but this network is not sufficient to overcome the surface tension forces generated at the gas-liquid interface. Alveolar collapse still does not occur, however, because the surfactant produced by the type II pneumocytes decreases the surface tension forces.

After it is synthesized, surfactant is stored as lamellar bodies and then secreted onto the alveolar surface. The upper right hand corner of Figure 1–9 shows a type II cell (EP2) containing lamellar bodies. A portion of the liquid layer that lines the alveoli is also seen (LL). The very thin layer of surfactant lying on top of this liquid layer is indicated by the arrows. Surfactant consists of several compounds, but its major component is phosphatidylcholine. Phosphatidylcholine has saturated fatty acids in both the one- and two-carbon po-

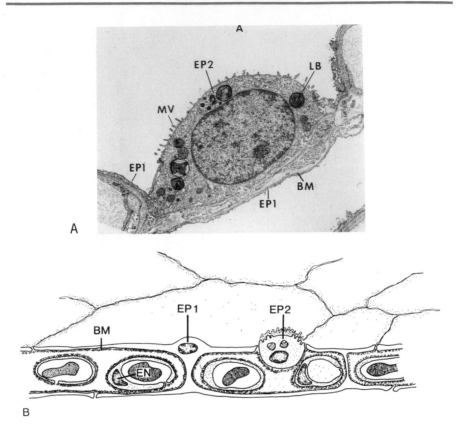

FIGURE 1–8. *A,* Electron micrograph showing epithelial type I *(EP1)* pneumocytes. Note the microvilli *(MV)* and lamellar bodies *(LB)* in the EP2. *B,* Schematic representation of the capillary endothelial *(EN)* barrier and alveolar membrane, showing the basement membrane *(BM)*, and the type I *(EP1)* and type II *(EP2)* cells. Note how type I pneumocytes cover an extensive area of the alveolar membrane. (Reprinted with permission from Weibel, E.R.: *The Pathway for Oxygen.* Cambridge: Harvard University Press, 1984, pp. 254, 256.)

sitions, allowing surfactant to undergo the configurational changes required to reduce surface tension. Several other lipid constituents are also present but in much smaller amounts. Protein is another major constituent of surfactant, representing approximately 11 per cent of its composition.

Surfactant forms a bilayer on the surface of the fluid that lines the alveoli. This bilayer acts to decrease the surface tension of the alveolar–liquid lining layer in much the same way as a detergent decreases the surface tension of water to aid in wetting cloth surfaces. Unlike detergent, the surface tension of surfactant is not constant but changes with area. As the area of the alveolar surface is reduced, the surfactant molecules come closer together, enhancing the surfactant's ability to lower surface tension. This prevents overdistention or collapse of alveoli during the respiratory cycle. Without surfactant, the alveoli tend to expand nonuniformly; some alveoli are larger, some are smaller, and

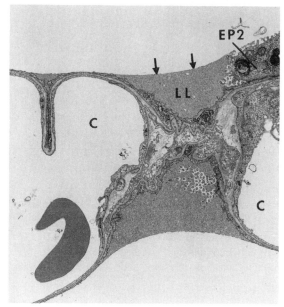

FIGURE 1–9. An electron micrograph of an alveolar septum of a human lung showing the lining layer *(LL)* between capillaries *(C)* covered by the thin layer of surfactant (arrows). (Reprinted with permission from Weibel, E.R.: *The Pathway for Oxygen.* Cambridge: Harvard University Press, 1984, p. 326.)

rather than exchanging gas with the environment, they tend to transfer gas only between themselves. This causes a severe deficiency in gas exchange, which is frequently seen in premature babies. Figure 1–10 shows the surface tension of sheep lung extracts obtained at various times during gestation. Note that surface tension drops precipitously at about 120 days' gestation. At the same time, the number of alveolar cells that contain lamellar bodies also increases, indicating that approximately 120 days is required before the alveolar type II cells begin surfactant production.

Prevention of Lung Collapse—Interdependence

There is another purely mechanical phenomenon that maintains the stability and surface area of the lung. Since the alveoli are held together by the surrounding tissue structures, the individual alveoli in the lungs are not totally independent of one another. The lung has an intricate mesh of interconnecting elastic and collagenous tissue fibers, which tends to oppose any nonuniform changes in regional volume. For example, the tendency to collapse in one area of the lung is opposed by the stretch from tissue fibers in surrounding areas. This phenomenon has been termed "interdependence" and is illustrated by the physical model shown in Figure 1–11. Assume that (1) a series of identical airtight balloons have been glued together; (2) all balloons are fully inflated at a pressure of $+20$ cmH$_2$O and would individually collapse at a pressure of 0 cmH$_2$O; and (3) the pressure in all except the central balloon is held constant at $+20$ cmH$_2$O. Now the pressure within the central balloon (Pcen) is gradually

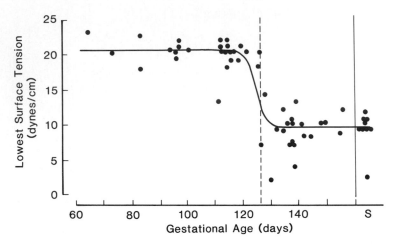

FIGURE 1–10. Surface tension of lung extracts as a function of gestational age in lambs. *S* = spontaneously delivered lambs. (Modified from Orzalesi, M.M., et al.: The development of the lungs of lambs. *Pediatrics 35*:373, 1965.)

decreased to 0 cmH$_2$O. As the pressure in the central balloon falls, the balloon does not collapse, since it is held open by the surrounding, interdependent balloons. Even if the pressure in the central balloon is lowered to −40 cmH$_2$O, total collapse will still not occur. The surrounding balloons are deformed as they oppose this collapse; note how their walls stretch inward. The overall result is an outward force from the peripheral balloons that holds the central balloon open. The tendency of any region of the lung to collapse is opposed by its interdependence with surrounding lung tissue in a similar fashion.

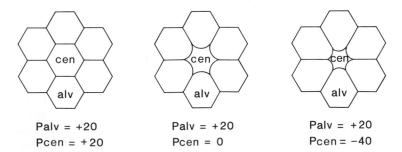

FIGURE 1–11. Cross-sectional shape and pressures in a centrally placed collapsible balloon attached to several other balloons inflated to a pressure of 20 cmH$_2$O. The pressure within the central balloon is decreased in steps from 20 to −40 cmH$_2$O. Note that the central balloon does not totally collapse since it is held open by the surrounding balloons. Palv is pressure in the surrounding balloons, and Pcen is pressure in the central balloon. (Modified from Mead, J., et al.: Stress distribution in lungs: A model of pulmonary elasticity. *J. Appl. Physiol., 28*:596, 1970.)

Matching of Ventilation to Perfusion

In the primary gas exchanging unit of the lung, pulmonary capillary blood is exposed to alveolar gas. The appropriate amount of blood must be brought into contact with the appropriate amount of fresh alveolar gas for adequate amounts of oxygen to be delivered to the body and for carbon dioxide to be removed from the body. This is referred to as matching ventilation to perfusion. Figure 1–12 schematically depicts the worst possible matching of ventilation to perfusion. In this two-alveoli lung model, all blood flow goes to one alveolus, which is not ventilated. Conversely, only the alveolus receiving no blood is ventilated. Clearly, no gas exchange can occur, even though total blood flow and ventilation may be normal.

Ventilation and perfusion must be reasonably well matched in all lung regions for adequate gas exchange to occur. The details of this matching are discussed in a later chapter. But briefly, the distribution of pulmonary blood flow is largely determined by gravity. When a person stands upright, blood flow goes preferentially, but not exclusively, to the lower lobes of the lungs. It is fortunate that most ventilation is also distributed to the bases in an upright individual. Therefore, the system is well engineered for maximal gas exchange by a structural design that matches ventilation to perfusion.

Provision of Collateral Air Channels

When the bronchi leading to a given region of the lung are occluded, the pores of Kohn (3 to 13 μm in diameter) between alveoli, the channels of Lambert (30 μm in diameter) that connect terminal bronchioles to alveoli, and the large

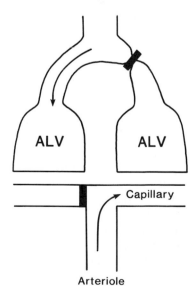

FIGURE 1–12. Schematic showing the worst possible ventilation-to-perfusion mismatch. The alveolus *(ALV)* on the left receives no blood flow but is ventilated. The alveolus on the right has all the blood flow (capillary) but no ventilation. Therefore, these alveoli cannot exchange gas between blood and the environment.

interbronchial connections (80 to 150 μm in diameter) in the terminal airways serve as passageways between the occluded and ventilated regions of the lung. The effectiveness of collateral ventilation varies greatly among species; it is highly developed in the dog, less well developed in man, and almost nonexistent in the lobulated lung of the pig.

NERVE SUPPLY OF THE RESPIRATORY SYSTEM

Motor Innervation

The motor innervation of the lung is derived from the sympathetic and parasympathetic divisions of the autonomic nervous system. Preganglionic parasympathetic fibers travel though the vagus nerve to ganglia located around and within the airways and blood vessels. Postganglionic parasympathetic fibers innervate the epithelial glands and the smooth muscle of the airways and the blood vessels. Postganglionic parasympathetic neurons, which release acetylcholine, represent the primary excitatory innervation of airway smooth muscle in all mammalian species. In the airways of man and other primates, a non-cholinergic-nonadrenergic nervous system provides the primary inhibitory innervation. Sympathetic and parasympathetic regulation of submucosal glands has been demonstrated.

The pulmonary vascular bed receives innervation from both sympathetic and parasympathetic fibers. The density of innervation gradually decreases as the size of the blood vessel decreases, and no nerve fibers are present in blood vessels smaller than 30 μm in diameter. It appears that sympathetic fibers constrict and parasympathetics dilate the blood vessels. However, the exact role of the autonomic system in the reflex control of the pulmonary vasculature has not been firmly established. It is well accepted, however, that the pulmonary arterial system does not exhibit the myogenic reflex seen in peripheral blood vessels. Lymphatic vessels and bronchial arteries and veins are also subject to both parasympathetic and sympathetic innervation.

Sensory Innervation

The upper airways, lungs, and chest wall contain several types of chemoreceptors and mechanoreceptors that respond to inhaled irritants and stresses placed on the respiratory system. These receptors protect the lung from inhaled irritants and help to stabilize alveolar ventilation and gas exchange. The upper airway receptors, which are located in the nose, pharynx, larynx, and trachea, are sensitive to both mechanical and chemical stimuli. Apnea and bradycardia, the "diving reflex," and sneezing are reflexes caused by the stimulation of nasal receptors. Stimulation of the tracheal irritant receptors causes coughing, which serves an important defense role in expulsion of irritant substances.

There are three basic types of receptors within the lung parenchyma: pulmonary stretch receptors, irritant receptors, and J-type receptors. The pulmonary stretch receptors are located within airway smooth muscle and are activated by lung distension. Their afferent neural fibers travel in the vagus nerve. Activation of these receptors causes the Hering-Breuer inflation reflex, which inhibits inspiration.

Irritant receptors lie between epithelial cells of the airways and respond to noxious agents such as particulate matter, cold air, and chemical irritants. Afferent impulses from these receptors travel in myelinated vagal fibers and produce reflex bronchoconstriction and increased ventilation.

The J-type receptors, or juxtapulmonary capillary receptors, lie in the interstitium between the alveoli and capillary walls. Innervation of these receptors is by nonmyelinated vagal fibers. J-type receptors are activated when pulmonary congestion causes an increase in pulmonary interstitial fluid volume. Stimulation of these receptors results in apnea, hypotension, bradycardia, bronchoconstriction, and dyspnea.

There are numerous muscle spindles and Golgi tendon organs located in the intercostal muscles of the chest wall and, to a lesser extent, in the diaphragm. The muscle spindles are arranged to detect changes in the length of these muscles. When they are stimulated, these receptors alter ventilation rate and depth. The muscle spindles and Golgi tendon organs are able to detect and compensate for changes in load imposed on the respiratory system.

SMOOTH MUSCLE OF THE RESPIRATORY SYSTEM

Smooth muscle extends from the trachea to the openings of the alveolar ducts. The fibers are arranged circumferentially in the trachea, connecting the ends of the horseshoe-shaped cartilages. The fibers become more spirally arranged and form a dense network in the intrapulmonary airways. Contraction of airway smooth muscle decreases airway diameter and increases the resistance to gas flow. Contraction of the alveolar duct smooth muscle causes a reduction in lung compliance, i.e., the lung becomes stiffer and more difficult to ventilate.

There is a great deal of interest in the factors responsible for airway smooth muscle tone. The normal functions of the airway smooth muscle are not well defined, but changes in tone are known to affect the volume of gas that does not exchange with the blood and to cause the airways to become more rigid, which alters the maximal rates of gas flow through the bronchi. Excessive contraction of airway smooth muscle is responsible for asthmatic attacks, a common but serious clinical entity. On the whole, however, little is known about the normal functional characteristics of the airway smooth muscle.

The characteristics of pulmonary vascular smooth muscle are also not firmly established. Airway and pulmonary arterial smooth muscle constrict during hypoxia, which results in the shunting of blood and gas away from poorly ventilated areas, thus helping to maintain better ventilation-perfusion matching. Hypoxia appears to cause pulmonary artery constriction by the release of humoral substances and/or a direct effect of hypoxia on the smooth muscle. Recent studies indicate that norepinephrine, epinephrine, angiotensin II, histamine, serotonin, and acetylcholine all constrict normal pulmonary blood vessels, but this effect is dependent on the existing smooth muscle tone of the vascular system. For example, histamine normally constricts pulmonary venules, but with increased vascular tone, such as that seen during alveolar hypoxia or in several forms of lung disease associated with release of vasoconstrictor substances, histamine causes these vessels to dilate. Similar findings have also been reported for epinephrine, i.e., constriction at low tone and dilatation at high tone.

SUMMARY

From this brief overview of lung structure and function it is obvious that the lung is designed to carry out very complex functions. There are a variety of mechanisms that bring about the optimal matching of alveolar ventilation to capillary perfusion to provide adequate gas exchange for a variety of metabolic needs. The lung also effectively defends itself, and consequently the body, against a potentially hostile environment. In addition, the lung performs important metabolic functions and allows us to communicate with each other through speech.

SUGGESTED READING

Cournand, A.: Air and blood. In Fishman, A.P., and Richards, D.W. (eds.): *Circulation of the Blood: Men and Ideas.* Bethesda: American Physiological Society, 1982, pp. 3–70.
Murray, J.F.: *The Normal Lung.* Philadelphia, W.B. Saunders Co., 1986.
Proctor, D.F.: The upper airways. I. Nasal physiology and defense of the lungs. *Am. Rev. Resp. Dis.,* 115:97, 1977.
Proctor, D.F.: The upper airways. II. The larynx and trachea. *Am. Rev. Resp. Dis.,* 115:315, 1977.
Weibel, E.R.: *The Pathway for Oxygen.* Cambridge: Harvard University Press, 1984.

QUESTIONS

1. The cross-sectional area of the bronchial tree increases approximately 500-fold between the 5th and 20th generations. True or false?

2. Pulmonary surfactant is produced by the type I alveolar lining cells. True or false?
3. The major component of pulmonary surfactant is phosphatidylcholine. True or false?
4. The postganglionic parasympathetic neurons constitute the primary inhibitory innervation to airway smooth muscle in man. True or false?

2

PULMONARY GAS VOLUMES AND VENTILATION

GAS VOLUMES

To study pulmonary physiology, the overall system should be defined in relation to the various volumes and capacities that are commonly used to describe lung function. Note that the term "capacity" is used to identify the sum of two or more volumes.

The various volumes and capacities are diagrammed in Figure 2–1. Many of the important volumes and capacities can be measured as shown by having the subject breathe into a spirometer, which consists of two inverted bells. The subject inhales and exhales into the movable inner bell, which is sealed by water. As the subject inhales, the gas volume in the inner bell decreases, and the pen linked by the pulley to the bell moves upward. The opposite occurs during exhalation. As the subject breathes, a tracing is obtained on paper mounted on a drum that revolves at a fixed rate; thus, a tracing of volume change versus time, i.e., a spirogram, is drawn. Reading the spirogram from left to right, the subject first breathes normally, defining the tidal volume (VT). Next the subject inhales maximally and then exhales maximally; this defines the vital capacity (VC). The person returns to tidal breathing and then inhales maximally after normal exhalation; this defines the inspiratory capacity (IC), the sum of the inspiratory reserve volume (IRV) and the tidal volume. After returning to tidal breathing, the subject is asked to exhale completely at the end of a normal expiration; this defines the expiratory reserve volume (ERV).

The block diagram to the left in Figure 2–1 indicates the various volumes and capacities discussed to this point; note that there is an additional volume that cannot be measured with a spirometer. This is the residual volume (RV), which is the amount of gas remaining in the lungs following a maximal expiration. If the residual volume is known, the total lung capacity (TLC) can be computed by adding RV and VC. TLC is the maximal amount of gas the lungs can hold. The residual volume in young adults amounts to about 25 per cent of the total lung capacity, and this fraction increases with age. Residual volume added to the expiratory reserve volume defines the functional residual capacity

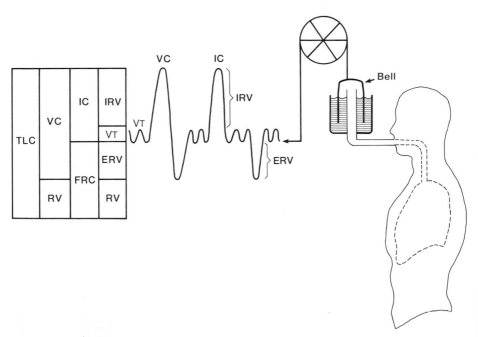

FIGURE 2–1. Diagram showing a human breathing into a spirometer. On expiration the inner bell rises, and on inspiration the inner bell falls. Measurements during normal tidal volume breathing (VT), maximum inspiration and expiration (vital capacity, VC), maximum inspiration (inspiratory reserve volume, IRV, and inspiratory capacity, IC), and maximum expiration (expiratory reserve volume, ERV) are shown. The resulting volumes and various lung capacities are shown in the block diagram on the left. TLC = total lung capacity, RV = residual volume, FRC = functional residual capacity.

(FRC). The FRC is a particularly important measurement because it is the amount of gas remaining in the lungs at the end of a normal, relaxed expiration. As will be seen in Chapter 6, FRC is determined by the balance between the tendencies of the lung to collapse and the chest wall to expand. In upright individuals, the FRC amounts to approximately 50 per cent of the total lung capacity, whereas in the supine position it is about 40 per cent of TLC. Normal values in upright subjects for these various volumes and capacities are given in Chapter 9, but here are some approximate values: TLC = 6 l, FRC = 3 l, RV = 1.5 l, V_T = 0.5 l, ERV = 1.5 l, IC = 3 l, IRV = 2.5 l, and VC = 4.5 l.

Measurement of Residual Volume

Very special techniques are needed to measure the residual volume. Usually the subject's FRC and expiratory reserve volume are measured separately and residual volume is calculated as:

$$RV = FRC - ERV \qquad (2-1)$$

The oldest method used to measure FRC is the *equilibration technique*. The subject is connected, at the end of a normal expiration, to a spirometer containing a known fractional concentration (C_1) of a test gas, such as helium, that is essentially insoluble in the body. The volume of gas in the spirometer (V_1) is known. The subject's FRC is unknown. The subject breathes into the spirometer until the concentration of the test gas in the lung equals that in the spirometer, reaching a fractional concentration of C_2. During the procedure, oxygen is added to the spirometer to match the subject's oxygen consumption, and CO_2 is removed to maintain a constant system volume. Since the initial amount of helium, $C_1 \times V_1$, becomes equally distributed between the spirometer and the subject, then $C_1 \times V_1 = C_2(V_1 + FRC)$. Solving for FRC:

$$FRC = [(C_1 \times V_1)/C_2] - V_1 \qquad (2-2)$$

Another well-established technique used to measure FRC is the *nitrogen washout procedure* (Fig. 2–2). The subject is connected by one-way valves to a bag containing 100% oxygen from which he inhales. The expired gas is collected in a previously evacuated bag. A nitrogen meter records the N_2 concentration at the mouth. Assume that the subject's lungs initially contain nitrogen at a fractional concentration of 0.80 (C_X). At the end of a normal breath, a valve is turned and the patient starts breathing into the system. With each inspiration, the nitrogen within the subject's lungs is diluted by the O_2 (Fig. 2–2B). For simplicity, assume that no nitrogen enters the system from the subject's body and that the subject clears all the nitrogen from his lungs. The

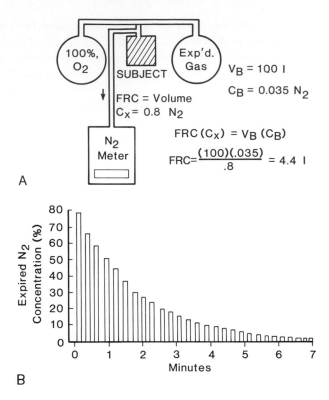

FIGURE 2–2. Measuring FRC using the nitrogen washout procedure. The subject (hatched box) breathes 100% O_2 and exhales into a bag past a N_2 meter. *A,* The expired gas volume (V_B = 100 l) and fractional nitrogen concentration (C_B = 0.035) are used to calculate FRC from the lung concentration of nitrogen (C_x = 0.80). *B,* The nitrogen measured at the mouth piece decreases to 0 with each inhalation of O_2 and rises to a progressively lower level after each breath, illustrating the washout of nitrogen from the lung.

exhaled nitrogen is collected in the expiratory bag; the volume, V_B, and fractional concentration of nitrogen in the bag, C_B, can now be measured:

$$FRC \times C_X = V_B \times C_B$$

or $$FRC = (V_B \times C_B)/C_X$$ (2–3)

if V_B = 100, C_B = 0.035, and C_X = 0.80

then $$FRC = \frac{(100)\ (0.035)}{0.80} = 4.4\ l$$

The pattern of the *nitrogen washout* is shown in Figure 2–2B. The nitrogen meter at the patient's mouth continuously records the N_2 concentration of inhaled and exhaled gas. With each breath of oxygen, the nitrogen meter reading goes to 0 per cent, and with each exhalation it rises. With each breath, the exhaled alveolar N_2 concentration falls until, at the end of 7 minutes, the usual length of the test, alveolar nitrogen has approached 0 per cent. The fact that it does not reach 0 can easily be corrected for, and a small correction is usually made for the amount of nitrogen that enters the lungs from the blood and body tissues.

A *body plethysmograph* is another device used to measure FRC. There are two types of body plethysmographs currently used. In one, the volume of the body plethysmograph is kept constant and pressure changes within the box are measured during respiration. In the other type of plethysmograph (Fig. 2–3), the pressure in the box remains atmospheric, and changes in gas volume during respiration are measured by a spirometer attached to the system. The subject is seated in an airtight box and, wearing a noseclip, breathes in and out through a mouthpiece connected to the atmosphere. As gas enters the lungs, the rib cage expands and displaces the gas from the box into the spirometer, which moves in an outward direction. The opposite occurs during expiration.

The principle involved in measuring lung volumes by the plethysmographic technique is the same regardless of which type of box is used. It is based on Boyle's Gas Law, which says that the product of the pressure and volume of a gas is constant, provided the temperature and number of moles of gas stay constant:

$$PV = P'V' \qquad\qquad (2\text{--}4)$$

Thus, there is an inverse relationship between the volume of a gas and the pressure to which it is exposed. Increasing the pressure causes a decreased

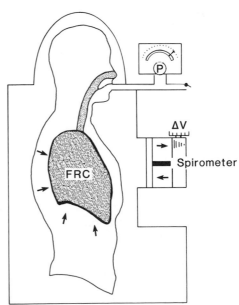

FIGURE 2–3. Diagram of a subject placed into a whole body plethysmograph. The box is airtight and the subject breathes in and out through a mouthpiece connected by a tube to a pressure meter *(P)* and to the atmosphere. The tube can be closed or opened by a flap-type valve. When gas enters the lung, the rib cage expands and displaces gas from the box into the spirometer, which moves in an outward direction to keep the box pressure equal to atmospheric pressure. FRC = functional residual capacity, ΔV, change in volume.

volume. It is important to recall that conditions must be isothermal to apply Boyle's Law. The gas in the lung is isothermal because the pulmonary capillary blood flow is large and serves as a heat sink. As gas is compressed, any increase in temperature is quickly absorbed by the blood flowing past the alveolar gas. Any tendency for temperature to fall during expansion is likewise counteracted by the flowing blood.

The basic procedure for measuring FRC with a body plethysmograph is as follows. With the subject sitting in the airtight plethysmograph, the motion of his chest is recorded by the spirometer attached to the box. At FRC, the airway is temporarily obstructed and the subject attempts to exhale. This maneuver compresses gas in the lungs and raises the airway pressure by ΔP. With no gas flow, airway pressure is equal to alveolar pressure. With the airway occluded and before any effort was made, the alveolar pressure was atmospheric, PB,* and the volume in the lungs was FRC. Upon expiration, the pressure increases by ΔP, whereas the volume of gas in the chest decreases. The change in volume, ΔV, is measured by the attached spirometer. The product of the original volume and its pressure (PB $\times$ FRC) must equal the product of the new volume (FRC $- \Delta V$) times its new pressure (PB $+ \Delta P$):

$$(FRC - \Delta V) (PB + \Delta P) = PB \times FRC$$

$$or\ FRC = (\Delta V/\Delta P)(PB + \Delta P) \qquad (2\text{--}5)$$

Compared with the other methods of determining FRC, the body plethysmographic method is quicker and can easily be repeated when desired. The other two commonly used methods require either washout of all the helium from the individual or reconstitution of the alveolar nitrogen before a repeat measurement can be made. This usually takes from 5 to 20 minutes, and in actual practice only one estimate is made by these methods. In contrast, it is possible to obtain several measurements of FRC in the same period using the body plethysmograph. Often in patients with airway disease, some regions of the lung communicate poorly with the trachea, and the helium dilution and nitrogen washout techniques tend to underestimate the FRC. In contrast, the body plethysmographic method always measures all of the gas contained in the lungs. Thus, it is not uncommon in obstructive lung disease for FRC as measured using the plethysmograph to be 0.5 to 1.0 l higher than that measured by the other techniques. However, the helium and nitrogen methods do give an index of ventilation distribution, which is not provided by the plethysmographic method. This is obtained by noting the time taken for the gas concentration to reach equilibrium in the helium dilution method, and by measuring the alveolar concentration of nitrogen at the end of 7 minutes in the nitrogen washout technique.

---

*Here PB is atmospheric pressure minus water vapor pressure (P_{H_2O}), which is 47 mmHg at body temperature. P_{H_2O} is subtracted because it remains constant throughout the volume and pressure changes during this measurement. Only the dry gases (O_2, N_2, CO_2) obey Boyle's law.

With appropriate correction factors, one can obtain a very good estimate of total lung capacity from *chest roentgenography.* This is a "poor man's" measurement of total lung capacity, but it has been used successfully, particularly in epidemiologic studies. One then need only measure the vital capacity separately to obtain the residual volume (RV = TLC − VC).

Alterations of Lung Volumes in Disease

Figure 2–4*A* shows the important volumes and capacities as a percentage of total lung capacity in a normal subject. Changes that occur in typical obstructive lung disease are shown in Figure 2–4*B*. Note that TLC is increased above the predicted value, VC is decreased, and RV and FRC are both markedly increased. Conversely, the pattern in Figure 2–4*C* illustrates severe restrictive disease, such as pulmonary fibrosis. Here, the VC is also reduced, but in addition there is a marked reduction in TLC, RV, and FRC. The reader is referred to Chapter 6, where these volume changes are related to changes in the elastic properties of the lung.

PULMONARY VENTILATION

Minute Ventilation

The easiest, but least useful, means of estimating ventilation is to collect expired gas over a given time interval, measure the volume, and express it as

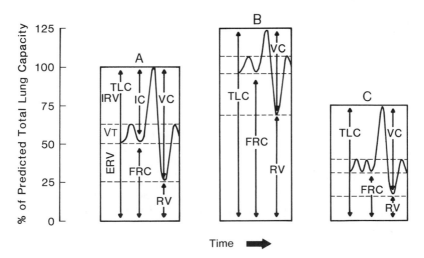

FIGURE 2–4. Various lung volumes and capacities as percentage of predicted total lung capacity for a normal subject *(A)* and in obstructive lung disease *(B)* and in restrictive lung disease *(C).*

liters per minute. Minute ventilation is denoted by the term $\dot{V}_E$, where E stands for expired gas.

Anatomic Dead Space

Although it is useful to know total ventilation, it is more important to know the volume of gas delivered to the alveoli, i.e., the alveolar ventilation ($\dot{V}_A$). This is illustrated in Figure 2–5. Gas that is inhaled into the alveoli passes through the anatomic dead space, namely the conducting airways, which have no alveoli and hence do not participate in gas exchange. As the subject takes a breath, the alveolar volume expands from V_{A_1} to V_{A_2} with little change in the dead space volume (V_D). During the breath, the alveolar gas remaining in the dead space at the end of the preceding breath is drawn into the alveoli along with the fresh gas. At the end of the breath, part of the inspired fresh gas resides in the dead space. It, of course, will be exhaled during expiration and does not contribute to ventilating the alveoli. Thus, the volume of the breath, V_T, is the sum of dead space volume, V_D, and the alveolar volume, V_A:

$$V_T = V_D + V_A \qquad (2\text{–}6)$$

Alveolar ventilation can therefore be calculated as:

$$\dot{V}_A = (V_T - V_D) \times N \qquad (2\text{–}7)$$

where N is the frequency of breathing in breaths per minute. For gas exchange, alveolar ventilation is the important parameter, since dead space ventilation plays no role in removing CO_2 from the body or adding O_2. However, dead space is important in humidification of inspired gas and in temperature conservation.

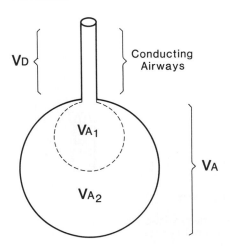

V_D

Conducting Airways

V_{A_1}

V_{A_2}

V_A

FIGURE 2–5. Changes in the volume of the gas spaces during a respiratory cycle. Note that the volume of the alveoli (V_A) increases significantly, from V_{A_1} to V_{A_2}, during inspiration and decreases on expiration, from V_{A_2} to V_{A_1}. The volume of the conducting airways (V_D) does not change significantly.

TABLE 2–1.   Effect of Dead Space Volume (VD) on Alveolar Ventilation

		Assume Constant V_D **= 150 ml**			
VT (ml)	× N =	$\dot{V}_E$ (ml/min)	(VT − VD)	× N =	$\dot{V}_A$ (ml/min)
250	32	8,000	100	32	3,200
500	16	8,000	350	16	5,600
1,000	8	8,000	850	8	6,800

Table 2–1 shows why the dead space must be considered when estimating alveolar ventilation. Three combinations are presented in which the minute ventilation equals 8,000 ml/min. The dead space is assumed constant, but the tidal volume varies from 250 to 1,000 ml, with the appropriate decreases in frequency (N) to produce a $\dot{V}_E$ of 8,000 ml/min. As shown in the table, with the same minute ventilation, the alveolar ventilation can vary from 3,200 to 6,800 ml/min, which is more than a two-fold difference.

One way to calculate alveolar ventilation is to estimate the anatomic dead space and subtract this from the tidal volume. The dead space volume can be estimated as 1 ml/lb body weight. For an average 70-kg man, $V_D = 70 \times 2.2 \times 1 \cong 150$ ml.

A more exact way to measure dead space is the Fowler technique, which involves using a respiratory circuit similar to that shown schematically in Figure 2–2. The subject inhales a breath of oxygen and then exhales, past a meter that measures N_2 very accurately, into a spirometer that measures the expired volume. A plot of expired nitrogen concentration versus expired volume is obtained (Fig. 2–6). The anatomic dead space is estimated under the assumption that dead space contains only oxygen, whereas the alveoli are filled with diluted nitrogen. During expiration, an N_2-free gas coming from the dead space is initially measured. A sudden step function should occur when alveolar gas

FIGURE 2–6. In the Fowler technique, used to estimate dead space, the subject takes a breath of 100% O_2 and exhales past a N_2 meter into a spirometer that measures expired volume. A curve relating expired nitrogen concentration (%) to the expired volume is generated. Phase I is pure dead space gas, phase III relates to the alveolar N_2 concentration, and phase II is a mixture of dead space and alveolar gas. By matching the shaded areas above and below the N_2 concentration curve in phase II, the anatomic dead space can be measured as 0.2 l. The pulsations occurring in the nitrogen concentration during phase III are called cardiogenic oscillations and are synchronous with the heartbeat.

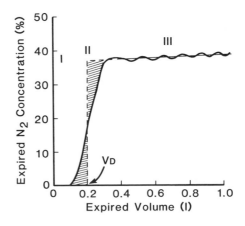

containing nitrogen reaches the N_2 meter as the alveoli start to empty. As can be seen from the tracing, this is not what happens. The curve obtained by this procedure is divided into three phases. Phase I is pure dead space gas containing no nitrogen, only 100% oxygen. During phase II, which has an S-shaped configuration, a mixture of alveolar gas and dead space gas is expired past the N_2 meter. Phase III is finally attained when pure alveolar gas is expired. The reason for the S-shaped rise in N_2 concentration during phase II is that molecular diffusive mixing occurs during the breath; oxygen diffuses from the dead space into the alveoli, whereas alveolar gas diffuses upward into the dead space. To analyze this curve, a perpendicular line is drawn such that the shaded areas of crosshatching in phase II are equal. The anatomic dead space is assumed to be the expired volume where the perpendicular line intersects the volume axis (0.2 l in Figure 2–6).

The Fowler technique is a clever method for measuring V_D, but if the subject holds his breath after inhaling O_2, continued mixing between V_D and V_A will cause an underestimation of V_D. In many diseased lung states, phase III does not plateau and Fowler's technique is inaccurate. Also, nonfunctioning, poorly perfused alveoli may be included as part of the anatomic dead space using the Fowler technique.

Direct Estimation of Alveolar Ventilation

Fortunately, there are more direct ways to estimate alveolar ventilation. The key is that little CO_2 is present in ambient air, its concentration being only about 0.03 per cent. Furthermore, since no gas exchange occurs in the anatomic dead space, all CO_2 collected during a given period of time is assumed to originate from the alveoli. If one measures the production of CO_2 ($\dot{V}_{CO_2}$) and knows the fractional concentration of CO_2 in the alveolar gas (F_{ACO_2}), one can compute alveolar ventilation from the following relationship:

$$\dot{V}_{CO_2} = \dot{V}_A \times F_{ACO_2}$$

(2–8)

$$\text{or } \dot{V}_A = \dot{V}_{CO_2}/F_{ACO_2}$$

In the study of gas exchange, it is more convenient to deal with the partial pressure (mmHg) of a gas rather than its fractional concentration. Partial pressure is proportional to the fractional concentration of a gas under dry conditions. For the partial pressure of alveolar CO_2:

$$P_{ACO_2} = F_{ACO_2} \times (P_B - 47)$$

(2–9)

where P_B is the barometric pressure. Conversion to dry gas requires that the partial pressure of water vapor (47 mmHg) be subtracted from barometric pressure. Substituting Equation 2–9 into Equation 2–8 yields:

$$\dot{V}_A = K(\dot{V}_{CO_2}/P_{ACO_2})$$

(2–10)

In normal lungs, arterial CO_2 (Pa_{CO_2}) is equivalent to alveolar CO_2 (PA_{CO_2}). Equation 2–10 can then be rewritten as:

$$\dot{V}_A = K(\dot{V}_{CO_2}/Pa_{CO_2}) \qquad\qquad (2\text{–}11)$$

where K is a factor that converts CO_2 concentrations to pressure (mmHg), alveolar ventilation to body temperature and pressure, saturated (BTPS), and CO_2 elimination to standard temperature, pressure dry (STPD). K is normally equal to 863 mmHg when $\dot{V}_A$ and $\dot{V}_{CO_2}$ are in milliliters per minute. If a subject has a $\dot{V}_{CO_2}$ of 200 ml/min and a Pa_{CO_2} of 43 mmHg, the alveolar ventilation is 4.0 l/min. The implications of Equation 2–11 will be discussed later, but note that at a fixed CO_2 production rate there is an inverse relationship between alveolar ventilation and arterial CO_2 tension. What is an appropriate alveolar ventilation? Generally speaking, it is an alveolar ventilation that maintains the Pa_{CO_2} in humans at about 40 mmHg regardless of activity level.

Physiologic Dead Space

The concept of a physiologic dead space evolved rather logically from the ideas previously considered to explain alveolar ventilation. The central idea is that the expired CO_2 comes from the alveoli. The physiologic dead space is the volume of gas that does not exchange with blood and includes the anatomic dead space and the gas in alveoli that does not exchange with blood (alveolar dead space). In normal subjects, the anatomic and physiologic dead spaces are the same. However, the physiologic dead space can be much larger than the anatomic dead space in some disease states. The derivation of the pertinent equations and the implications of this concept are discussed in Chapter 8.

INTERRELATIONS AMONG VENTILATION AND ALVEOLAR PARTIAL PRESSURES

It was shown in Table 2–1 that, for a given minute ventilation and dead space, a considerable variation in alveolar ventilation can occur depending on the tidal volume and respiratory frequency. The effect of alveolar ventilation on PA_{CO_2} is defined by Equation 2–10. At a constant rate of CO_2 production, increased alveolar ventilation leads to a reduction in PA_{CO_2}, and vice versa. Changes in alveolar ventilation also affect the alveolar O_2 tension, PA_{O_2}. Basically, PA_{O_2} reflects the balance between oxygen supplied by ventilation and that removed by the blood. For example, a low alveolar ventilation will lead to an increase in PA_{CO_2} but a decrease in PA_{O_2}.

The interrelations between ventilation and O_2 tension are best appreciated from the alveolar gas equation (see Eq. 8–10). Whereas it is quite difficult to measure PA_{O_2} from expired gas, this equation allows us to calculate mean PA_{O_2}

accurately. The alveolar equation is found in Chapter 8, and its derivation is shown in the appendix. The student should consult Chapter 8 for a more detailed discussion of the relationship between P_{ACO_2} and P_{AO_2}.

PATHOLOGIC FACTORS AFFECTING ALVEOLAR VENTILATION AND DEAD SPACE

There are several situations associated with *alveolar hyperventilation*. In the presence of an increased inspired CO_2, there will be stimulation of the chemoreceptors with increased ventilation. Hyperventilation can also occur with anxiety and at high altitudes, where the low O_2 tension leads to hypoxic stimulation of the peripheral chemoreceptors. In these latter two cases, the arterial P_{CO_2} will fall and can lead to symptoms of acute hypocarbia, such as tinnitus, numbness, and tingling of lips and extremities.

Alveolar hypoventilation can occur in a number of situations. Diseases of the central nervous system can cause hypoventilation, as can drugs, weakness or paralysis of respiratory muscles, and breathing through a high resistance airway with resultant respiratory muscle fatigue. Alveolar hypoventilation resulting in CO_2 retention commonly occurs in chronic obstructive pulmonary disease. In this type of lung disease, there is a severe mismatch between the ventilation and perfusion of various lung areas such that CO_2 is not effectively removed, resulting in hypercarbia.

An increase in physiologic dead space is commonly encountered in patients with chronic obstructive lung disease. Pulmonary emboli also cause an increase in the physiologic dead space. In these cases, there are many areas that function poorly in terms of gas exchange, and their continued ventilation leads to an increase in the physiologic dead space.

SUGGESTED READING

DuBois, A.B., Botelho, S.Y., Bedell, G.N., Marshall, R., and Comroe, J.H., Jr.: A rapid ple-thysmographic method for measuring thoracic gas volume: A comparison with a nitrogen washout method for measuring functional residual capacity in normal subjects. *J. Clin. Invest.*, 35:322–326, 1956.
Fowler, W.S.: Intrapulmonary distribution of inspired gas. *Physiol. Rev.*, 32:1–20, 1952.

QUESTIONS

1. Which of the following lung capacities cannot be measured by a spirometer? a. total lung capacity; b. inspiratory capacity; c. vital capacity; d. functional residual capacity.
2. In the helium dilution method for estimating FRC, the spirometer con-

tains 4 l of helium at 10% concentration, and the equilibrium concentration is 5 per cent. What is the subject's FRC?

3. If a subject has a $\dot{V}_{CO_2}$ of 400 ml/min and a Pa_{CO_2} of 40 mmHg, what is the alveolar ventilation ($\dot{V}_A$)?

DIFFUSION AND ITS APPLICATION TO THE LUNG
Gas Diffusion Through a Liquid
Fick's Law of Diffusion

CAPILLARY EXCHANGE OF O_2 and CO_2 IN THE LUNG
The Diffusion Path
Perfusion-Limitation Versus Diffusion-Limitation

RELATIONSHIP OF ERYTHROCYTE TRANSIT TO DIFFUSIVE TRANSFER OF O_2 AND CO_2
Oxygen
Carbon Dioxide

DIFFUSING CAPACITY
Definition of Diffusing Capacity
O_2 Diffusing Capacity
CO Diffusing Capacity
Single-Breath Method for Measurement of Diffusing Capacity
Steady-State Method for Measurement of Diffusing Capacity

PHYSIOLOGIC AND PATHOLOGIC FACTORS THAT ALTER DIFFUSING CAPACITY
Physiologic Factors
Pathologic Factors

3

DIFFUSIVE
TRANSFER OF
RESPIRATORY
GASES

DIFFUSION AND ITS APPLICATION TO THE LUNG

Chapter 1 dealt with the structure of the lungs. It described the remarkable increase in total airway cross-sectional area from the trachea to the respiratory bronchioles. Because of this increase in cross-sectional area, flow velocity decreases as gas moves peripherally into the respiratory unit. In the respiratory unit, bulk flow is virtually absent, and gas transport occurs primarily by molecular diffusion. This is a process whereby gas molecules move from a zone where the gas exerts a high partial pressure to a zone where it exerts a lower partial pressure. This molecular diffusion within the respiratory unit is sufficiently rapid to mix the inspired gas with the resident gas.

This chapter addresses the transfer of gas from the respiratory unit across the alveolar-capillary membrane and into the pulmonary capillary blood and vice versa. Historically, Haldane and Bohr believed that this gas transfer was accomplished by active secretion, whereas Krogh and Barcroft thought that the transfer occurred by molecular diffusion. Today, the latter view is believed to be correct. However, it has been postulated by some that the presence of enzyme systems such as P-450 in the cell membrane may facilitate O_2 transfer across the alveolar-capillary membrane, and CO_2 transport may also be facilitated because of the high levels of carbonic anhydrase in the membrane.

Because molecular diffusion involves the movement of gas molecules from a region with a high concentration or partial pressure to a region with a low concentration or partial pressure, molecular diffusion results in equal concentrations in both regions if sufficient time elapses. Light gases achieve equilibrium faster than heavy gases. This is expressed mathematically by Graham's Law, which states that the relative rates of molecular diffusion of two gases are inversely related to the square roots of their molecular weights:

$$\frac{\text{rate of gas 1 diffusion}}{\text{rate of gas 2 diffusion}} = \sqrt{\frac{MW_2}{MW_1}} \tag{3-1}$$

For example, since the molecular weight of O_2 is 32 and the molecular weight of CO_2 is 44, the rate of diffusion of CO_2 relative to that of O_2 in a gas phase is:

$$\frac{\text{rate of } CO_2 \text{ diffusion}}{\text{rate of } O_2 \text{ diffusion}} = \sqrt{\frac{32}{44}} = \frac{5.66}{6.63} = 0.85$$

Thus, in a gaseous phase, CO_2 diffusion is 15 per cent slower than O_2 diffusion.

Gas Diffusion Through a Liquid

The alveolar-capillary membrane consists, to a large extent, of water. When a gas is in contact with a liquid, the partial pressure in the gas phase equilibrates with the partial pressure in the fluid phase. This increases the concentration of the gas in the fluid and provides the driving force for the diffusion of the gas through the liquid phase. The rate of diffusion of gas through a liquid depends on its solubility in the particular liquid. The greater the solubility, the greater its concentration in the liquid and the more rapid the rate of diffusion through the liquid.

The relative rate of diffusion of two gases from a gas phase through a liquid is directly proportional to the solvent solubilities and inversely proportional to the square roots of their molecular weights:

$$\frac{\text{rate of gas 1 diffusion}}{\text{rate of gas 2 diffusion}} = \sqrt{\frac{MW_2}{MW_1}} \times \frac{\text{solubility gas 1}}{\text{solubility gas 2}} \tag{3-2}$$

As an example, consider CO_2 and O_2, which have water solubilities of 0.567 and 0.0244, respectively, diffusing through water:

$$\frac{\text{rate of CO}_2 \text{ diffusion}}{\text{rate of O}_2 \text{ diffusion}} = \sqrt{\frac{32}{44}} \times \frac{0.567}{0.0244} = 0.85 \times 23.24 \cong 20$$

Therefore, even though the diffusion of CO_2 in gas is 15 per cent slower than that of O_2, CO_2 diffuses 20 times faster through a watery medium such as the alveolar-capillary membrane.

Fick's Law of Diffusion

The rate of diffusion across a membrane is quantitatively expressed by Fick's First Law of Diffusion. This law states that the volume of gas that diffuses per unit time $(\dot{V})$ across a membrane is directly proportional to the surface area of the membrane (A), the partial pressure difference of the gas on either side of the membrane $(P_1 - P_2)$, and the diffusion coefficient for a particular gas (D) and inversely proportional to the thickness of the membrane (ΔX):

$$\dot{V} = \frac{D \times A \times (P_1 - P_2)}{\Delta X} \tag{3–3}$$

The magnitude of the diffusion coefficient (D) depends on the square root of the gas's molecular weight and the solubility of the gas in the alveolar-capillary membrane.

CAPILLARY EXCHANGE OF O_2 AND CO_2 IN THE LUNG

The Diffusion Path

In the lung, gas transport to and from the blood occurs through the alveolar-capillary membrane. This membrane consists of several layers of tissue. The alveoli are lined by type I and type II epithelium attached to a basement membrane. Between this basement membrane and the pulmonary capillary endothelial basement membrane is a thin interstitial space. The total thickness of the alveolar-capillary membrane is approximately 0.35 μm (1/3000 of a millimeter). The diameter of the pulmonary capillaries is approximately equal to the diameter of the erythrocytes (7 to 8 μm). Because of this close match between the size of the erythrocyte and the capillary, the diffusion path through the plasma to the erythrocyte is relatively short. In fact, the length of the diffusion path across the surface membrane of the erythrocyte into its interior is considerably greater than that of the alveolar-capillary membrane; this contributes significantly to the total diffusion resistance for any gas entering or leaving the interior of the red cell.

Perfusion-Limitation Versus Diffusion-Limitation

Hemoglobin has an extremely high affinity for carbon monoxide (CO). Therefore, large amounts of CO bind to hemoglobin even at low partial pressures. With a normal pulmonary blood flow, CO will continue to diffuse through the alveolar-capillary membrane to combine with hemoglobin. Hence, the amount of CO that crosses the alveolar-capillary membrane is limited only by the properties of the membrane and not by the pulmonary blood flow, i.e., *transfer of CO is diffusion-limited*. By contrast, the diffusion of gases that bind poorly with hemoglobin, such as nitrous oxide (N_2O), is limited by the pulmonary blood flow, i.e., *transfer of N_2O is perfusion-limited*. Gases that are perfusion-limited can be used to measure pulmonary blood flow, whereas gases that are diffusion-limited, such as CO, can be used to measure pulmonary diffusing capacity.

The affinity of hemoglobin for O_2 is less than that for CO but greater than that for N_2O such that pulmonary capillary O_2 tension is in equilibrium with alveolar O_2 tension. Under these resting conditions, the transfer of O_2 is perfusion-limited. However, if the diffusion properties of the alveolar-capillary membrane are altered by disease, the transfer of O_2 can become diffusion-limited.

RELATIONSHIP OF ERYTHROCYTE TRANSIT TO DIFFUSIVE TRANSFER OF O_2 AND CO_2

Oxygen

The rate at which the chemical reaction between O_2 and hemoglobin occurs is an important factor in the uptake of O_2 by the blood. The transfer of O_2 can be considered to consist of two phases (Fig. 3–1). In the first phase, O_2 diffuses across the alveolar-capillary membrane, through the plasma, and across the erythrocyte membrane. The resistance to gas diffusion across the alveolar-capillary-plasma-erythrocyte membrane is defined as $1/D_M$, where D_M is the diffusing capacity of the alveolar-capillary-plasma-erythrocyte membrane. In the second phase, O_2 chemically combines with hemoglobin. θ is defined as the volume of O_2 (ml) combining in 1 minute with the erythrocytes contained in 1 ml of blood (assuming a normal hemoglobin concentration) at a partial pressure of 1 mmHg. Therefore, θ multiplied by the entire pulmonary capillary blood volume (Vc) defines the chemical reaction rate between hemoglobin and O_2 for the entire lung. The inverse of this product, $1/\theta Vc$, has the units of resistance. Because the resistances to gas diffusion across the alveolar-capillary-plasma-erythrocyte membrane and to chemical binding of O_2 to hemoglobin are in series, their sum equals the total resistance that O_2 encounters as it moves from the alveoli to combine with hemoglobin:

$$\frac{1}{D_L} = \frac{1}{D_M} + \frac{1}{\theta Vc} \qquad (3\text{–}4)$$

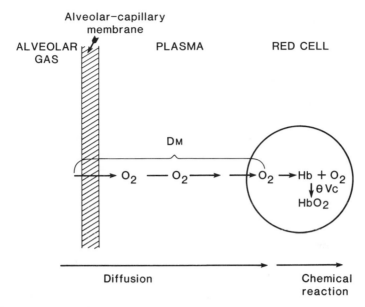

FIGURE 3–1. Transfer of O_2 in the lung. O_2 diffuses from the alveolar gas through the alveolar-capillary membrane through the plasma and then through the erythrocyte membrane (D_M). In the red cells, O_2 reacts chemically with hemoglobin to form HbO_2. θ represents the reaction rate. Vc is the pulmonary capillary blood volume. θVc is the reaction rate for O_2 with hemoglobin for the entire lung. The distance between the alveolar-capillary membrane and the erythrocyte membrane has been greatly increased on this diagram for illustrative purposes.

where $1/D_L$ is the total resistance. The membrane resistance, $1/D_M$, and the chemical reaction resistance, $1/\theta Vc$, are approximately equal in magnitude. However, the rate of reaction of O_2 with hemoglobin depends on the O_2 saturation of hemoglobin. If the O_2 saturation of hemoglobin is low, the reaction rate is fast ($\theta > 1$); conversely, if the saturation is high, the reaction rate is slow ($\theta < 1$). Therefore, the chemical reaction resistance is large compared with the membrane resistance at high hemoglobin saturation; by contrast, the membrane resistance is large compared with the reaction rate at low hemoglobin saturation.

The mean time required for a red blood cell to traverse the pulmonary capillary is 0.75 sec in a normal resting subject (Fig. 3–2A), whereas equilibration with alveolar gas occurs within 0.25 sec. Thus, there is an excess amount of time for oxygenation to occur. The transit time for red blood cells decreases considerably during exercise or hard work, but, in all but the most extreme cases, the transit time remains greater than the time required for complete equilibration. The pulmonary capillary blood volume for gas exchange is 60 ml in normal resting subjects and increases only by approximately 50 per cent, to 95 ml, during exercise.

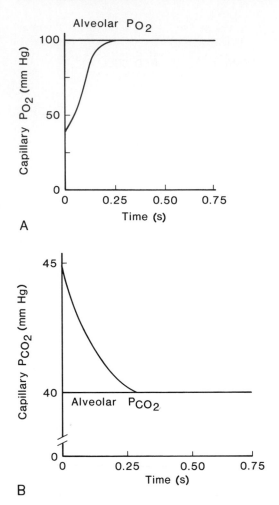

FIGURE 3–2. *A,* Mean transit time for an erythrocyte passing through the pulmonary capillaries is 0.75 second at rest, but equilibration between alveolar and capillary O_2 tensions occurs much more quickly (0.25 s). *B,* The time for equilibration between alveolar and capillary CO_2 tensions is similar to that for O_2. Even though the diffusivity of CO_2 across the alveolar-capillary membrane is approximately 20 times greater than that of O_2, equilibration of CO_2 between alveolar gas and blood is retarded by the relatively slow rate of the chemical reactions of CO_2 in the plasma.

Carbon Dioxide

The diffusivity of CO_2 across the alveolar-capillary membrane is approximately 20 times greater than that of O_2. Therefore, one would expect the rate of transfer of CO_2 to exceed that of O_2. But the rates of transfer for CO_2 and O_2 are similar (see Fig. 3–2). This is because the rates of the chemical reactions involving CO_2 in the blood are much slower than those for reactions involving O_2.

DIFFUSING CAPACITY

Definition of Diffusing Capacity

To accurately explain gas exchange using Fick's Law, it is necessary to know the surface area and thickness of the alveolar-capillary membrane and the diffusion coefficients for the gases. At present, this information remains unknown, since the thickness and surface area of the alveolar-capillary membrane cannot be measured in a living subject. By rearranging Equation 3–3 and defining D_L as $(D \times A/\Delta X)$, the equation can be rewritten as:

$$D_L = \frac{D \times A}{\Delta X} = \frac{\dot{V}}{(P_A - P_c)} \tag{3–5}$$

where P_A is the mean alveolar partial pressure of the diffusing gas and P_c is the mean capillary partial pressure. All terms on the right side of Equation 3–5 can be determined experimentally. The diffusing capacity (D_L) is defined as the uptake of gas per minute $(\dot{V})$ per mmHg pressure difference $(P_A - P_c)$ and has the units of conductance (ml/min/mmHg), which is the inverse of resistance. From Equation 3–5 it is apparent that the diffusing capacity can be altered by changes in surface area, thickness, or the diffusion coefficient of the membrane or any combination of these factors. It is possible that a normal diffusing capacity may be associated with an increased membrane thickness if its effect is counterbalanced by an increased surface area.

O$_2$ Diffusing Capacity

The diffusing capacity of the lung for O_2 is difficult to measure because no method to directly determine the mean pulmonary capillary O_2 tension is available. Because of this problem, O_2 diffusing capacity is frequently calculated from the CO diffusing capacity using an appropriate correction factor (see following section).

CO Diffusing Capacity

Because the transfer of CO across the alveolar-capillary membrane is diffusion-limited, it is an ideal gas for determining the diffusing capacity of the lung. The affinity of hemoglobin for CO is so high (240 times that of O_2) that the mean capillary CO partial pressure $(P_{c_{CO}})$ remains near 0 and can usually be ignored. Therefore, Equation 3–5 is expressed as:

$$D_{L_{CO}} = \frac{\dot{V}_{CO}}{P_{A_{CO}}} \tag{3–6}$$

The diffusing capacity of the lung for CO can be converted into that for O_2 by multiplying by 1.23. This factor is determined from the relative diffusivities of CO and O_2 using Equation 3–2 and 0.0184 for the solubility of CO in water:

$$\frac{\text{rate of } O_2 \text{ diffusion}}{\text{rate of CO diffusion}} = \sqrt{\frac{28}{32}} \times \frac{0.0244}{0.0184} = 1.23$$

Several methods are currently used to measure the CO diffusing capacity. In clinical practice the most widely used techniques are the single-breath method and the steady-state method.

Single-Breath Method for Measurement of Diffusing Capacity

In the single-breath technique, the subject exhales completely. He then rapidly and maximally inhales a gas mixture containing CO and helium (He). At total lung capacity the subject holds his breath for a short period. During the subsequent exhalation, the first 500 ml of the expirate are discarded; the remaining expired gas is collected, and the fractional alveolar CO concentration (FA_{CO}) is determined. Assuming that no appreciable amount of He passes into the blood, and using the helium dilution (FA_{He}/FI_{He}) and the inspired fractional CO concentration (FI_{CO}), the fractional alveolar CO concentration at the beginning of breath-holding ($(FA_{CO})_0$) can be calculated as:

$$(FA_{CO})_0 = \frac{FA_{He}}{FI_{He}} \times FI_{CO} \tag{3-7}$$

The alveolar gas volume (VA) can also be calculated from the He dilution:

$$VA = \frac{VI \times FI_{He}}{FA_{He}} \tag{3-8}$$

where VI is the inspired volume and FI_{He} and FA_{He} are the fractional inspired and alveolar He concentrations, respectively. During the period of breath-holding, CO diffuses through the alveolar-capillary membrane into the blood. The alveolar CO concentration decreases exponentially during the breath-holding. The rate of decrease in alveolar CO concentration depends on the diffusing capacity and the alveolar gas volume:

$$(FA_{CO})_t = (FA_{CO})_0 \exp - \frac{DL_{CO} \times 713 \times t}{VA \times 60} \tag{3-9}$$

where $(FA_{CO})_t$ is the fractional alveolar CO concentration during breath-holding at time t. Equation 3–9 can be solved for DL_{CO}:

$$DL_{CO} = \frac{VA \times 60}{713 \times t} \times \ln \frac{(FA_{CO})_0}{(FA_{CO})_t} \tag{3-10}$$

To determine the CO diffusing capacity using the single-breath method, one must know the inspired gas volume (VI), the fractional alveolar He concentration at the end of the breath-holding (FA_{He}), the fractional inspired He concentration (FI_{He}), the fractional inspired CO concentration (FI_{CO}), and the time of breath-holding (t).

The advantage of the single-breath technique is its rapidity, which allows the measurement to be repeated every few minutes. The disadvantage of this technique is that breath-holding is not a normal physiologic state, and some subjects may experience difficulty holding their breath for the required 10 seconds. The normal value for CO diffusing capacity as determined by the single-breath method for a resting subject is 31 ml/min/mmHg, standard temperature, pressure dry (STPD).

Steady-State Method for Measurement of Diffusing Capacity

Using this method to measure the CO diffusing capacity, a subject breathes a gas mixture containing CO for a 3-minute period. To improve reproducibility of measurements and to amplify abnormalities in the diffusing capacity, subjects are sometimes asked to perform moderate exercise (to increase their cardiac output) during the test.

Uptake of CO from alveolar gas into pulmonary capillary blood ($\dot{V}_{CO}$) is determined from the minute ventilation ($\dot{V}_E$) and the difference between the inspired (FI_{CO}) and mean expired ($F\overline{E}_{CO}$) fractional CO concentrations. Alveolar partial pressure of CO (PA_{CO}) is estimated from the end-tidal CO tension. The CO diffusing capacity (DL_{CO}) is then calculated using Equation 3–6.

The advantage of the steady-state method is that it requires little subject cooperation and can be performed on exercising subjects. The disadvantage of this method is that alveolar CO tension must be determined from an end-tidal gas sample. The normal value for the CO diffusing capacity determined by the steady-state method measured at moderate exercise is 31 ml/min/mmHg (STPD), the same value obtained using the single-breath method.

An important advantage of the steady-state method over the single-breath method is that fractional uptake of CO, which is another index of pulmonary diffusion, can be calculated from the available information:

$$\text{Fractional CO uptake} = \frac{V_{CO}}{FI_{CO} \times VI} \tag{3–11}$$

The normal fractional CO uptake is 0.5 and can decrease to values smaller than 0.3 with diffusion impairment.

PHYSIOLOGIC AND PATHOLOGIC FACTORS THAT ALTER DIFFUSING CAPACITY

Physiologic Factors

The diffusing capacity increases with body surface area because larger individuals have a larger pulmonary capillary surface area. This is not unexpected, since large individuals must transfer larger amounts of O_2 and CO_2. Age has a minimal effect on the diffusing capacity for CO, decreasing it by only about 1 ml/min/mmHg per decade. Exercise increases the diffusing capacity, presumably through dilation and/or opening of previously unperfused capillaries (recruitment), which increases the surface area for diffusion. With very strenuous exercise, the diffusing capacity may reach a plateau value, which has been identified as the maximal diffusing capacity.

In the supine position, both at exercise and at rest, diffusing capacity increases with lung volume as shown in Figure 3–3. However, for the erect subject, diffusing capacity is a function of lung volume only during exercise. This difference in erect subjects is due to an increased capillary surface area and volume during exercise. Because of this effect, the supine position may be the best body position for measuring the diffusing capacity.

The diffusing capacity is also affected by the partial pressures of O_2 and CO_2 in the alveolar gas. Low alveolar O_2 tension increases the CO diffusing capacity, whereas high alveolar O_2 tension decreases it. This effect is possibly due to changes in the rate of CO uptake by the erythrocyte. Increases in alveolar CO_2 tensions slightly increase the diffusing capacity, due to either an increased pulmonary blood flow or a dilation of pulmonary capillaries.

Pathologic Factors

Any condition that alters the membrane component of the diffusing capacity or the reaction rate between carbon monoxide and hemoglobin can

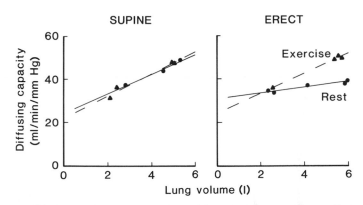

FIGURE 3–3. Effect of lung volume on CO diffusing capacity in supine and erect subjects as measured by the single-breath method during rest (solid line) and exercise (dashed line). The diffusing capacity increases with lung volume in supine subjects. But, for a given lung volume, the diffusing capacities are similar at rest and exercise. Presumably this is because the pulmonary capillaries are maximally filled with blood in the supine position such that the increase in pulmonary vascular pressure caused by exercise cannot further expand the capillary volume. The diffusing capacity does not greatly increase with increased lung volume in erect subjects at rest. In contrast to the supine position, the diffusing capacity in erect subjects increases markedly with exercise at any lung volume, apparently because the pulmonary capillaries are not maximally dilated at rest. (Adapted from Gurtner, G.H., and Fowler, W.S.: Interrelationships of factors affecting pulmonary diffusing capacity. *J. Appl. Physiol., 30*:619–624, 1971.)

change the diffusing capacity. Thickening of the alveolar-capillary membrane increases the diffusion path length and thus decreases the diffusing capacity by directly increasing the resistance of the membrane component. Conditions associated with thickening of the alveolar membrane include pulmonary fibrosis, interstitial edema, and intra-alveolar edema. But in most forms of lung pathology, a surface area reduction is the most common factor causing a decreased diffusion capacity.

Although the CO diffusing capacity does not distinguish between an increased diffusion path length and a decreased surface area, it is still an extremely important pulmonary function test. Measurement of CO diffusing capacity is particularly useful as a tool to follow the response of a pulmonary disease to a particular treatment and as an indicator of the natural progression of the disease process. Early in the course of pulmonary interstitial and vascular disease, the CO diffusing capacity is frequently the only pulmonary function test that is abnormal. In obstructive lung disease, a low CO diffusing capacity indicates the presence of emphysema, a disease associated with destruction of alveolar-capillary units, long before a positive diagnosis can be made using chest roentgenograms. By contrast, the CO diffusing capacity is usually normal in obstructive airway disease such as bronchitis and asthma. The cause of the high CO diffusing capacity occasionally observed in patients with asthma is not understood. In anemic patients the CO diffusing capacity is decreased, presumably owing to a reduction in the hemoglobin concentration. This reduction in diffusion capacity may be counterbalanced, in part, by a compensatory increase in cardiac output. Polycythemia has the opposite effect of anemia, i.e., it increases the hemoglobin concentration.

SUGGESTED READING

Forster, R.E.: Exchange of gases between air and pulmonary capillary blood: Pulmonary diffusing capacity. *Physiol. Rev.*, 37:391–452, 1957.
Wagner, P.D.: Diffusion and chemical reaction in pulmonary gas exchange. *Physiol. Rev.*, 57:257–312, 1977.

QUESTIONS

1. Why are the rates of transfer for O_2 and CO_2 across the alveolar-capillary membrane similar?
2. Why is the transfer of CO diffusion-limited?
3. What is the most common cause of a reduction in the CO diffusing capacity of the lung?

OXYGEN
O$_2$ Consumption
O$_2$ Stores
O$_2$ Transport
Oxygen Dissolved in Blood
Hemoglobin
Chemically Combined Oxygen
Oxyhemoglobin Dissociation Curve

FACTORS AFFECTING THE OXYHEMOGLOBIN DISSOCIATION CURVE
Carboxyhemoglobin

CARBON DIOXIDE
CO$_2$ Production
CO$_2$ Stores
CO$_2$ Transport
CO$_2$ Dissociation Curve

GAS TRANSPORT
IN THE BLOOD

OXYGEN

O$_2$ Consumption

Aerobic metabolism is totally dependent on O$_2$ uptake from the inspired gas and its subsequent delivery to the tissues. The volume of oxygen inhaled per unit time equals the volume of gas inhaled ($\dot{V}_I$) multiplied by the fractional concentration of inspired oxygen ($F_{I_{O_2}}$). The volume of oxygen exhaled per unit time equals the volume of gas exhaled in this time ($\dot{V}_E$) multiplied by the fractional concentration of expired oxygen ($F_{E_{O_2}}$). The difference between the inspired and expired oxygen equals the O$_2$ uptake ($\dot{V}_{O_2}$):

$$\dot{V}_{O_2} = (\dot{V}_I \times F_{I_{O_2}}) - (\dot{V}_E \times F_{E_{O_2}}) \qquad (4\text{--}1)$$

To calculate O$_2$ uptake using Equation 4–1, four measurements are needed.

Simultaneous measurement of both $\dot{V}_I$ and $\dot{V}_E$ is impractical; therefore, O_2 uptake is usually determined by considering the rate of N_2 exchange in the lungs. In a steady state, there is no net uptake or elimination of nitrogen. Therefore, the volume of inhaled nitrogen per unit time ($\dot{V}_I \times F_{I_{N_2}}$) equals the volume of exhaled nitrogen per unit time ($\dot{V}_E \times F_{E_{N_2}}$):

$$\dot{V}_I \times F_{I_{N_2}} = \dot{V}_E \times F_{E_{N_2}} \tag{4-2}$$

Solving Equation 4–2 for $\dot{V}_I$ results in:

$$\dot{V}_I = \dot{V}_E \times F_{E_{N_2}}/F_{I_{N_2}} \tag{4-3}$$

Substituting Equation 4–3 into Equation 4–1 yields:

$$\dot{V}_{O_2} = \{[(F_{E_{N_2}}/F_{I_{N_2}}) \times F_{I_{O_2}}] - F_{E_{O_2}}\} \times \dot{V}_E \tag{4-4}$$

Even though Equation 4–4 is more complex than Equation 4–1, all variables can be easily obtained.

When considering O_2 uptake, recall that the volume occupied by a gas depends on both temperature and pressure. To normalize for differences in temperature and pressure, it is conventional to define O_2 uptake in terms of defined physical conditions of standard temperature, pressure dry (STPD). This standardization allows a comparison to be made between measurements of O_2 uptake in Denver (5,000 feet) and San Francisco (sea level) (see appendix). $\dot{V}_{O_2}$ for a normal human at rest is usually about 250 ml/min.

O_2 Stores

O_2 uptake can be equated to O_2 consumption only in a steady state. When uptake is less than consumption, oxygen body stores are depleted. Conversely, when uptake exceeds consumption, oxygen is added to the body's stores, but the capacity for storing oxygen in the body is small. If O_2 intake from the environment is interrupted, these limited O_2 stores are quickly depleted, and hypoxemia, unconsciousness, and death ensue in a few minutes.

Oxygen is stored at several sites in the body. When a subject breathes room air, the major reservoir of available oxygen is in combination with hemoglobin. For a subject with normal blood volume and hemoglobin content, 850 ml of oxygen are stored in the blood. At sea level, this amount is only minimally increased by breathing 100% oxygen, because the hemoglobin is nearly fully saturated when the subject is breathing air. Approximately 500 ml of oxygen are contained in the lungs of an adult breathing air at end-expiration. This amount of O_2 can be increased to 2.5 l when breathing 100% oxygen. The remaining stores of O_2 are bound to myoglobin (in the muscles) and contribute less than 100 ml of oxygen. Because of the hyperbolic shape of the myoglobin dissociation curve, oxygen bound to myoglobin is only available for local consumption because it is released only at the low oxygen tensions prevailing in working muscle.

O₂ Transport

The hemoglobin in the red blood cell provides the major vehicle for oxygen transport by the blood. Oxygen dissolved in plasma is less important in terms of O_2 transport but is still significant since oxygen must be dissolved in plasma to pass to and from hemoglobin.

OXYGEN DISSOLVED IN BLOOD

According to Henry's Law, the volume of oxygen dissolved in plasma is directly proportional to its partial pressure and solubility in plasma. The solubility of oxygen is defined by the absorption coefficient for oxygen (αO_2), which is the volume of oxygen dissolved in one volume of blood at 0°C and 760 mmHg oxygen partial pressure; αO_2 is equal to 2.3 ml/100 ml of blood. For an O_2 partial pressure of 100 mmHg, only 0.3 ml (2.3 × 100/760) of oxygen is dissolved in each 100 ml of blood. In normally functioning lungs, the volume of oxygen in solution can be increased about six-fold by breathing 100% oxygen at 1 atmosphere of pressure.

HEMOGLOBIN

Hemoglobin is a chromoprotein that consists of four polypeptide chains. Each chain contains a protoporphyrin, consisting of four pyrrole rings linked by methane bridges, and a central bivalent ferrous (Fe^{++}) ion (heme group). The ferrous ion is attached by covalent bonds to the four pyrrole groups. A fifth covalent bond attaches the ferrous ion to a protein moiety, globin, which constitutes the bulk of the hemoglobin molecule. The linkage between the ferrous ion and the globin moiety allows the ferrous ion to bind oxygen reversibly. Because hemoglobin has a tetrameric structure, 1 mole of hemoglobin can maximally combine with 4 moles of oxygen. One g of hemoglobin theoretically can combine with 1.38 ml of oxygen. The actual amount is less, presumably because a small fraction of the hemoglobin is in an inactive form.

The valency of the ferrous ion of the hemoglobin does not change when it combines with oxygen. The binding of O_2 to Fe^{++} is therefore referred to as oxygenation rather than oxidation. Oxygenation of hemoglobin transforms it to *oxyhemoglobin (HbO₂)*, which has a bright red color. Deoxygenation transforms oxyhemoglobin to *deoxygenated hemoglobin (Hb)*, which has a purple color. Changes in the oxygenation of Hb are responsible for the color differences between arterial and venous blood. Under certain pathologic conditions, oxidation of the heme group occurs, and the ferrous ion is converted to the ferric state (Fe^{+++}). The *oxidized form of hemoglobin, methemoglobin,* is unable to release its oxygen to the tissues.

Adult human hemoglobin (HbA) contains two types of polypeptide chains, α-chains and β-chains. In *fetal hemoglobin (HbF)*, the two β-chains of adult hemoglobin are replaced by two δ-chains. This difference provides HbF with a much stronger affinity for oxygen than HbA. *Sickle cell hemoglobin (HbS)* has altered β-chains such that the solubility of HbS at low P_{O_2} is reduced, allowing it to crystallize within the erythrocyte. This causes the sickling of red cells seen in this disease. Sickled erythrocytes may occlude blood vessels, causing "thrombotic" episodes associated with pain. When the sickled cells are subsequently released after stasis, they are more fragile, causing increased hemolysis and anemia.

CHEMICALLY COMBINED OXYGEN

Most of the oxygen in blood is not carried in solution but is combined with hemoglobin. The total volume of oxygen carried in the blood, the O_2 content (C_{O_2}), is the oxygen in solution plus that combined with hemoglobin. The maximal volume of oxygen that can be bound by hemoglobin is called the O_2 capacity. The O_2 saturation of hemoglobin (S_{O_2}) is expressed as a percentage of the O_2 capacity.

Assume that a subject has an O_2 content of 19 ml per 100 ml of blood, a hemoglobin concentration of 15 g/100 ml of blood, and a partial pressure of oxygen (P_{O_2}) of 70 mmHg. The oxygen in solution in 100 ml of blood is calculated below:

$$(P_{O_2}/760) \times \alpha O_2 = 70/760 \times 2.3 = 0.21 \text{ ml/100 ml}$$

Thus, the oxygen chemically bound to hemoglobin is $19 - 0.21 = 18.79$ ml/100 ml. Since the O_2 capacity of hemoglobin is 1.38 ml/g, 15 g of hemoglobin can combine maximally with 20.70 ml of oxygen. The O_2 saturation of hemoglobin in this example is 90.8 per cent [$(18.79/20.70) \times 100$].

The partial pressure of oxygen in arterial blood for a healthy, young subject breathing room air at sea level is 100 mmHg, and this partial pressure results in an arterial blood hemoglobin saturation of approximately 97.5 per cent and an arterial O_2 content (Ca_{O_2}) of 20 ml/100 ml of blood. The normal partial pressure of oxygen in mixed venous blood ($P\bar{v}_{O_2}$) is 40 mmHg, which results in a mixed venous saturation ($S\bar{v}_{O_2}$) of 70 per cent and an O_2 content ($C\bar{v}_{O_2}$) of 15 ml/100 ml of blood. The difference between arterial and mixed venous O_2 contents ($Ca_{O_2} - C\bar{v}_{O_2}$) is, therefore, $20 - 15$, or 5 ml/100 ml of blood. Since each 100 ml of blood loses 5 ml of oxygen to the tissues, a total blood flow ($\dot{Q}$) of 5,000 ml/min would be necessary to satisfy an O_2 uptake ($\dot{V}_{O_2}$) of 250 ml/

min. This relationship among blood flow, O_2 uptake, and arteriovenous O_2 difference is expressed in the classic Fick equation:

$$\dot{V}_{O_2} = \dot{Q}(Ca_{O_2} - C\bar{v}_{O_2}) \tag{4-5}$$

OXYHEMOGLOBIN DISSOCIATION CURVE

The oxyhemoglobin dissociation curve (Fig. 4–1) defines the relationship between O_2 content and the partial pressure of oxygen. This relationship can be determined experimentally by equilibrating small quantities of blood with gas mixtures containing different partial pressures of oxygen.

The oxyhemoglobin dissociation curve has a sigmoid shape because the four molecules of oxygen combine with the ferrous ion in a series of steps. The addition of successive molecules of oxygen produces a different affinity. This sigmoid shape of the oxyhemoglobin dissociation curve has several important functional implications. Since the curve is flat at high O_2 tensions, it provides a protective effect against fluctuations in C_{O_2} when alveolar O_2 tension is changed. For instance, a reduction in P_{O_2} from 100 to 70 mmHg reduces the O_2 content only minimally. However, at a P_{O_2} of less than 70 mmHg, small changes in O_2 tension greatly decrease hemoglobin oxygen content. This latter factor facilitates the unloading of oxygen from hemoglobin in the tissues, where P_{O_2} is lower than in blood.

The partial pressure of oxygen required to produce a 50 per cent saturation of hemoglobin is defined as the P_{50}. Under normal physiologic conditions (pH 7.4, temperature 37°C, P_{CO_2} 40 mmHg), the P_{50} is 26 mmHg; i.e., 50 per cent of the hemoglobin is saturated at a P_{O_2} of 26 mmHg. An increase in the P_{50} is termed a right shift of the oxyhemoglobin dissociation curve, whereas a reduction in P_{50} characterizes a shift to the left. The *right or left shifts* of the

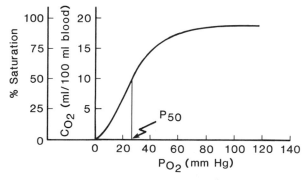

FIGURE 4–1. Oxyhemoglobin dissociation curve for hemoglobin. The partial pressure of oxygen that results in a 50% saturation of hemoglobin is called the P_{50}. The normal P_{50} is 26 mmHg. C_{O_2} represents O_2 content, and P_{O_2} represents the oxygen partial pressure.

oxyhemoglobin dissociation have important physiologic implications as described hereafter.

FACTORS AFFECTING THE OXYHEMOGLOBIN DISSOCIATION CURVE

Numerous factors affect the position of the oxyhemoglobin dissociation curve. Increases in P_{CO_2}, hydrogen ion concentration (decreased pH), or both cause a right shift of the oxyhemoglobin dissociation curve (Fig. 4–2A and B). Therefore, the O_2 content of hemoglobin at a given O_2 tension is less when P_{CO_2} is elevated (*Bohr effect*) or when pH is decreased. The effect of P_{CO_2} on the dissociation curve is independent of the effect of pH. An increase in blood temperature also shifts the oxyhemoglobin dissociation curve to the right, and a reduction in temperature shifts the curve to the left (Fig. 4–2C). Therefore, the conditions that exist in the tissues (i.e., increased temperature, high P_{CO_2}, and low pH) facilitate the release of oxygen from hemoglobin. These shifts of the oxyhemoglobin dissociation curve have a relatively small overall effect on oxygen delivery, and recruitment of capillaries and increases in blood flow are considered to be the most important mechanisms of increasing the delivery of oxygen to the tissues.

An increase in the concentration of 2,3-DPG in the red blood cell decreases the affinity of hemoglobin for O_2. This decrease is associated with a right shift of the oxyhemoglobin dissociation curve. 2,3-DPG is normally synthesized in red blood cells, and high levels of 2,3-DPG occur in conditions in which O_2 delivery is impaired, e.g., anemia, thyrotoxicosis, and chronic hypoxemia.

The physiologic value of a right shift of the oxyhemoglobin dissociation

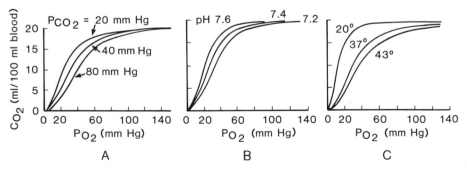

FIGURE 4–2. *A,* The oxyhemoglobin dissociation curve is shifted to the right by an increase in P_{CO_2} and to the left by a reduction in P_{CO_2} (Bohr effect). *B,* The oxyhemoglobin dissociation curve is shifted to the right by a decrease in pH and to the left by an increase in pH. *C,* Increasing blood temperature shifts the oxyhemoglobin dissociation curve to the right, whereas a reduction in temperature shifts the curve to the left. C_{O_2} refers to O_2 content, and P_{O_2} is partial pressure of O_2.

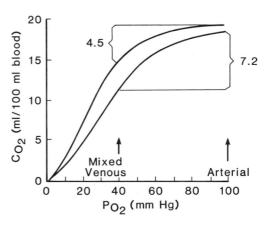

FIGURE 4–3. Hypothetical example of a right shift of the oxyhemoglobin dissociation curve. Both blood samples have equal O_2 capacities, but one curve is shifted to the right, which increases O_2 release from 4.5 to 7.2 ml/100 ml of blood.

curve is based on the reduction in the slope of the curve. This effect is illustrated in Figure 4–3. The figure shows two oxyhemoglobin dissociation curves for two blood samples with the same O_2 capacities. For the normal dissociation curve (left curve), a reduction in P_{O_2} from 100 (arterial) to 40 mmHg (mixed venous) results in the release of 4.5 ml of oxygen from 100 ml of blood. With the right-shifted curve, the O_2 content at a P_{O_2} of 100 mmHg (arterial) is nearly the same as that of the normal blood represented by the left curve. Therefore, the loading of oxygen in the lung is unchanged. However, the O_2 content of the right-shifted curve at a P_{O_2} of 40 mmHg is considerably less than that of the normal curve, meaning that more oxygen is released from the blood for a given arteriovenous difference in P_{O_2}. In this example, 7.2 ml of O_2 per 100 ml of blood is released, representing an increase of approximately 50 per cent in oxygen delivery.

The change in O_2 affinity is much more pronounced in patients with chronic anemia. In the lower curve of Figure 4–4, the O_2 capacity has been reduced by half to simulate anemia. Even though the oxygen content has been halved,

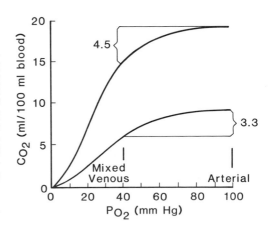

FIGURE 4–4. Diagrammatic representation of O_2 content of blood with a normal hemoglobin concentration of 15 g/100 ml of blood (upper curve) and anemic blood with a hemoglobin concentration of 7.5 g/100 ml of blood (lower curve). Although this is a drastic reduction in hemoglobin concentration, the right shift in the oxyhemoglobin dissociation curve would cause 75% of the normal amount of oxygen to be delivered without reducing mixed venous O_2 tension.

the arterial hemoglobin saturation is the same in both conditions. Even with this reduction in O_2 capacity, 75 per cent of the normal oxygen delivery still occurs without reducing mixed venous O_2 tension. Because this change in hemoglobin-O_2 affinity does not require energy expenditure, it is a very economical way to improve O_2 delivery. However, this compensatory mechanism is ineffective when an anemic patient becomes hypoxemic, because the right-shifted oxyhemoglobin dissociation curve impairs O_2 loading in the lungs.

Carboxyhemoglobin

Carbon monoxide, an odorless and colorless gas, is a product of incomplete combustion. Each of the four ferrous ions of the hemoglobin molecule can combine with 1 molecule of carbon monoxide. In fact, the affinity of hemoglobin for carbon monoxide is 240 times greater than that for oxygen. The combination of CO with hemoglobin forms *carboxyhemoglobin*, which is unable to transport oxygen to the tissues.

Common sources of carbon monoxide in our environment include the exhaust of combustion engines and tobacco smoke. Heavy smokers commonly have 10 per cent of their hemoglobin combined with carbon monoxide, and smoking during pregnancy can result in measurable amounts of carboxyhemoglobin in fetal blood. Hyperbaric oxygenation or 100% oxygen is used therapeutically for carbon monoxide poisoning to facilitate carbon monoxide displacement from hemoglobin.

CARBON DIOXIDE

CO_2 Production

The volume of carbon dioxide exhaled per unit time can be calculated from the volume of gas exhaled per unit time ($\dot{V}E$) and the fractional concentration of carbon dioxide in the exhaled gas (FE_{CO_2}). Similarly, the volume of carbon dioxide inhaled per unit time equals the volume of gas inhaled in this time ($\dot{V}I$) multiplied by the fractional concentration of inspired carbon dioxide (FI_{CO_2}). The difference between the amount exhaled and the amount inhaled equals the carbon dioxide eliminated per unit time ($\dot{V}_{CO_2}$):

$$\dot{V}_{CO_2} = (\dot{V}E \times FE_{CO_2}) - (\dot{V}I \times FI_{CO_2}) \qquad (4\text{–}6)$$

Since the inspired gas mixture contains negligible amounts of carbon dioxide (0.03 per cent), Equation 4–6 reduces to:

$$\dot{V}_{CO_2} = FE_{CO_2} \times \dot{V}E \qquad (4\text{–}7)$$

CO_2 Stores

In a steady state, CO_2 elimination equals CO_2 production. Whenever elimination is less than production, carbon dioxide is retained and body CO_2

stores increase. Conversely, if CO_2 elimination is greater than its production, body CO_2 stores are depleted. In complete respiratory arrest, the arterial P_{CO_2} increases by 3 to 6 mmHg per minute. The CO_2 *storage capacity* is much larger than that for oxygen, and an adult person can store as much as 120 l of CO_2 in the tissues. Most carbon dioxide is stored in the form of bicarbonate in bone, with only a small fraction present in solution in body water. The other major storage sites for carbon dioxide are blood, lung, and soft tissues. The rate of release or buildup in these tissues is different: bone exchanges carbon dioxide slowly, whereas blood and lungs exchange CO_2 very rapidly.

CO_2 stores and their different clearance rates are of clinical importance. Patients retaining carbon dioxide may become unconscious (CO_2 narcosis) if arterial P_{CO_2} increases to a level of 100 mmHg. Because of the slow elimination of CO_2 from the brain, these patients may remain in CO_2 narcosis even when the partial pressure of carbon dioxide in the arterial blood has been reduced by vigorous hyperventilation. The time courses of changes in Pa_{CO_2} after acute hypoventilation or hyperventilation are different; the rate of reduction of Pa_{CO_2} with hyperventilation is considerably faster than the rate of increase of Pa_{CO_2} with hypoventilation.

CO_2 Transport

Carbon dioxide is transported in plasma and red blood cells in the form of several reversible chemical combinations (Fig. 4–5). In plasma, carbon di-

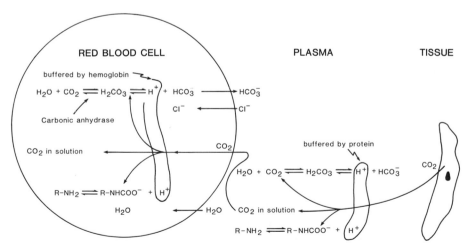

FIGURE 4–5. Diagrammatic representation of CO_2 transport in plasma and in the red blood cell. Hydration of carbon dioxide is much faster in red blood cells than in plasma because of the presence of carbonic anhydrase within the red blood cell. Hemoglobin is a weaker acid when deoxygenated, which facilitates the buffering of hydrogen ions released during hydration. Bicarbonate ions leave the red blood cell, and chloride ions diffuse inward to maintain electrical neutrality.

oxide exists in three forms. A negligible amount reacts with plasma proteins to form carbamino compounds according to the equation:

$$R - NH_2 + CO_2 \rightarrow R - NHCOO^- + H^+$$

A small fraction of carbon dioxide remains in solution and combines with water (is hydrated) to form carbonic acid:

$$H_2O + CO_2 \rightarrow H_2CO_3$$

This process is slow in plasma since carbonic anhydrase, the enzyme that catalyzes this reaction, is not present. The concentration of carbon dioxide in plasma is approximately 1,000 times greater than that of carbonic acid. However, the small amount of carbonic acid that is formed dissociates into hydrogen and bicarbonate ions:

$$H_2CO_3 \rightarrow H^+ + HCO_3^-$$

Most carbon dioxide entering the plasma passes into the red blood cells, where it is also carried in three forms. Some carbon dioxide remains in solution, but a much larger fraction combines with hemoglobin to form carbamino-hemoglobin. The hydrogen ion that is formed in this process is buffered by hemoglobin in the red blood cell. This reaction is facilitated by the release of oxygen from hemoglobin, which makes hemoglobin a weaker acid.

The largest fraction of carbon dioxide in the red blood cell is hydrated to form carbonic acid, which dissociates into bicarbonate and hydrogen ions. The rate of hydration in the red blood cell is accelerated by the presence of the enzyme *carbonic anhydrase*, which allows this reaction to proceed about 10,000 times faster in red blood cells than in plasma. (However, when carbonic anhydrase is inhibited, blood can still adequately transport the carbon dioxide produced by the tissues.) The negatively charged bicarbonate ion diffuses out of the red blood cell into the plasma. This process would unbalance the electrical neutrality within the red blood cell unless an equal number of positively charged ions (cations) accompanied the outward diffusion of the bicarbonate ion into plasma. Alternatively, an equal number of negatively charged ions (anions) could diffuse from the plasma into the red blood cell to maintain electroneutrality. Since the membrane of the red blood cell has a low permeability for cations, the electrical neutrality is maintained by the diffusion of chloride ions from plasma into the red blood cell. This process is called the *Hamburger* or *chloride shift*. The net result of this shift in anions is that the major fraction of carbon dioxide produced in the tissues is carried in the plasma as bicarbonate ion. The chloride shift increases the osmotic pressure in the red blood cell; consequently, water moves from the plasma into the red blood cell. This results in an increased red blood cell volume in venous blood.

In a steady state, a normal person produces approximately 200 ml of carbon dioxide each minute. Assuming a cardiac output ($\dot{Q}$) of 5 l/min and a $\dot{V}_{CO_2}$ of 200 ml/min, each 100 ml of blood must transport 4 ml of carbon dioxide [(200/

5,000) $\times$ 100]; that is, the venous-arterial difference in CO_2 content ($C\bar{v}_{CO_2}$ $-$ Ca_{CO_2}) is 4 ml/100 ml of blood. Slightly more than 50 per cent of the carbon dioxide is in the blood as plasma bicarbonate, and 25 per cent exists as carbaminohemoglobin. The remaining 25 per cent of the carbon dioxide is dissolved in blood (5 per cent), combined with carbamino compounds (5 per cent) in plasma, or exists as bicarbonate in the red blood cells (15 per cent).

The ratio of $\dot{V}_{CO_2}/\dot{V}_{O_2}$ is the respiratory exchange ratio (R). In a steady state, R varies between 0.7 and 1.0, depending on the food source being metabolized. If lipids are primarily consumed, R approaches 0.7, whereas with carbohydrate as a predominant component of the diet, R approaches 1.0. R values significantly less than 0.7 or in excess of 1.0 indicate that the subject is not in a steady state. For instance, hyperventilation increases CO_2 elimination much more than O_2 uptake; that is, the R value will transiently exceed 1.0.

CO_2 Dissociation Curve

The relationship between chemically bound carbon dioxide and the partial pressure of carbon dioxide is defined by the CO_2 dissociation curve (Fig. 4–6A).

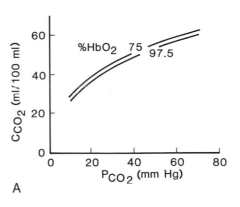

FIGURE 4–6. *A,* CO_2 dissociation curve. The state of oxygenation of hemoglobin affects the position of the CO_2 dissociation curve (Haldane effect). C_{CO_2} represents the CO_2 content of blood, and P_{CO_2} represents the partial pressure of carbon dioxide. *B,* Comparison of the shape of the oxyhemoglobin and CO_2 dissociation curves. The slope of the CO_2 dissociation curve is about three times steeper than that of the oxyhemoglobin dissociation curve. C_{CO_2} represents CO_2 content of blood, C_{O_2} represents oxygen content of blood, and P_{CO_2} and P_{O_2} are the partial pressures of CO_2 and O_2 in blood, respectively. (Adapted from West, J.B.: *Respiratory Physiology.* Baltimore: Williams & Wilkins, 1985.)

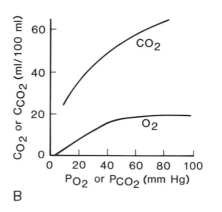

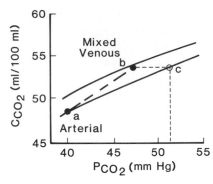

FIGURE 4–7. The Haldane effect, as illustrated here, is of physiologic importance in carbon dioxide transport. Deoxygenated blood (mixed venous) has a greater capacity to carry CO_2 than does oxygenated blood (arterial). In the absence of this shift in the CO_2 dissociation curve, tissue P_{CO_2} would need to increase considerably to load the same amount of CO_2.

Important differences exist between the oxyhemoglobin dissociation curve and the CO_2 dissociation curve (Fig. 4–6B). First, in contrast to the oxyhemoglobin dissociation curve, the CO_2 dissociation curve is nearly linear in the physiologically important range of P_{CO_2} (20 to 55 mmHg). Second, the slope of the CO_2 dissociation curve is steeper than that of the oxyhemoglobin dissociation curve. This means that, for a given change in partial pressure, significantly more carbon dioxide can be transported in blood as compared with oxygen.

The degree of hemoglobin oxygenation affects the position of the CO_2 dissociation curve (*Haldane effect*) (Fig. 4–7). The reason for this effect is that deoxygenated hemoglobin has a higher affinity for H^+ and a greater ability to form carbaminohemoglobin than does oxygenated hemoglobin. When oxygen is released from hemoglobin in the tissues, the capacity of the blood to carry carbon dioxide increases (point a → point b). With O_2 loading of hemoglobin, the reverse process occurs in the lung (point b → point a). In the absence of the Haldane effect, tissue P_{CO_2} would need to increase to 51 mmHg (point a → point c) to produce the same C_{CO_2} found in mixed venous blood at a P_{CO_2} of 46 mmHg in the presence of the Haldane effect.

SUGGESTED READING

Farhi, L. E.: Gas stores of the body. In Fenn, W.O., and Rahn, H. (eds.): *Handbook of Physiology*: Section 3: Respiration, Volume 1. Bethesda: American Physiological Society, 1964, pp. 873–885.

Roughton, F.J.W.: Transport of oxygen and carbon dioxide. In Fenn, W.O., and Rahn, H. (eds.): *Handbook of Physiology*: Section 3: Respiration, Volume 1. Bethesda: American Physiological Society, 1964, pp. 767–825.

QUESTIONS

1. What is the difference between oxygen content, oxygen saturation, and oxygen capacity?
2. What is the functional importance of the sigmoid shape of the oxyhemoglobin dissociation curve?

3. Why is the Haldane effect important?
4. What are the major storage sites for CO_2 and O_2?
5. O_2 uptake is usually determined from the rate of N_2 exchange in the lungs. If $FE_{N_2} = 0.5103$, $FI_{N_2} = 0.5059$, $FI_{O_2} = 0.4941$, $FE_{O_2} = 0.4672$, and $\dot{V}E = 7,500$ ml/min, what is $\dot{V}_{O_2}$?
6. Assume that a subject has an arterial O_2 content of 22 ml/100 ml of blood, a hemoglobin concentration of 16 g/100 ml of blood, and a P_{O_2} of 85 mmHg. A. What is the amount of oxygen in solution in 100 ml of blood? B. What is the O_2 saturation of hemoglobin?
7. If Ca_{O_2} is 19 ml/100 ml of blood and $C\bar{v}_{O_2}$ is 16 ml/100 ml of blood, what blood flow is necessary to sustain a $\dot{V}_{O_2}$ of 400 ml/min?
8. If a subject breathes room air and has an FE_{CO_2} of 0.05 and a $\dot{V}E$ of 7,500 ml/min, what is $\dot{V}_{CO_2}$?

5

PULMONARY AND BRONCHIAL CIRCULATIONS

INTRODUCTION

The pulmonary circulation is a low pressure, low resistance system containing highly compliant blood vessels in comparison with the systemic circulation, which is a high pressure, high resistance, and low compliance system. The pulmonary blood vessels generally have a passive role in the control of pulmonary blood flow because the primary function of the pulmonary circulation is to transport blood to the lung for oxygenation and carbon dioxide elimination. Consequently, the pulmonary circulation must accept whatever cardiac output is required to meet the metabolic demands of the body tissues while maintaining low pulmonary vascular pressures. This can again be contrasted with blood flow in the systemic circulation, which is closely controlled to meet the local metabolic demands of individual organ tissues over a wide range of perfusion pressures.

Vascular Anatomy

The anatomy of the right heart and pulmonary vessels reflects the low pressures and resistances in the pulmonary circulation. The wall thickness of the right ventricle is only 4 to 5 mm or about one-third that of the more muscular left ventricle and the right ventricle forms a crescent shape around the left ventricle. The wall of the main pulmonary artery consists of eight elastic layers with a thin medial layer of smooth muscle and is only one-fifth as thick as the wall of the ascending aorta. This means that the larger pulmonary arteries are primarily elastic and are well suited to accommodate changes in intravascular volume with little change in vascular pressure. Smooth muscle fibers constitute only about 2 per cent of the pulmonary artery wall thickness, but they provide a larger fraction of the wall thickness after several generations of branching. Therefore, the smaller arteries (with diameters of 1 mm down to 100 μm) are relatively more muscular. The maximum relative amount of smooth muscle occurs in arteries between 100 and 200 μm in diameter, which are located near the respiratory bronchioles. In subsequent branchings, the spiral muscular layer diminishes as the arterial vessels approach the alveolar ducts. Muscle fibers are completely absent within the wall of arterioles with diameters of less than 30 μm; thus, pulmonary arterioles differ significantly in appearance from the small muscular arterioles of the systemic circulation. As the pulmonary arterioles further divide, they branch into single 13 μm diameter blood vessels, one of which supplies each of the 300 million alveoli. These vessels divide into approximately 100 billion pulmonary capillaries, each about 12 μm long and 7 to 8 μm in diameter. Alveolar capillaries form such a dense array that alveolar septa are often described as a sheet of flowing blood pierced by intercapillary posts of interstitial connective tissue (Fig. 5–1). In contrast to the small arteries, the small veins (100 μm to 1 mm in diameter) have a thin, poorly organized muscular layer but contain substantial amounts of collagen.

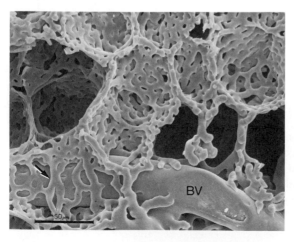

FIGURE 5–1. A scanning electron micrograph of a latex cast of alveolar capillaries and an extra-alveolar blood vessel (BV) in dog lung. The dense network of capillaries is punctured by small posts of tissue. The arrow indicates capillaries not within an alveolar septa. The bar indicates scale. (Reproduced courtesy of Luchtel D.: *J. Appl. Physiol., 53*:510–515, 1982.)

Pulmonary arteries generally accompany bronchi, whereas pulmonary veins course through interlobular septa and join the pulmonary arteries and bronchi only near the hilus. Exceptions to this branching pattern are seen in the supernumerary pulmonary arteries, which supply 25 per cent of the blood flow at the level of the respiratory bronchioles. These supernumerary vessels may provide a source of collateral blood flow in the event of occlusion of the primary blood supply.

There are approximately 3.6 branches from each parent stem in the 17 generations of the arterial tree. Vessel diameter and length both decrease by approximately 40 per cent with successive branchings. This leads to an increase in the total cross-sectional area of successive vascular generations (Fig. 5–2, solid line). Since velocity (dashed line) and cross-sectional area are inversely related, blood velocity is high in the large conducting vessels but slows abruptly as the red cells approach and enter the alveolar capillaries. Blood velocity in the capillaries is sufficiently slow to allow ample time for exchange of respiratory gases (see Fig. 3–2A). The time required for red cells to pass through the capillaries is approximately 0.75 sec, but longer transit times occur within regions of the lung where blood flow is reduced and in the longer capillaries of the pleural surface.

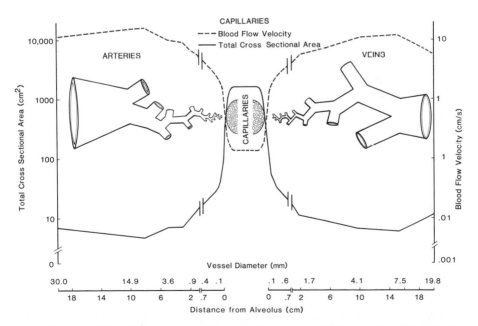

FIGURE 5–2. Relationship between total cross-sectional area (solid line) and blood flow velocity (dashed line) in the pulmonary circulation as a function of vessel diameter and distance from the alveoli. Note that the scale is expanded four times from 0 to 0.7 cm distance from the alveoli to depict details, and a logarithmic scale is used for area and velocity. Diagram of arterial and venous vessel branchings represents approximate proportions of lengths and diameters.

Alveolar and Extra-alveolar Vessels

Pulmonary vessels are also classified according to how their resistance responds to lung inflation. Large extraparenchymal pulmonary arteries and veins are directly exposed to the subatmospheric intrathoracic pressure that acts on their outer surface. The smaller arteries and veins within the lung parenchyma are surrounded by connective tissue sheaths on which the alveolar walls attach. These attachments exert an outward radial traction on the sheaths and increase the vessel diameters when the lung is inflated. These vessels are called *extra-alveolar vessels*. The pressure surrounding vessels smaller than approximately 50 μm in diameter is determined by alveolar gas pressure and alveolar fluid surface tensional forces. These vessels, which are exposed to alveolar gas pressures, may close at high alveolar pressures and are termed *alveolar vessels*. However, mechanical forces acting on alveolar *corner vessels* actually cause them to remain open, rather than close, even at high alveolar gas pressures. Therefore, these corner vessels behave as extra-alveolar vessels.

Pressures surrounding the blood vessels contribute to the *transmural pressure* (Ptm), which is the distending pressure of the vessel. Transmural pressure is equal to the difference between vascular (Pvas) and perivascular interstitial (Pis) pressures:

$$Ptm = Pvas - Pis \qquad (5\text{--}1)$$

When transmural pressure is increased by a more subatmospheric perivascular interstitial pressure, vessel diameter is increased. Since resistance decreases in proportion to the fourth power of the vessel radius, blood flow will be greatly increased. Conversely, a less subatmospheric perivascular pressure decreases both Ptm and vessel diameter, resulting in an increased vascular resistance and a reduction in blood flow. The transmural pressure for alveolar capillaries is approximately equal to capillary intravascular pressure minus the alveolar pressure, whereas the transmural pressure of extra-alveolar vessels is equal to vascular pressure minus pleural pressure.

Transmural distending pressures are different from the *driving pressure* responsible for producing blood flow. The driving pressure is the difference between intravascular pressures at the arterial and venous ends of the blood vessel. The relationship between driving pressure and pulmonary blood flow ($\dot{Q}$) is given by:

$$(Ppa - Pla) = \dot{Q} \times Rvas \qquad (5\text{--}2)$$

where Ppa is mean pulmonary arterial pressure, Pla is mean left atrial pressure, and Rvas is pulmonary vascular resistance. Perivascular pressures significantly affect pulmonary blood flow by altering pulmonary vascular resistance but usually do not change the driving pressure between pulmonary artery and left atrium.

PULMONARY VASCULAR PRESSURES

As a consequence of the low vascular resistance in the pulmonary circulation, the mean pulmonary arterial pressure is only about one-seventh that needed to force the same amount of blood through the high resistance systemic circulation (Table 5–1). Normal systolic/diastolic pulmonary artery pressures are about 24/8 mmHg in human lungs, producing a mean arterial pressure of 13.3 mmHg. Mean left atrial pressure is normally 6 mmHg. Therefore, the driving pressure between the pulmonary artery and left atrium (7.3 mmHg) is approximately 1/12 that of the systemic circulation. Since the same cardiac output passes through both circulations, the total pulmonary vascular resistance is about 1/12 that of the systemic circulation.

The lack of small muscular arterioles in the pulmonary circuit results in the longitudinal pressure profile in the pulmonary circulation, as shown schematically in Figure 5–3. Because flow pulsations and pressure are not damped in the lung's small arterioles, pulsatile flow and pressure are transmitted along the entire length of the pulmonary circulation. In fact, the resistance is so low that pulmonary artery diastolic pressures can approach pulmonary venous pressure. Indeed, diastolic pressure is often used to approximate left atrial pressure in patients. Because of this low arteriolar resistance and the viscous drag of the blood within the capillaries, as much as 40 per cent of the total pressure drop may occur across the pulmonary capillaries at normal vascular pressures and flows. However, with respect to the average capillary pressure, the total vascular resistance is approximately equally divided between pre- and postcapillary resistance blood vessels.

Pulmonary artery and pulmonary wedge pressures are frequently measured in selected patients using a catheter placed into the pulmonary artery (Swan-Ganz balloon catheter). Advancing the catheter and inflating its balloon occludes a small artery, producing a continuous channel of static fluid between the catheter tip and the pulmonary veins. Since the pressure drop between the pulmonary veins and left atrium is normally small, the *pulmonary artery*

TABLE 5–1.   Comparison of Pulmonary and Systemic Vascular Pressures and Blood Flows

	Pulmonary Circulation	Systemic Circulation
Arterial (systolic/diastolic) pressure	24/8 mmHg	120/80 mmHg
Mean arterial pressure	13.3 mmHg*	93.3 mmHg
Mean atrial pressure	(left) 6 mmHg	(right) 2 mmHg
Mean capillary pressure	10 mmHg	18 mmHg
Driving pressure	7.3 mmHg	91.3 mmHg
Blood flow	5 l/min	5 l/min
Vascular resistance	1.5 mmHg/l/min	18.3 mmHg/l/min

*Calculated as 1/3 (difference between systolic and diastolic pressures) + diastolic pressure, e.g., mean pulmonary arterial = 1/3(24 − 8) + 8 = 5.3 + 8 = 13.3.

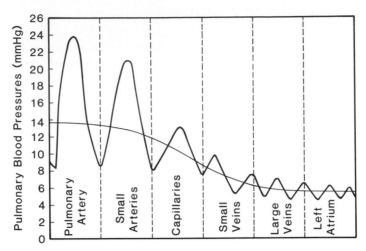

FIGURE 5–3. Mean (light solid line) and pulsatile (heavy solid line) blood pressures in different segments of the pulmonary circulation. Note the significant pulsatile pressures throughout the pulmonary circulation and the similarity of pulmonary artery diastolic and left atrial pressures.

wedge pressure is a good estimate of left atrial pressure, provided that the veins are not completely collapsed (which could occur during pulmonary vascular hypotension or with mechanical ventilation using high airway pressures).

PULMONARY BLOOD VOLUME

Of the total circulating blood volume (70 to 80 ml/kg body weight), approximately 10 per cent is present within the pulmonary circulation (480 ml). This blood volume is divided approximately equally between arteries (150 ml), microvessels (180 ml), and veins (150 ml). However, these volumes can change considerably with vascular pressure changes.

The pressure-volume relationship of the pulmonary circulation is shown in Figure 5–4. As pulmonary blood volume doubles, the vascular pressure increases four-fold from point A to point B. This means that the pulmonary blood volume can increase by about 500 ml in human adults, and pulmonary vascular pressure increases only by about 35 mmHg.

Volume changes in the pulmonary circulation are a function of the vascular compliance (Cvas), which is the change in blood volume (ΔVvas) for a given change in vascular pressure (ΔPvas):

$$Cvas = \Delta Vvas/\Delta Pvas \qquad (5-3)$$

Pulmonary vascular compliance is normally about 30 ml/mmHg for the entire human lung (point C, which is derived by calculating the slope of the pressure volume curve at point A). Approximately 70 per cent of the total compliance

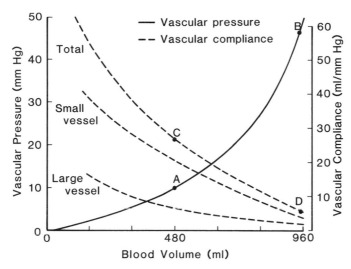

FIGURE 5–4. Pressure-volume relationship of the pulmonary circulation showing vascular pressure (solid line). Total vascular compliance, compliance of small blood vessels (< 100 μm diameter), and the compliance of larger blood vessels (> 100 μm diameter) are shown as dashed lines. At a normal pulmonary blood volume of 480 ml and a vascular pressure of 11 mmHg (point A), the compliance of the total vasculature is about 30 ml/mmHg (point C). When the volume doubles to 960 ml, vascular pressure increases four-fold (point B), and the compliance of all components decreases to point D.

is located in the small vessels. Compliance is higher in the alveolar vessels (small vessel) because they are surrounded by gas and can be easily distended, whereas extra-alveolar vessels (large vessel) are tethered to the alveolar walls and are more rigid and less compliant. As pulmonary vascular volume doubles, total compliance falls from 30 to about 6 ml/mmHg (point C→point D).

Pulmonary blood volume is estimated in humans by analyzing the passage of a substance confined to the vascular compartment of the pulmonary circulation (see Appendix C). Pulmonary blood volume is decreased by any disease that destroys parenchymal tissue, such as emphysema, or occludes vessels, such as pulmonary embolization. Pulmonary vascular volumes increase during left heart failure and mitral insufficiency because of the high pulmonary vascular pressures associated with these conditions.

PULMONARY BLOOD FLOW

Pulmonary blood flow is most often measured using the *thermal-dilution method*. A small bolus of cold saline is injected through a catheter into the right atrium. The time required for the bolus to pass from the injection site to a thermistor located on the catheter tip in the pulmonary artery is used to calculate pulmonary blood flow. This technique is now widely used to measure pulmonary blood flow in patients, and its application has been further simplified by modern catheter and computer technologies. The method for calculation of pulmonary blood flow using the thermal-dilution method is found in Appendix C.

The following methods can also be used to measure pulmonary blood flow. The *Fick principle* uses oxygen uptake ($\dot{V}_{O_2}$) and mixed venous ($C\bar{v}_{O_2}$) and arterial (Ca_{O_2}) oxygen contents to calculate blood flow as $\dot{Q} = \dot{V}_{O_2}/(Ca_{O_2} - C\bar{v}_{O_2})$. Another technique used to measure pulmonary blood flow involves the use of a body plethysmograph. A subject in a plethysmograph breathes a mixture of N_2O and O_2 from a bag. Since N_2O rapidly equilibrates across the alveolar-capillary membrane, N_2O uptake by the lung is perfusion-limited (see Chapter 3). The plethysmograph gas volume decreases with time as the pulmonary blood absorbs N_2O, and this decrease is directly related to blood flow. By integrating the decrease in plethysmograph gas volume, the pulmonary blood flow can be estimated. In yet another technique, a subject inspires a gas mixture containing a low concentration of acetylene (0.5 per cent). Since acetylene uptake is also perfusion-limited, the exponential decrease in its concentration in alveolar gas is proportional to blood flow.

In many instances the regional distribution of pulmonary blood flow can be quite useful in the detection of perfusion defects associated with conditions such as pulmonary embolization. The regional distribution of pulmonary blood flow can be evaluated by injecting either radioactive xenon or microspheres of albumin labeled with radioactive iodine. The radioactivity of these substances is subsequently measured using external detectors placed over the lung. The measured radioactivity is proportional to the regional blood flow.

FACTORS AFFECTING VASCULAR RESISTANCE

Vascular Pressure

Pulmonary vascular resistance decreases when blood flow and pressure are increased, as shown in Figure 5–5. When cardiac output increases from 5 to 15 l/min, the rise in pulmonary artery pressure (solid line, point A→point C) is attenuated by the concurrent reduction in pulmonary vascular resistance (dashed line, point A→point B). However, once resistance reaches a minimum value (point B), any additional increase in cardiac output will cause a greater increase in pulmonary artery pressure. When left atrial pressure is low (6.0 mmHg), pronounced decreases in vascular resistance occur with increased pulmonary arterial pressure (Fig. 5–6). Recruitment of additional capillaries and distension of microvessels account for these large decreases in vascular resistance. By contrast, pulmonary artery pressure has little effect on vascular resistance when left atrial pressure is high (14.8 mmHg). Once all vessels have

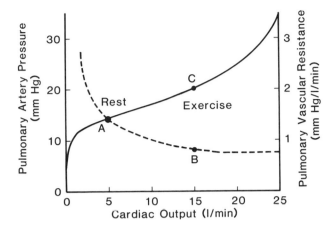

FIGURE 5–5. Relationship of pulmonary artery pressure (solid line) and vascular resistance (dashed line) to cardiac output. At rest (point A), cardiac output is 5 l/min and pulmonary vascular resistance is 1.5 mmHg/l/min. During exercise, if cardiac output triples to 15 l/min, pulmonary vascular resistance decreases by one-half (point B), and pulmonary arterial pressure increases by only 6 mmHg (point C).

been fully recruited and are maximally distended, as seen with high left atrial pressure, no further decrease in resistance can occur.

Hematocrit

Since the pressure drop between the pulmonary artery and the capillaries is small, the viscous drag of the blood in the capillaries contributes significantly to pulmonary vascular resistance. When hematocrit is below 40 per cent, the pulmonary vascular resistance decreases by 0.5 per cent for each per cent decrease in hematocrit. However, for hematocrits greater than 40 per cent, the relative resistance change is much greater (4 per cent per hematocrit unit). A large increase in pulmonary vascular resistance is seen in polycythemia, in which hematocrits can increase to 55 to 60 per cent.

Lung Volume

The relationship between total pulmonary vascular resistance and lung volume is "U" shaped, i.e., vascular resistance increases at both high and very low lung volumes as shown in Figure 5–7. At low lung volumes, the extra-alveolar vessels are distorted and have a knarled appearance due to the reduction in radial wall traction. This distortion causes an increase in vascular resistance by decreasing the cross-sectional area of the extra-alveolar vessels (dashed line). At higher lung volumes, the extra-alveolar vessels are surrounded by a more subatmospheric perivascular pressure, so that their resistance decreases. At the same time, however, the alveolar walls are stretched and the

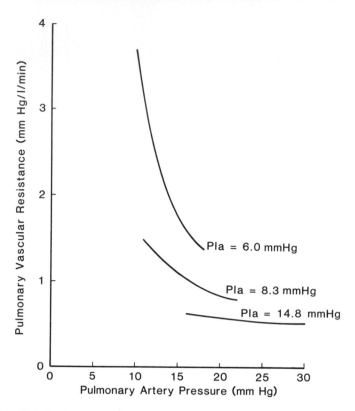

FIGURE 5–6. Plot of pulmonary vascular resistances as a function of pulmonary artery pressure at three different left atrial (Pla) pressures (6.0, 8.3, and 14.8 mmHg). Lower resistance values are associated with the higher left atrial pressures.

alveolar vessels are compressed, increasing their contribution to pulmonary vascular resistance (dashed-dotted line). It is of interest to note that vascular resistance reaches its minimum value at functional residual capacity (FRC).

REGIONAL BLOOD FLOW DIFFERENCES

Vascular Waterfall

Because the alveolar vessels are exposed to alveolar gas pressure, their blood flow is greatly affected by this pressure. Figure 5–8 shows a model depicting the effects of surrounding pressure. As long as the pressure surrounding the alveolar vessels (Palv) is less than the intravascular pressure, the pulmonary blood flow is determined by the difference between pulmonary arterial (Ppa) and pulmonary venous (Ppv) pressures (Fig. 5–8A). But when the pressure surrounding the alveolar vessels is greater than the intravascular

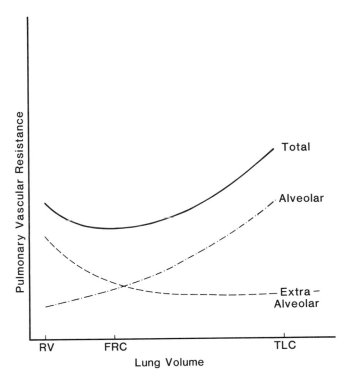

FIGURE 5–7. Effect of lung volume on total pulmonary vascular resistance (solid line), extra-alveolar vessel resistance (dashed line), and alveolar vessel resistance (dashed-dotted line). Note that the total resistance is minimal at functional residual capacity *(FRC)*. *TLC* = total lung capacity, *RV* = residual volume.

FIGURE 5–8. Model depicting the effects of surrounding pressure (Palv) on pulmonary blood flow. Ppa, Palv, and Ppv refer to pulmonary arterial, alveolar and venous pressures, respectively. (Redrawn from Fishman, A.P.: Pulmonary circulation. In Fishman, A.P., and Fisher, A.B. (eds.): *Handbook of Physiology:* Section 3: The Respiratory System, Volume 1. Circulation and Non-respiratory Function. Bethesda: American Physiological Society, 1985, p. 101.)

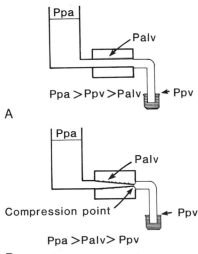

pressure, the alveolar vessels will collapse (Fig. 5–8B). Because of the pressure drop associated with flow of blood through the tube, the pressure within the tube is less in its more distal segment. When the pressure in the tube falls below the alveolar pressure, the driving pressure for flow abruptly becomes Ppa-Palv, and changes in the outflow pressure (Ppv) have no effect on flow. This effect has been described as similar to that seen in a waterfall (or a sluice), where the height of the fall does not affect the flow over the lip of the fall. A similar mechanism is responsible for expiratory airflow limitation as discussed in Chapter 7.

Blood Flow Zones

Figure 5–9 shows that a vertical distance of 30 cm separates the apices from the bases of the lungs. This allows gravity to markedly affect the vertical distribution of regional vascular pressures and blood flows; vascular pressures and blood flows are less at the top of the lung than at the bottom. A hydrostatic pressure gradient of 1 cmH₂O/cm vertical height exists for the intravascular

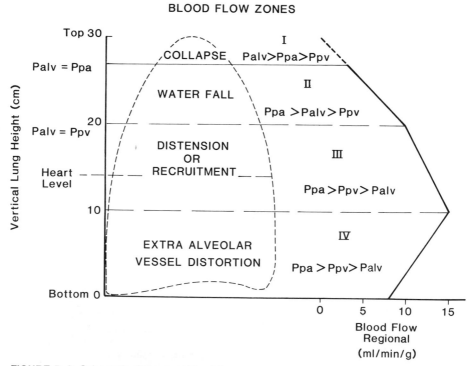

FIGURE 5–9. Schematic diagram of blood flow zones in an idealized upright lung. The figure shows an upright lung of 30 cm height, demonstrating zones I, II, III, and IV, and the pressure relationships within these zones. The regional blood flow from top to bottom of the lung is shown in the right portion of the figure.

pressures in both arteries and veins. In this example, the mean pulmonary venous (left atrial) pressure (Ppv) is assumed to be 6 cmH$_2$O and the mean pulmonary artery pressure (Ppa) is assumed to be 14 cmH$_2$O at heart level. The resultant driving pressure for flow at the level of the heart is 8 cmH$_2$O. In contrast to vascular pressures, alveolar gas pressure is the same at all vertical lung heights and equals atmospheric pressure (0 cmH$_2$O) at rest. Since Ppv decreases by 1 cmH$_2$O/cm vertical distance above the heart, it equals alveolar gas pressure at a height of 6 cm above heart level. Similarly, *mean* Ppa equals alveolar gas pressure at 14 cmH$_2$O above heart level. Although intravascular pressures are different at each lung level, the driving pressure for blood flow varies only when Palv exceeds Ppv.

Four blood flow zones are defined within the lung based on the relationship among mean pulmonary arterial (Ppa), pulmonary venous (Ppv), and alveolar gas (Palv) pressures as shown in Figure 5–9. In zone I, at the very top of the lung, alveolar gas pressure exceeds mean arterial pressure (Palv > Ppa > Ppv), and perfusion occurs only during systole when pulsatile pressure in the alveolar capillaries exceeds alveolar gas pressure (as shown by the dashed line in blood flow at the right uppermost part of Figure 5–9). Mechanical distending forces on capillaries located at alveolar wall junctions (corner vessels) tend to maintain patency of these vessels, even when alveolar gas pressure exceeds intravascular pressure. In these corner capillaries, blood flow occurs even higher in the lung than predicted from average vascular and alveolar pressures (dashed portion of blood flow line in zone I).

The next region down the lung is defined as zone II. In this zone, alveolar gas pressure exceeds venous outflow pressures (Ppa > Palv > Ppv), and blood flow is determined by the arterial to alveolar pressure gradient (Ppa-Palv). Compression of alveolar vessels (or waterfall conditions) occurs at the point where intravascular pressure equals alveolar gas pressure. Since pulmonary artery pressure increases by 1 cmH$_2$O/cm vertical distance down the lung, the driving pressure also increases by 1 cmH$_2$O/cm vertical height down the lung.

In zone III, Ppa > Ppv > Palv, and the driving pressure for blood flow is Ppa-Ppv. Since arterial and venous intravascular pressures are equally affected by gravity, blood flow increases down this zone, although the mean driving pressure remains constant. The increased blood flow in this zone occurs because the increased intravascular pressures (both arterial and venous) reduce pulmonary vascular resistances by distension and/or recruitment of microvessels.

In zone IV, Ppa > Ppv > Palv, and blood flow decreases down the lung even though the driving pressure for flow does not change. This phenomenon can be understood by recalling the effects of lung volume on vascular resistance as shown in Figure 5–6. At very low lung volumes, resistance in extra-alveolar vessels increases owing to a decrease in the distending forces exerted on the vessel sheaths by alveolar attachments. This causes vessel distortion and increased vascular resistance. In the vertical lung, regional gas volume is greater at the top of the lung than at the bottom. This is because pleural pressure is more subatmospheric at the top, creating a greater regional transpulmonary pressure. Conversely, pleural pressure is less subatmospheric at the lung bases and may actually exceed atmospheric pressure. This results in a decreased regional lung volume and a tendency for extra-alveolar vessels to be distorted in the lower portion of the lung. Zone IV conditions exist in the entire lower one-half to one-third of the lung during quiet respiration in the upright posture.

Changes in lung volume can alter this fraction, as seen in Figure 5–10. Expiration to residual volume (RV) increases the area of zone IV such that flows at the top of the lung can actually exceed those at the bottom. These effects are attributable to the more positive pleural pressures at low lung volumes, which increase the tendency for extra-alveolar distortion at the lung bases. Conversely, inspiration to total lung capacity (TLC) reduces the zone IV area owing to increased distension of these extra-alveolar vessels.

Distribution of regional blood flow is markedly affected by body position and cardiac output. In a recumbent subject, zone I is essentially abolished, resulting in a more uniform perfusion of lung as compared with an upright subject. Flow gradients between dorsal and ventral regions of the lung exist in the recumbent subject. Exercise increases vascular pressures at all vertical levels such that all lung regions are more uniformly perfused and the gas exchange area of the lung is maximized. Pulmonary arterial hypotension produces the opposite effect, causing an increased amount of the lung to be perfused under zone I and II conditions. During mechanical ventilation, the higher mean airway pressure increases Palv, causing the amount of lung perfused in zones I and II to increase.

CONTROL OF PULMONARY VASCULAR TONE

Although predominantly passive mechanical forces determine regional blood flow distribution in the lung, the smooth muscle in arteries and veins as well as contractile elements of interstitial cells and myofibroblasts respond to

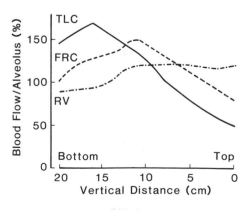

FIGURE 5–10. Blood flow as a function of lung height when human lungs are maintained at total lung capacity (TLC), functional residual capacity (FRC), or residual volume (RV). Note that zone IV (the decreasing flow toward the bottom of the lung) becomes progressively smaller as lung volume increases. (Adapted from Hughes, J.M., Glazier, J.B., Maloney, J.E., et al.: Effect of lung volume on the distribution of pulmonary blood flow in man. *Resp. Physiol.,* 4:58–72, 1968.)

many vasoactive compounds that actively influence regional blood flow distribution. Various receptors and reflexes have been identified in the pulmonary circulation, but their contributions to the control of either total or regional blood flow under normal conditions are not known. A modest autonomic innervation, with both adrenergic and cholinergic components, is found in the muscular vessels of the pulmonary circulation. Stimulation of the sympathetic nervous system constricts the blood vessels of the lung, whereas parasympathetic stimulation causes vasodilatation. There are both α and β adrenergic receptors, but sympathetic tone is usually very low.

Vasoactive Compounds

Table 5–2 lists numerous compounds that affect pulmonary vascular resistance and their sites of action. With only a few exceptions, the same vasoactive agents that constrict systemic blood vessels cause similar responses in the

TABLE 5–2. Vasoactive Agents in the Adult Pulmonary Circulation

Agent	Proposed Site of Action
Vasoconstriction	
Sympathetic stimulation	Muscular arteries
Epinephrine	Arteries and veins (α and β receptors)
Norepinephrine	Arteries, α receptors
Serotonin	Small arteries (veins)
Histamine	Venules, H_1 receptors (blocked by Benadryl)
Vasoactive intestinal peptide	—
Hypoxia	Small arteries
Hypercapnia	Arteries
Acidemia	Arteries
Arachidonic acid	Small veins
Thromboxane A_2	
Angiotensin II	
Leukotrienes	LTD_4 small arteries, veins, and bronchi
$PGF_{2\alpha}$	Veins
PGE_2	Veins
Substance P	Veins
PGD_2	—
PGH_2	—
*Vasodilation**	
Parasympathetic stimulation	—
Isoproterenol	— (β receptors)
Bradykinin	—
Acetylcholine	—
PGE_1	Arteries
PGI_2	Small arteries and veins
Dopamine	
Phentolamine	
Histamine	H_2 receptors (blocked with cimetidine)

*Many of these compounds cause different effects in different species. The response is dependent on pulmonary vascular tone, e.g., histamine constricts vessels with normal tone but dilates vessels with high vascular tone.

pulmonary circulation. Histamine is a notable exception to the rule, since it is a potent constrictor of the venules in the pulmonary circulation but a vasodilator in the systemic circulation. Interestingly, under experimental conditions in which pulmonary vascular tone has been increased, histamine can actually cause vasodilation. Serotonin (5-hydroxytryptamine), released during allergic responses, causes intense pulmonary vasoconstriction, platelet aggregation, and bronchoconstriction. Several arachidonate products increase pulmonary vascular resistance; these products include prostaglandins $F_{2\alpha}$ and E_2, thromboxane A_2, and the leukotrienes (some of which are the slow reacting substances associated with the bronchoconstriction of asthma).

Because the pulmonary circulation normally maintains a low vascular tone, many vasodilators have a more pronounced effect when the initial pulmonary vascular tone is high. Prostacyclin (PGI_2) is a potent vasodilator of the pulmonary circulation and is released by the vascular endothelial cells in response to a variety of stimuli. It is currently thought that the balance between the levels of PGI_2 and thromboxane A_2 sets the normal pulmonary vascular tone.

Hypoxia, Hypercapnia, and pH Effects

The pulmonary hypoxic vasoconstrictor response is considered to be a means of reducing pulmonary blood flow to poorly ventilated lung regions. In lung regions with low O_2 tensions, the vascular resistances are high, resulting in a redistribution of blood flow to regions with higher O_2 tensions. This results is better matching of ventilation to perfusion and more efficient overall gas exchange. This vascular response occurs largely as a result of alveolar hypoxia rather than arterial hypoxemia. The response of lobar pulmonary blood flow to graded changes in alveolar oxygen tension is shown in Figure 5–11A. There is little decrease in lobar pulmonary blood flow until the P_{AO_2} falls below 90 mmHg. This vasoconstriction occurs almost exclusively at the small muscular arteries. When alveolar P_{CO_2} is altered in the range of 20 to 50 mmHg, no consistent change in blood flow is observed (Fig. 5–11B). However, at higher P_{ACO_2} values, blood flow is reduced.

Vascular resistance increases by 50 per cent for each reduction in pH of 0.1 unit below normal. Of more importance is the multiplicative effect of a decreased pH on the hypoxic vasoconstrictor response to low alveolar O_2 tensions. The hypoxic vasoconstrictor response is three times more potent when there is a simultaneous decrease in pH of 0.1 to 0.2 unit. Hypercapnia also enhances the hypoxic vasoconstrictor response to low alveolar O_2 tensions, whereas alkalosis and hypocapnia generally oppose the response. The enhancement of the hypoxic vasoconstrictor response by both regional hypercapnia and acidemia may be of considerable importance, since these conditions usually occur together in poorly ventilated lung regions.

The mechanism responsible for the hypoxic vasoconstriction is still unknown. The vasoconstriction is precapillary and calcium dependent and appears

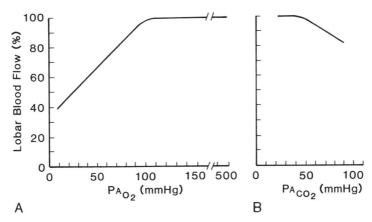

FIGURE 5–11. Effect of gradual changes in alveolar oxygen tension *(A)* and CO_2 tension *(B)* on lobar blood flow. Note that a marked reduction in blood flow occurs at alveolar (P_{AO_2}) levels below 90 mmHg or alveolar (P_{ACO_2}) levels above 46 mmHg. (Adapted from Barer, G.R., Howard, P., Shaw, J.W.: Stimulus-response curves for the pulmonary vascular bed to hypoxia and hypercapnia. *J. Physiol., 211*:139–155, 1970.)

to be mediated by a locally released and locally active substance. Oxygen-free radicals and leukotrienes have been suggested as local mediators. Cyclo-oxygenase blockers such as indomethacin, aspirin, and meclofenamate enhance the hypoxic response, whereas cromolyn, PGE_1, and calcium channel blockers attenuate the response. Volatile anesthetics attenuate the response, whereas intravenous anesthetics have little or no effect.

PULMONARY HYPERTENSION

Increases in pulmonary vascular resistance usually result in increased pulmonary arterial pressure. Diseases that produce destruction of small arterial vessels produce pulmonary hypertension, which is further aggravated if cardiac output also increases. Emphysema, scleroderma, interstitial fibrosis, and granulomatous diseases increase pulmonary vascular resistance because they destroy blood vessels. Persistent hypoxia, especially in the presence of acidosis, leads to hypertension because of intense vasoconstriction. Pulmonary emboli also increase pulmonary arterial pressure and vascular resistance by obstructing flow through embolized portions of the lung. The ultimate pathophysiologic consequences of pulmonary hypertension are right heart hypertrophy (*cor pulmonale*) and right heart failure leading to death if the hypertension is not relieved.

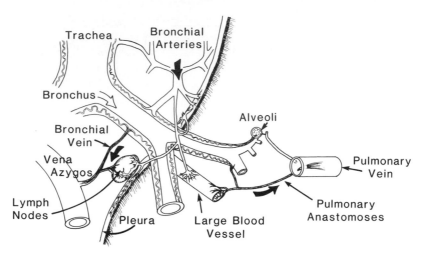

FIGURE 5–12. Diagram of bronchial circulation showing the distribution of blood flow to the bronchi, pleura, lymph nodes, and large blood vessels. Note that venous drainage of the larger bronchi returns to the right atrium via the azygous vein but blood from smaller bronchi flows to the left atrium via bronchopulmonary anastomoses. (From Deffebach, M.E., Charan, N.B., Lakshminarayan, S., and Butler, J.: The bronchial circulation. *Am. Rev. Resp. Dis., 135*:463–481, 1987.)

BRONCHIAL CIRCULATION

The bronchial circulation provides the primary nutrient blood flow to the trachea, large and small bronchi, adventitia of large pulmonary blood vessels, visceral pleura, sympathetic ganglia, and hilar lymph nodes (Fig. 5–12). Total bronchial blood flow is small and normally constitutes only 1 to 2 per cent of total cardiac output (50 to 100 ml/min). The dense submucosal vascular plexuses in the trachea and bronchi warm and provide fluid to humidify the inspired gas. Bronchopulmonary anastomoses provide an important collateral source of blood supply to the lung parenchyma. This blood can also participate in gas exchange.

In humans, there are usually two bronchial arterial branches to the left lung and one or two to the right lung. These vessels are small (1.5 mm in diameter) and arise from the aorta and intercostal arteries. Rarely, branches from the internal mammary, subclavian, or coronary arteries are seen. Bronchial arteries follow the outside of the airways down to the terminal bronchioles. Small arterial branches penetrate inward through the muscle layers and anastomose to form the submucosal vascular plexus that extends all the way to the level of the terminal bronchioles. Nutrient vessels supply the walls of the bronchi. In respiratory bronchioles and alveoli, the bronchial vessels can anastomose directly with small pulmonary arteries, capillaries, and veins. Bronchial veins draining the large extrapulmonary airways join the azygous vein, which empties into the right atrium. Venous drainage from the intraparenchymal airways exits through bronchopulmonary anastomoses to the pulmonary veins and left atrium. Addition of this deoxygenated bronchial blood to the oxygenated pulmonary venous blood contributes to the *venous admixture* of arterial blood. Bronchopulmonary anastomotic flow and the resulting venous admixture are reduced by both high pulmonary vascular pressures and high alveolar gas pressures. These high pressures cause venous drainage to be shunted away from the pulmonary veins to the systemic venous system.

Systemic arterial hypoxemia and alveolar hypoxia can increase anastomotic bronchial blood flow. An increased Pa_{CO_2} increases total and anastomotic bronchial blood flow, whereas an increased PA_{CO_2} has little effect. Dilation of anastomotic vessels due to changes in Pa_{CO_2} or Pa_{O_2} is blocked by indomethacin (which blocks the formation of prostaglandins), whereas $PGF_{2\alpha}$ increases anastomotic blood flow. Positive pressure ventilation decreases anastomotic flow by compressing the bronchopulmonary anastomoses.

The bronchial capillaries are fenestrated and respond to agents such as histamine similarly to other systemic vessels. Histamine causes an increased microvascular permeability to fluid and macromolecules because of endothelial contraction. Mucosal edema results, and bronchial blood flow is increased. Recall that in the pulmonary circulation, histamine can produce venous constriction but causes no change in capillary wall permeability to macromolecules.

The bronchial circulation undergoes a remarkable hypertrophy in response to inflammatory diseases of the lung. Chronic bronchitis, bronchiolitis, and bronchiectasis may result in bronchopulmonary anastomotic blood flow as high as 30 per cent of cardiac output. This may cause a significant portion of the cardiac output to bypass the gas-exchanging units of the lung and a decrease in the O_2 saturation of arterial hemoglobin. Granulomas and neoplasms of the lung are supplied by the bronchial circulation, and the hemoptysis seen in these diseases often results from rupture of these bronchial blood vessels.

PULMONARY CIRCULATION IN THE FETUS AND NEWBORN

Remarkable changes occur in the circulation at birth that cause a dramatic reduction in pulmonary vascular resistance. Figure 5–13 is a diagrammatic representation of the fetal circulation. Fetal blood is oxygenated at the placenta by diffusion of O_2 from maternal sinus blood to fetal blood. Gradients for CO_2 and pH between maternal (Pa_{CO_2} = 37 mmHg, pH = 7.48) and fetal blood (Pa_{CO_2} = 42 mmHg, pH = 7.3) provide the driving force for CO_2 and hydrogen ion exchange across the placenta. In the fetus, oxygenated blood in the umbilical vein, with a Pa_{O_2} of only 30 mmHg but a hemoglobin saturation of 75 per cent, courses primarily through a liver bypass, the ductus venosus, with a small portion passing through the liver. This oxygenated blood, representing 75 per cent of total cardiac output, enters the right atrium, where it mixes with blood

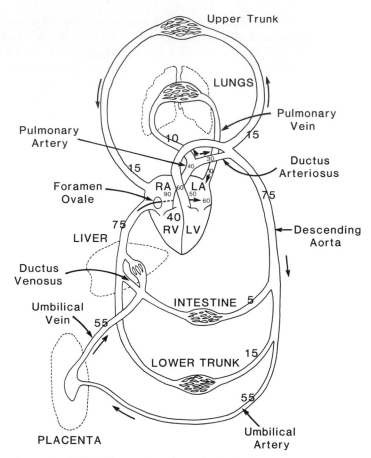

FIGURE 5–13. Diagram of the human fetal circulation showing the direction of blood flow (arrows) and percentage of cardiac output at each point. (Redrawn from Murray, J.F.: *The Normal Lung.* Philadelphia: W.B. Saunders, 1976, p. 9.)

from the upper trunk (15 per cent of cardiac output). Together this flow makes up 90 per cent of the cardiac output, which enters the right atrium. A portion of the blood in the right atrium (40 per cent of cardiac output) passes into the right ventricle and is pumped into the pulmonary artery. The remaining portion (50 per cent of cardiac output) flows through the foramen ovale into the left atrium and mixes with blood returning from the lung (representing 10 per cent of cardiac output). Therefore, 60 per cent of the cardiac output flows through the left atrium. This blood flows into the left ventricle and is pumped into the ascending aorta. The blood in the pulmonary artery is distributed to the lungs (10 per cent of cardiac output) or flows through the ductus arteriosus (30 per cent of cardiac output) to enter the descending aorta. Fifteen per cent of the cardiac output leaves the aorta and goes to the upper trunk, whereas the remaining 75 per cent of the cardiac output is distributed to the other body tissues and placenta as shown in Figure 5–13.

Note in Figure 5–13 that the blood going to the upper trunk (15 per cent of cardiac output) leaves the aorta before the blood from the ductus arteriosus is added. Because of a special ridge in the right atrium, the *eustachian valve*, that preferentially shunts oxygen-rich blood from the inferior vena cava through the foramen ovale, the blood in the left side of the heart and ascending aorta has a higher oxygen saturation than that in the pulmonary artery. Therefore, oxygen-rich blood perfuses the brain. Most of the blood in the pulmonary artery, which has a low oxygen saturation, bypasses the high resistance pulmonary circulation *via* the ductus arteriosus to enter the descending aorta. The blood in the descending aorta is distributed to the intestine (5 per cent of cardiac output), lower trunk (15 per cent of cardiac output), and placenta (55 per cent of cardiac output).

After birth, the fluid-filled lungs of the fetus expand with gas and the ductus venosus and ductus arteriosus close. These events promote pulmonary gas exchange, which did not exist before birth. When the lungs expand at birth, pulmonary vascular resistance decreases markedly in response to (1) the filling of alveoli with gas rather than liquid, which allows alveolar blood vessels to fill; (2) the increased P_{AO_2}, which causes vasodilation of pulmonary blood vessels; and (3) the decreased P_{ACO_2} and increased arterial pH, which also favor vasodilation of pulmonary vessels. Because of the decreased pulmonary vascular resistance, pulmonary arterial pressure decreases and pulmonary blood flow greatly increases. Since aortic pressure and systemic vascular resistance increase at the same time that pulmonary artery pressure decreases, blood flow through the ductus arteriosus actually reverses and moves from the aorta into the pulmonary artery. This left-to-right shunt usually continues for a few days after birth until the ductus arteriosus closes.

At birth, the foramen ovale closes spontaneously because the pressure becomes higher in the left atrium than in the right atrium. In addition, the ductus venosus closes after birth.

When the ductus arteriosus does not close, the left-to-right shunt causes the infant's right ventricle to work harder. Since only oxygenated blood passes through this shunt, cyanosis is not present. In the past, it was felt that the sudden increase in Pa_{O_2} caused ductal closure. It is now known that a product of arachidonic acid metabolism maintains patency of the ductus. For many years a persistent patent ductus arteriosus was closed surgically, but indomethacin, which blocks the formation of arachidonic acid metabolites, is now used to close the patent ductus arteriosus.

Infant Respiratory Distress Syndrome

In premature infants delivered before adequate surfactant has been formed or in cases of meconium aspiration during delivery, pulmonary edema, arterial hypoxemia, and respiratory failure may develop. The lungs of these infants are characterized by focal areas of atelectasis, edema, and a protein-rich exudate (hyaline membrane). The high surface tension in the alveoli leads to regional collapse and prevents homogeneous inflation of the lungs. Formation of pulmonary edema is promoted by regional stresses that damage capillaries and increase their permeability to macromolecules. In addition, high surface tensional forces can promote transport of fluid into the alveoli. A glassy pink (hyaline) appearance of the proteinaceous fluid layer in the alveoli is seen in stained histologic sections and has led to the use of the term "hyaline membrane disease" for this condition.

Tetralogy of Fallot

In this congenital malformation, four congenital abnormalities exist: (1) the aorta originates from the right ventricle or overrides the ventricular septum; (2) the pulmonary artery is stenosed and the majority of blood flow from the right ventricle bypasses the lungs to enter the aorta; (3) a ventricular septal defect is present that allows blood to pass from the left ventricle into the right ventricle; and (4) the right ventricle hypertrophies since it must pump blood against a high aortic pressure. In this condition, as much as 75 per cent of the blood can bypass the lungs and cyanosis will be obvious owing to the large quantity of deoxygenated blood reaching the periphery.

Atrial Septal Defect

Sometimes an opening exists between the left and right atrium that allows blood to be shunted from the left to the right atrium. This is the most common congenital lesion of the heart, ranging from an open foramen ovale to complete absence of the atrioventricular (AV) septum. The foramen ovale may not close in 5 to 20 per cent of the population, but, because the left atrial pressure exceeds the right atrial pressure, the valve-like flap closes the opening and prevents left-to-right shunting. As a consequence of an atrial septal defect, the right ventricle must pump an abnormally large quantity of blood. This may lead to right ventricular hypertrophy and subsequent heart failure if not surgically corrected.

SUGGESTED READING

Deffebach, M.E., Charan, N.B., Lakshminarayan, S., and Butler, J.: The bronchial circulation. Am. Rev. Resp. Dis., 135:463–481, 1987.

Fishman, A.P.: Dynamics of the pulmonary circulation. In Hamilton, W.F. (ed.): Handbook of Physiology: Section 2: Circulation, Volume II. Bethesda: American Physiological Society, 1963, pp. 1667–1743.

Fishman, A.P.: Pulmonary circulation. In Fishman, A.P., and Fisher, A.B. (eds.): Handbook of

Physiology: Section 3: The Respiratory System, Volume 1. Circulation and Non-respiratory Function. Bethesda: American Physiological Society, 1985, pp. 93–165.

QUESTIONS

1. If cardiac output is 4 l/min, pulmonary artery pressure is 15 cmH_2O, and left atrial pressure is 5 cmH_2O, what is pulmonary vascular resistance?

2. Blood flow through a collapsible tube is 100 ml/min when inflow pressure is 20 mmHg, outflow pressure is 5 mmHg, and surrounding pressure is 0 mmHg. If the surrounding pressure is increased to 15 mmHg, what will be the approximate blood flow that results?

3. In a normal subject, total peripheral resistance is about how many times the pulmonary vascular resistance?

4. Why does regional blood flow increase down zone III but decrease down zone IV when estimated driving pressure is about the same in both zones?

THE RESPIRATORY PUMP
Inspiration
Expiration
Respiratory Muscle Strength

ELASTIC PROPERTIES OF THE LUNG
Static Pressure-Volume Curve
Static Compliance
Surface Tension

ELASTIC PROPERTIES OF THE CHEST WALL

VERTICAL GRADIENT OF PLEURAL PRESSURE
Effect on Regional Ventilation
Single-Breath Nitrogen Washout Test
Interregional Nonuniformity
Intraregional Nonuniformity

6

MECHANICS OF BREATHING: STATIC

The respiratory system consists of two parts: a pump (the chest wall) and a gas exchanger (the lungs). The study of lung mechanics deals with the pressures acting on this system and the changes in volume that they produce. The pressures developed by the respiratory muscles are necessary to overcome (1) the elastic properties of the lung and the chest wall, and (2) the flow-resistive properties of the airways. The major gas flow-resistive pressure losses occur in the airways and define the *dynamic behavior* of the respiratory system, whereas the *static behavior* is a function of the elastic properties of the respiratory system.

THE RESPIRATORY PUMP

The respiratory pump consists of three parts: the rib cage and its associated muscles, the diaphragm, and the abdomen and its muscles.

89

Inspiration

The major muscle of inspiration is the *diaphragm*. The diaphragm actually consists of two functionally distinct parts that have different segmental innervations and embryologic origins. The crural portion of the diaphragm extends from the spinal column to the central tendon and lies in the posterior portion of the thoracic cavity. The costal portion of the diaphragm attaches to the ribs at one extreme and to the central tendon at the other. As the costal portion contracts, the dome of the diaphragm descends, displacing the abdominal contents downward. The abdominal contents resist displacement and act as a fulcrum. Thus, as the diaphragm shortens, the ribs are lifted up, increasing the transverse diameter of the thoracic cavity. Contraction of the crural portion only displaces the abdomen, since it lacks attachments to the rib cage.

During exercise and vigorous breathing maneuvers, the accessory inspiratory muscles are brought into play. These are the scalene muscles, which elevate the first two ribs and the sternum, and the sternomastoids, which elevate the sternum. In recent years, the role of the internal and external intercostal muscles in the breathing process has been questioned. These muscles are now believed to play more of a role in posture than in breathing. The parasternal intercostal muscles, however, do act in concert with the scalene muscles to elevate the sternum, causing the anterior-posterior diameter of the rib cage to increase during inspiration.

Expiration

Expiration is normally a *passive* event. This is because the elastic energy stored in the system during inspiration is generally sufficient to produce a normal expiration with no further energy requirement, like a balloon deflating. But with either exercise or increased demands on the system, which can occur in various forms of lung disease, expiration becomes an active process. In conditions that require active expiration, the major expiratory muscles are those of the *abdominal wall*: the rectus abdominis, the internal and external oblique muscles, and the transversus abdominis. Contraction of the abdominal muscles increases the intra-abdominal pressure, forcing the diaphragm upward. The internal intercostal muscles, which displace the ribs down and backward, also assist in expiration.

Respiratory Muscle Strength

It is often useful to measure the strength of the respiratory muscles. This is done by having the individual either inhale or exhale with maximal effort against an occluded airway. The resulting airway pressures are then measured at various lung volumes (Fig. 6–1). Positive, or expiratory, pressures are plotted to the right on the diagram, and negative, or inspiratory, pressures are plotted

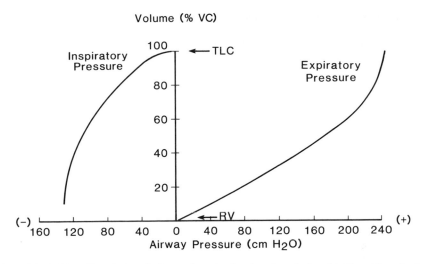

Volume (% VC)

FIGURE 6–1. Plot of inspiratory (left negative abscissa) and expiratory (right positive abscissa) pressures. The volumes are plotted as a percentage of vital capacity (VC). Note that the expiratory muscles produce greater pressures (i.e., are stronger).

on the left. Volume is plotted as a percentage of the vital capacity. As Figure 6–1 illustrates, expiratory pressure changes more than inspiratory pressure, indicating that the expiratory muscles are stronger than the inspiratory muscles. Maximal expiratory muscle strength occurs near total lung capacity, whereas the inspiratory muscles are strongest near residual volume. These plots are similar to skeletal muscle length-tension diagrams if volume is equated to muscle length and pressure is equated to tension. There is an optimal length for both inspiratory and expiratory muscles, just as there is an optimal length for skeletal muscle. As the muscles shorten, during either expiration or inspiration, the maximal available tension decreases.

The average maximal expiratory pressure (MEP) for adult males measured near TLC is 230 cmH_2O, whereas MEP for females averages 150 cmH_2O. Maximum inspiratory pressures (MIP) measured near residual volume average 125 cmH_2O for males and 90 cmH_2O for females (see Chapter 9). These pressures greatly exceed those needed for normal respiratory function. This large reserve of respiratory muscle strength is rarely used except during a cough (when high pressures are needed to generate high velocities of flow in the airways) or defecation and parturition (when high intra-abdominal pressures are necessary).

ELASTIC PROPERTIES OF THE LUNG

The lung is an elastic organ, and if the chest is opened it collapses much as a balloon collapses when opened to the atmosphere.

Static Pressure-Volume Curve

The elastic properties of the lung are measured by determining the pressure required to maintain the lung inflation at various volumes. A simple model that represents the lung parenchyma as a bellows and the airways as a tube is shown in Figure 6–2A. The bellows can be inflated in two ways: (1) pressure can be applied to the opening of the tube, with a resulting volume change, or (2) the bellows can be placed in an airtight chamber such that when the chamber pressure is lowered, the bellows will expand. In each case, the pressure inside the bellows is greater than the surrounding pressure. In Figure 6–2A, the pressure surrounding the bellows is −5 cmH_2O, i.e., 5 cmH_2O below atmospheric, and that inside the bellows is 0 cmH_2O, or atmospheric pressure. Thus, the *distending pressure* of the bellows (pressure inside minus pressure outside) is +5 cmH_2O. If the bellows is removed from the chamber (exposed to atmospheric pressure) and inflated to 5 cmH_2O, the distending pressure would again be 5 cmH_2O, and the volume of the bellows would be the same. In both cases, the bellows expands because the internal pressure is higher than the surrounding pressure. The example of subatmospheric surrounding pressures is more similar to that of the lung in the chest, since pleural pressures become more subatmospheric during inflation.

When the lung is inflated step-wise from RV (0.4 l) to TLC (3.2 l) and then deflated step-wise back to RV, Figure 6–2B is generated. Volume is plotted

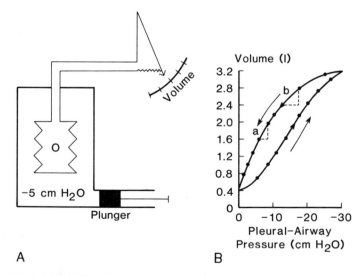

FIGURE 6–2. *A,* Model of the lung as represented by a bellows placed in an airtight box. The bellows can be expanded by creating a subatmospheric pressure (−5 cm H₂O) in the box (analogous to decreasing pleural pressure). When this is done, the pressure-volume curve in *B* is generated. The lower curve represents inspiration, whereas the upper curve represents expiration. The dotted lines at points a and b are used to calculate static lung compliance, as explained in the text.

as a function of the distending pressure, i.e., pleural-minus-airway pressure or transpulmonary pressure as presented previously. Note that the resulting curves are not linear and that the inflation portion of the plot (lower curve) is different than the deflation portion (upper curve). The difference between the inflation and deflation curves is due to a phenomenon called *hysteresis*. Hysteresis is caused by (1) the gradual recruitment or opening of alveoli that are collapsed at residual volume, and (2) changes in the surface tension characteristics of the lungs as their volume changes (see discussion hereafter). In the absence of these two factors, the inspiratory and expiratory curves would be almost identical.

Static Compliance

Static compliance ($\Delta V/\Delta P$) is the change in volume for a unit change in pressure under conditions of no flow. The units of compliance are liters per cmH_2O. Compliance depends on the lung volume at which it is measured. For instance, the compliance measured from the descending (expiratory) limb of the plot in Figure 6–2B as lung volume decreases from 2 l to 1.6 l is 0.4 l/3 $cmH_2O = 0.133$ l/cmH_2O (point a). In contrast, if compliance is measured as lung volume decreases from 2.8 to 2.4 l, compliance is 0.4 l/6 $cmH_2O = 0.067$ l/cmH_2O (point b).

Because of this volume dependency, compliance is usually measured at functional residual capacity (FRC). This is done to normalize the lung's compliance to the same portion of the pressure-volume curve for all subjects. Compliance varies with lung size, being much higher in large individuals as compared with small individuals, e.g., the compliance of whale lungs is larger than that of bat lungs because the TLC of whale lungs is huge as compared with that of bat lungs. However, compliance is normalized to eliminate the effects of different lung capacities when it is divided by FRC. Compliance divided by FRC is termed *specific compliance* and is fairly constant from person to person and from species to species, since the static transpulmonary pressures at total lung capacity (TLC) and residual volume (RV) are the same regardless of lung size. In the example above, the compliance at FRC was 0.133 l/cmH_2O; if the FRC is 1.6 l, then the specific compliance is 0.083 cmH_2O^{-1} (0.133/1.6). Specific compliance values of this magnitude are found in species ranging from bats to whales.

Surface Tension

You may recall from physics that an air-liquid interface tries to diminish its free energy by decreasing the area of the interface. This generates surface tension, a contractile force acting parallel to the surface, since forces between molecules in a liquid pull the surface molecules toward the interior. Such a surface force is generated in the gas-filled lung and tends to cause the small liquid-lined alveoli to collapse.

Consider the pressure-volume plots for an isolated lung shown in Figure 6–3. The solid line represents the inflation and deflation curves for a lung ventilated with air, whereas the dashed line represents a lung ventilated with saline. The behavior of the collagen and elastin fibers has not changed, so why is less pressure required to expand the saline-filled lung? The answer is that the surface tension of the lung has been changed. When an air-liquid interface is replaced by a liquid-liquid interface, surface tension is abolished and the resistance to inflation (lung *recoil*) decreases considerably. The contribution of surface tension to the overall lung recoil pressure is very important, as can be seen from the horizontal displacement between the air and saline curves of Figure 6–3.

The tendency of the lung to collapse is opposed by the connective tissue network described in Chapter 1, but this opposing force is not sufficient to overcome the forces generated by surface tension. Nevertheless, collapse does not occur. The reason is that the lung produces a material, called *surfactant*, that decreases surface tension forces.

Figure 6–4A shows the classic measurement of surface tension. A platinum strip is suspended in a fluid-filled trough. The surface tension at the air-fluid interface pulls the platinum strip into the fluid, and this force is measured. One can also determine if surface area alters surface tension by moving the barrier to change the film area. In Figure 6–4B, surface tension is plotted against surface area. First, consider what happens with water in the trough (upper dashed line). Water has a surface tension of approximately 70 dynes/cm, which does not change with changing film area. Adding a detergent lowers the surface tension to about 30 dynes/cm, but again there is no effect of surface area on surface tension (lower dashed line). The loop in Figure 6–4B shows the behavior of material containing surfactant that has been washed from the

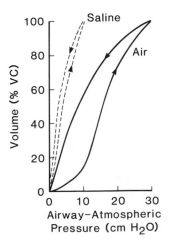

FIGURE 6–3. Plot of airway − atmospheric pressure for an isolated lung inflated with air (solid line) or saline (dashed line). Note that the saline-filled lung is more compliant owing to a reduction in surface tension.

WILHELMY BALANCE

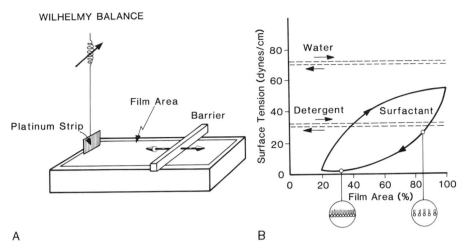

FIGURE 6–4. Illustration of how the surface tension of a fluid can be measured. The surface area can be altered by moving the barrier in the Wilhelmy balance as depicted in *A,* and the force generated on the fluid at the platinum strip (surface tension) can be measured. This force is plotted in *B* as a function of film area. Surface tensions for water and a detergent (dashed lines) remain constant as the film area changes, but with surfactant, surface tension increases with area and exhibits hysteresis (solid line). Insets show distances between surfactant molecules at different film areas. (Redrawn from Weibel, E.R.: *The Pathway for Oxygen.* Cambridge: Harvard University Press, 1984, p. 321.)

alveolar surface of the lungs. The surface tension of this alveolar substance is much lower than that of water. But, importantly, the surface tension of surfactant does change as a function of surface area. Unlike detergent, surface tension increases with surface area (as shown in the inset) because the surfactant molecules are pulled farther apart (as shown in the insets). Conversely, surface tension falls with a decrease in area because the molecules are closer to each other. Thus, surfactant has two striking effects on surface tension: (1) it decreases the overall surface tension of water or plasma, and (2) it causes surface tension to fall as area decreases.

The importance of surface tension changing with area is illustrated in Figure 6–5. Assume that an alveolus is like a small soap bubble (Fig. 6–5A). The pressure required to inflate such a bubble is directly proportional to four times the surface tension (T) and inversely related to the radius (r). If surface tension remained constant as the radius decreased, the pressure required to keep the bubble inflated would increase dramatically. Now consider the situation where two bubbles with different radii but the same surface tension are connected, as shown in Figure 6–5B. The smaller bubble (1), which is similar to an alveolus with a small radius, will have a higher pressure and, consequently, will empty into the larger bubble (2) until the smaller bubble collapses.

In the lung, alveoli are of different sizes, and if collapse occurred, alveolar surface area would fall, with disastrous consequences on gas exchange. That this could happen in the absence of surfactant can be shown functionally and

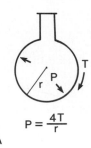

$$P = \frac{4T}{r}$$

A

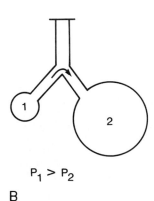

$P_1 > P_2$

B

FIGURE 6–5. *A,* The pressure (P) required to inflate the bubble is equal to four times the surface tension (T) and divided by its radius (r). In *B,* soap bubbles representing small (1) and large (2) alveoli with the same surface tensions are connected by a common tube. Because the small bubble has a higher pressure (P_1), it will empty into the larger bubble.

anatomically. Figure 6–6 shows electron micrographs of a normal lung (A) and a surfactant-depleted lung (B). Note that in the surfactant-depleted lung, the smaller alveoli have collapsed into an adjacent large alveolus. In Figure 6–7, a pressure-volume curve of a normal air-filled lung is shown as the solid line. As the pressure across the lung (the transpulmonary pressure) increases, the lung inflates to its maximum volume. As transpulmonary pressure is gradually lowered, the lung empties along the deflation limb to the left until it reaches its resting volume at 0 transpulmonary pressure. Note on the deflation limb of the curve that at a transpulmonary pressure of about 4 cmH$_2$O, the lung is still 60 per cent expanded (solid arrow). If all surfactant is removed from the lung, the pressure-volume curve shown by the dashed line is generated. The inflation limb is similar to that of the normal lung, but there is a striking difference on deflation. Lung volume is much less at each transpulmonary pressure for the surfactant-depleted lung. In the surfactant-depleted lung, a pressure of 14 cmH$_2$O is required to maintain a volume of 60 per cent of total lung capacity (open arrow). A lung such as this, which is seen in the respiratory distress syndrome of infants, requires abnormally high pressures to maintain inflation.

To further illustrate the importance of surfactant, consider the fetal lung. Before birth, the fetal lung is filled, to approximately 40 per cent of TLC, with fluid that contains little surfactant. During parturition, most of this fluid is squeezed out of the lungs. However, a significant volume of fluid with a low

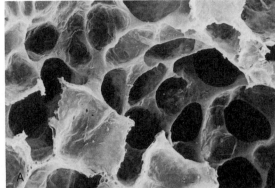
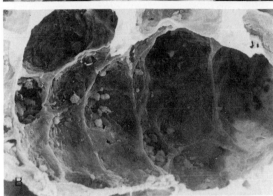

FIGURE 6–6. Electron micrograph showing a normal lung *(A)* and a surfactant-depleted lung *(B)*. Note the collapse of small alveoli and the overdistension of larger alveoli in the surfactant-depleted lung. (Courtesy of Dr. T.A. Wilson, University of Minnesota.)

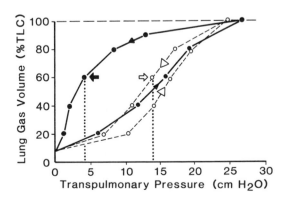

FIGURE 6–7. Pressure-volume curves of a normal lung (solid line) and a surfactant-depleted lung (dashed line). (Adapted from Clements, J.A., and Tierney, D.F.: In Fenn, W.O., and Rahn H. (eds.): *Handbook of Physiology:* Section 3. Respiration, Volume 2. Alveolar stability associated with altered surface tension. Bethesda: American Physiological Society, 1964, pp. 1565–1583.)

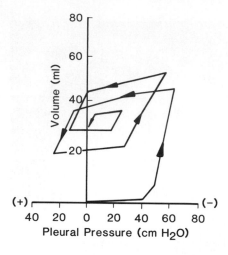

FIGURE 6-8. Pressure-volume curves of the lung in the normal infant at the onset of respiration. (Adapted from Avery, M.E.: *The Lung and Its Disorders in the Newborn Infant.* Philadelphia: W.B. Saunders, 1968, p. 29.)

concentration of surfactant remains in the lung. Figure 6–8 shows the pressure-volume curves generated in the first moments of life. During the first breath sufficient force must be generated to (1) move air and a column of viscous fluid into the lungs, (2) overcome the surface tension forces at the air-fluid interfaces, and (3) distend the elastic lung tissues. As shown in the figure, pleural pressure may fall to -40 cmH$_2$O before air enters the lung, and peak pressures as great as -100 cmH$_2$O have been recorded during the first few breaths. Since a significant volume of air is accumulated in the lung with the first few breaths, each successive breath requires a lower distending pressure until the normal functional residual capacity is reached.

In addition, ventilation of the newborn lung is uneven because the surface tension opposes expansion of the lung. Pulmonary surfactant helps to stabilize the alveoli by decreasing this surface tension. This reduces the pleural pressure required for lung expansion and allows for more uniform ventilation of the lung. Shortly after birth, the FRC is near its normal value and gas exchange is sufficient to sustain life. The fluid remaining in the lungs is rapidly absorbed by active and passive processes that transport the fluid into the pulmonary interstitium. The fluid is then reabsorbed into the capillaries or carried away by the pulmonary lymphatics. This process concentrates the surfactant in the lung, reduces surface tension forces, and promotes more even ventilation. Premature infants whose lungs lack surfactant require large transpulmonary pressures to adequately expand their lungs and, therefore, experience serious difficulty with gas exchange. This situation is similar to that shown in Figure 6–7 (dashed line) for the adult lung that lacks surfactant.

ELASTIC PROPERTIES OF THE CHEST WALL

In the preceding section, the elastic properties of the lung were discussed, but it is important to remember that the chest wall also has elastic properties.

Therefore, the pertinent applied pressure for the chest wall is the difference between pleural pressure and body surface or atmospheric pressure, i.e., the transthoracic pressure. Since contraction of the respiratory muscles can alter the elastic properties of the chest wall, a pressure-volume measurement must be made not only during 0 flow but also during relaxation of the muscles. To generate a pressure-volume curve for the lung and chest wall, pleural and airway pressures are measured as a subject inhales to total lung capacity and relaxes against an occluded airway. A volume of gas is exhaled, the airway occluded again, and the new pressures noted. This procedure is repeated until residual volume is reached. For simplicity, only the deflation portion of the pressure-volume curves are shown in Figure 6–9.

The lungs and chest wall work in concert but clearly have different elastic properties. In Figure 6–9, the applied pressure to the lung is the difference between alveolar and pleural pressures, whereas that to the chest wall is the difference between pleural and atmospheric pressures. The applied pressure of the total system is the difference between alveolar and atmospheric pressures. The chest wall pressure-volume curve (w) can be measured directly or computed as the difference between the lung and total curves. The chest wall curve has a resting volume (at 0 applied pressure) of about 78 per cent of total lung capacity. Above this volume, the chest wall tends to collapse, whereas below this volume the chest wall recoils in an outward direction. Thus, a subatmospheric pressure must be applied to decrease the volume of the chest wall below its resting volume. In contrast, the isolated lung has a collapse tendency over its entire volume range. During a normal relaxed expiration, deflation stops at FRC, which is the volume at which the collapsing pressure of the lung (point a) is balanced by the expanding pressure of the chest wall (point b), i.e., the total system pressure is at 0 (dashed line).

When an individual changes from the sitting to the supine position, the

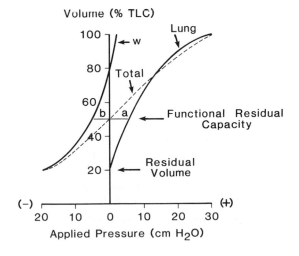

FIGURE 6–9. Plots of deflation pressure-volume curves of the lung, chest wall (w), and the total respiratory system (dashed line). Note that at FRC the outward recoil tendency of the chest wall (point b) exactly balances the tendency of the lung to collapse (point a).

abdominal contents push the diaphragm up, which leads to a shift to the right of the chest wall pressure-volume curve but does not change the lung pressure-volume curve. Therefore, the balance point between the lung and chest wall decreases, and FRC falls. You can test this phenomenon very easily; simply hold your breath at FRC in the upright position, lie down, and then open your mouth. Note that you exhale gas as your FRC decreases.

VERTICAL GRADIENT OF PLEURAL PRESSURE

Until this point, ventilation has been considered to be uniform throughout the lung. However, the situation becomes more complex when the interaction of the chest wall with the lung is considered. There is a vertical gradient in pleural pressure, i.e., the pressure acting on the upper portions of the lung is more subatmospheric than that acting on the lower lung. In the upright position, the bases of the lung are termed *dependent*, whereas the upper lungs or apices are termed *nondependent*. In the supine position, the dorsal surface becomes dependent. In the right lateral decubitus position, the right lung becomes dependent relative to the left lung. There is considerable argument over the factors, such as gravity and chest wall shape, responsible for the generation of this vertical gradient of pleural pressure, but there is no doubt that it exists.

Effect on Regional Ventilation

Since the pleural pressure acting on the nondependent regions of the lung is more subatmospheric, the nondependent regions of the lung are more inflated than the dependent regions. The change in pleural pressure with distance up and down the lung is fairly uniform, averaging about 0.4 cmH$_2$O/cm lung height, causing the regional lung volume to decrease gradually from apex to base in the upright position. To appreciate the importance of this fact, *regional vital capacities (VC)* and *regional pressure-volume curves* must be considered. In normal subjects, the pressure-volume curve of each lung region, expressed as a percentage of regional VC, is identical.

Consider an upright lung that is 30 cm in height. When overall volume is at FRC, the pressure at the apex (point c in Figure 6–10A) is -14 cmH$_2$O. The volume of this region is 71 per cent of its regional VC. The pressure at the most dependent portion (point a) is 12 cmH$_2$O less (30 cm $\times$ 0.4 cmH$_2$O/cm), which corresponds to 13 per cent of its regional VC. Thus, in the upright position, when the overall lung is at FRC, the nondependent portion of the lung is more distended than the lower portion. If the subject takes a breath that increases the transpulmonary pressure (pleural-minus-airway) at both sites by 2.5 cmH$_2$O, the volume of the dependent portion increases from point a to point b, an 18 per cent change in its regional VC. However, the nondependent region changes from point c to point d, only an 8 per cent increase in its regional

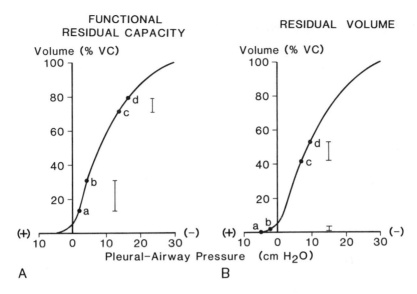

FIGURE 6–10. Pressure-volume curves showing dependent (point a) and nondependent (point c) lung regions. If the distending pressure is increased by 2.5 cmH₂O at FRC *(A)*, the lung volume changes from point a to point b and point c to point d for the dependent and nondependent lung regions, respectively. At RV *(B)*, the dependent portion of the lung is little affected by inflation (point a to point b), and the independent region receives most of the ventilation (point c to point d).

VC. Clearly, at FRC, ventilation is greater to the dependent portion of the lung. If the subject exhales to residual volume as shown in Figure 6–10B, the volume of the dependent portion of the lung is now at point a (0 per cent of its regional VC), whereas the volume of the nondependent portion is at point c (42 per cent of its regional VC). When the transpulmonary pressure is changed by 2.5 cmH₂O on inspiration, almost no gas enters the dependent portion (point a to point b); most of the inspired gas goes to the nondependent portion as its volume changes from point c to point d.

These regional differences in ventilation are very important determinants in matching ventilation to blood perfusion during normal FRC breathing. This phenomenon will be considered in more detail in Chapter 8. Briefly, the bases of the lung are better perfused than the apices owing to the weight of the column of blood in the upright position at FRC, and ventilation to the lung bases is also better (see Fig. 6–10A). Thus, there is an excellent matching of ventilation to perfusion; higher ventilation and blood flow go to the bases, whereas lower ventilation matches the lower flow to the top of the lungs. [Remember that the pleural pressure gradient depends on position. If the subject lies on his right side (right lateral decubitus position), the right (dependent) lung will ventilate better than the left lung. This can be confirmed by comparing the breath sounds over the dependent and nondependent lungs of a colleague in the right lateral decubitus position.]

Single-Breath Nitrogen Washout Test

The single-breath nitrogen washout test is a useful index of the distribution of ventilation and is also an important measurement for detecting early lung disease. The test is performed as follows. The subject exhales completely and then inhales a full vital capacity breath of 100% oxygen. Upon reaching total lung capacity, the subject exhales steadily and slowly to residual volume. The volume and instantaneous nitrogen concentration of the expired gas are measured. When nitrogen concentration is plotted against exhaled volume, Figure 6–11 is generated. The curve is usually divided into four distinct phases. Phase I represents pure dead space gas that contains only 100% oxygen. Phase II contains a mixture of partly diluted gas from the anatomic dead space plus gas from the alveoli. This portion of the curve was analyzed in Figure 1–6. During phase III, the so-called alveolar plateau, there is still a gradual rise in nitrogen concentration caused by two factors: (1) *inter*regional differences in ventilation, and (2) *intra*regional differences in N_2 concentrations. Phase IV is termed the closing volume of the lung.

Interregional Nonuniformity

Interregional differences in ventilation are shown in Figure 6–10. At residual volume in the upright position, the upper portions of the lung have a larger volume as compared with the dependent portions. Since the apices contain a large volume of gas, there is a larger volume of N_2 in the apices than in the dependent portions of the lung. As a subject inhales 100% O_2 from residual volume, very little of the inspired oxygen initially goes to the dependent portion of the lung, most going to the nondependent portion. Later in inspiration, however, the dependent portion receives the majority of the inspired volume. As inspiration continues, more and more oxygen flows to the dependent zones. The dependent regions, therefore, start with a small volume of N_2 and end up with a low N_2 concentration, whereas the nondependent regions start with a large volume of N_2 and end up with a higher N_2 concen-

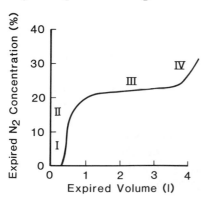

FIGURE 6–11. Single-breath nitrogen washout. Phase I is pure dead space gas. Phase II is a mixture of dead space and alveolar gas. Phase III is alveolar gas, and the slight upward slope represents an increasing N_2 concentration due to inter- and intraregional nonuniform emptying of lung regions. Phase IV occurs at low lung volumes when the upper regions suddenly increase their relative contribution to expired gas.

tration. Thus, a concentration gradient of nitrogen is established between the nondependent and dependent portions of the lung.

As the subject exhales from total lung capacity, the initial expired gas comes predominantly from the dependent portions of the lung, where the N_2 concentration is lowest. As expiration continues, more gas comes from the nondependent portions, which have higher N_2 concentrations, producing the gradual increase in the slope of phase III. As the dependent regions reach low lung volumes, their emptying rates decrease very rapidly, and the upper regions increase their contribution to the expired gas. This results in a rather sharp rise in nitrogen concentration (phase IV of Figure 6–11) toward the end of expiration, designated as the closing volume. There is some debate as to whether phase IV actually reflects airway closure in dependent regions of the lung or whether it is the result of a marked slowing of dependent lung emptying. The closing volume, or phase IV, was once believed to be an especially useful indicator of early airway disease, i.e., an increased closing volume would indicate the early stages of lung disease. However, as evidence accumulated, phase IV was found to be very variable and is no longer thought to be a reliable measure of early lung disease. However, the slope of phase III does appear to be a very sensitive indicator of early airway disease; the larger the slope, the greater the degree of lung disease. Normally, phase III shows cardiogenic oscillations, which, for simplicity, have been eliminated in Figure 6–11.

Intraregional Nonuniformity

In addition to the *inter*regional differences in the distribution of ventilation, a nongravity dependent contribution to the phase III slope of the N_2 washout curve also occurs. This contribution is due to *intra*regional variations in ventilation. The filling and emptying of an elastic body, such as a lung region, through an airway is similar to the charging (filling) and discharging (emptying) of a capacitor (C) through a resistor (R). The time constant of a resistance-capacitance circuit is defined as the time required for the capacitor to alter its charge by 63 per cent of its initial value. This time constant is equal to the product of the resistance times the capacitance, or, in the lung, to resistance times compliance. The product of resistance and compliance has the units of time; i.e., R ($cmH_2O/l/sec$) $\times$ C (l/cmH_2O) = seconds. An increased time constant indicates a decreased rate of discharging or charging.

Figure 6–12A shows two bellows (representing lungs) connected in parallel. Each bellows has a resistance, in its connection to the main tube, and a compliance, which is a function of the bellows wall. Since the bellows have the same resistances and compliances (equal time constants), they participate equally in ventilation. Therefore, the two bellows fill and empty uniformly and synchronously, even at high ventilation rates. Two bellows with different time constants are shown in Figure 6–12B. The diameter of the airway leading to one of the units is reduced, which increases its resistance. Its time constant is

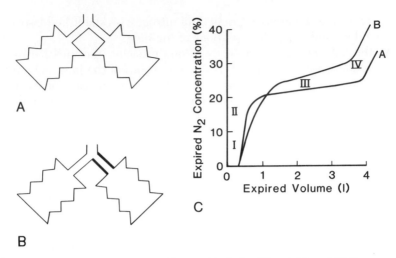

FIGURE 6–12. Plot of two different sets of lungs with similar *(A)* and different *(B)* time constants. Curve A represents the single-breath nitrogen washout curve for lung units with equal time constants. Curve B shows the single-breath nitrogen washout curve for lung units with different time constants. Note the larger phase III slope of curve B.

longer than that of its companion unit. During the single-breath N_2 washout test, the lung with the longer time constant fills more slowly and receives less oxygen than its parallel partner. Therefore, its nitrogen concentration is less diluted with oxygen. The unit with the higher N_2 concentration empties more slowly and contributes its higher nitrogen gas later in expiration, causing a steeper phase III, as shown in Figure 6–12C.

SUGGESTED READING

Black, L.F., and Hyatt, R.E.: Maximal respiratory pressures: Normal values and relationship to age and sex. *Am. Rev. Resp. Dis.*, 99:696–702, 1969.

Mead, J., and Martin, H.: Principles of respiratory mechanics. *Phys. Ther.*, 48:478–494, 1968.

Otis, A.B., McKerrow, C.B., Bartlett, R.A., Mead, J., McIlroy, M.B., Selverstone, N.J., and Radford, E.P., Jr.: Mechanical factors in distribution of pulmonary ventilation. *J. Appl. Physiol.*, 8:427–443, 1956.

Roussos, C., and Macklem, P.T.: The respiratory muscles. *N. Eng. J. Med.*, 307:786–797, 1982.

QUESTIONS

1. During a very slow deflation of the lung from 1.8 to 1.0 l, the trans-pulmonary pressure decreases from 12 to 8 cmH_2O. The compliance of this lung is: a. 0.2 l/cmH_2O; b. 5.0 cm/l.

2. The patient cannot sit up. You wish to evaluate the breath sounds in

the right lung. You should have the patient lie on: a. the right side; b. the left side.

3. Consider two lung regions of equal compliance. Region A has three times the airway resistance of region B. Region B will empty three times faster than region A. True or false?

FLOW-RESISTIVE PRESSURE LOSSES
Types of Flow
Measurement of Airway Flow Resistance
Factors Affecting Resistance
Upper Airway Resistance
Distribution of Airway Resistance

MAXIMAL EXPIRATORY FLOW
Expiratory Flow Limitation
Dynamic Compression
Determinants of Maximal Expiratory Flow (MEF)

WORK OF BREATHING

LUNG MECHANICS IN DISEASE
Alterations in FRC
Frequency Dependence of Compliance
Maximal Respiratory Pressures

7

MECHANICS OF BREATHING: DYNAMICS

FLOW-RESISTIVE PRESSURE LOSSES

The changes in pleural pressure that occur during the respiratory cycle are required to oppose both the elastic properties of the pulmonary system and the flow-resistive properties of the airways. The elastic pressures that counteract the elastic properties of the respiratory system were discussed in Chapter 6, but they were analyzed at times of zero flow; that is, they reflect static, not dynamic, behavior. The pressures that overcome resistance to gas flow can be measured only during breathing and depend primarily on the rate at which volume is changing and less on absolute lung volume per se.

Types of Flow

The predominant type of gas flow in the lung is *laminar* flow, an orderly pattern in which flow is linearly related to pressure. The pressure loss during laminar flow is described mathematically by the classical Poiseuille equation:

$$\Delta P = \frac{8\mu l \dot{V}}{\pi r^4} \qquad (7-1)$$

and since $R = \Delta P/\dot{V}$,

$$R = \frac{8\mu l}{\pi r^4} \qquad (7-2)$$

ΔP is the hydrostatic pressure drop, $\dot{V}$ is the gas flow, μ is gas viscosity, l is path length, and r is the radius of the tube. Note that for a given tube radius and length, resistance is constant. Therefore, laminar pressure-flow relations are linear, i.e., changes in $\dot{V}$ are linearly related to changes in ΔP. However, note that the resistance is inversely related to the radius of the tube. For example, if the radius (r) decreases by one-half, then the resistance will increase 16-fold, i.e., $1/(\frac{1}{2})^4$. Laminar flow is also dependent on viscosity and length but is not affected by changes in density. The difference between viscosity and density sometimes confuses the student, but recall that a very viscous oil may float on water, demonstrating the difference between viscosity and density.

Turbulent flow, on the other hand, is chaotic, with vortices and eddies occurring in a flowing stream. As flow increases under conditions of turbulence, so does resistance; that is, the pressure-flow relationship in turbulent flow is nonlinear. Viscosity (μ) is of minor importance, whereas density (ρ) assumes a more important role in determining the pressure drop (ΔP) during turbulent flow, as shown in Equation 7–3.

$$\Delta P = \frac{l\mu^{1/4}\rho^{3/4}\dot{V}^{3/4}}{r^{19/4}} \qquad (7-3)$$

The Reynolds number (Re) is the ratio of the pressure loss due to density-dependent or inertial flow (radius times density) versus the pressure loss due to viscous flow (viscosity times tube area):

$$Re = \frac{2\rho r \dot{V}}{\mu A} \qquad (7-4)$$

The Reynolds number is used to predict the nature of a particular flow. There is a gradual transition from laminar to turbulent flow at a Reynolds number of 2,000. Turbulence exists at a Reynolds number greater than 2,000.

A pressure loss also occurs owing to *convective acceleration*. This pressure loss is due to an effect named for Bernoulli, the famous physiologist-physicist. This effect is illustrated in the left panel of Figure 7–1. When a fluid, either liquid or gas, flows from a tube of large cross-sectional area (A) into a tube of

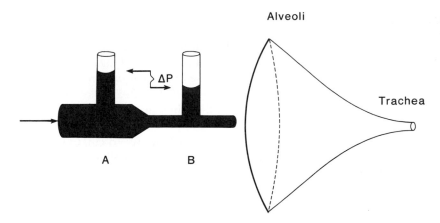

FIGURE 7–1. The left panel shows flow from a large tube into a smaller one. If flow is maintained at a constant rate, a ΔP will be produced owing to the Bernoulli effect (convective acceleration). The right panel depicts how a similar effect occurs when gas flows out of the large cross-sectional area of the small airways (alveoli) into the smaller cross-sectional area of the trachea. A large pressure drop can occur as gas flows from the alveoli to the trachea, as seen in the physical model depicted in the left panel.

smaller cross-sectional area (*B*), the velocity of the fluid must increase greatly to maintain the same volume flow. This acceleration creates a pressure difference (ΔP), illustrated in the model by the difference in the heights of the two water columns, due to conversion of potential energy (pressure) to kinetic energy (flow velocity). This pressure drop occurs even under conditions of completely frictionless flow and is given by:

$$\Delta P \sim \frac{\rho \dot{V}^2}{A^2} \qquad (7\text{–}5)$$

$$R \sim \frac{\rho \dot{V}}{A^2}$$

Thus, the resistance (R) is directly proportional to the flow and density of the fluid, and the pressure-flow relationship is nonlinear.

The right panel of Figure 7–1 shows why the Bernoulli effect is important during gas flow in the lung. During expiration, gas moves through the small peripheral airways, which have a huge total cross-sectional area. The velocity here is quite low. At the tracheal end of the system, where the total cross-sectional area is 1/1,000 that of the peripheral airways, a marked increase in the velocity must occur to deliver the same volume of gas. This causes a significant pressure drop at high flow.

Measurement of Airway Flow Resistance

How can the individual components of pressure due to gas flow–resistive and elastic properties of the lung be separated in intact lungs? To evaluate this problem, a simple bellows-box model is used in which the pressure, flow, and volume changes of the system can be measured (Fig. 7–2). Gas flow is 0 at two points during the respiratory cycle, end-expiration and end-inspiration. The cycle starts at end-expiration (E), where the pressure difference between the airway opening and the outer surface of the bellows is -5 cmH$_2$O. Since flow is 0, this pressure difference is required to keep the bellows inflated at this volume. At the end of a 0.4 l tidal volume inspiration (I), the pressure at zero

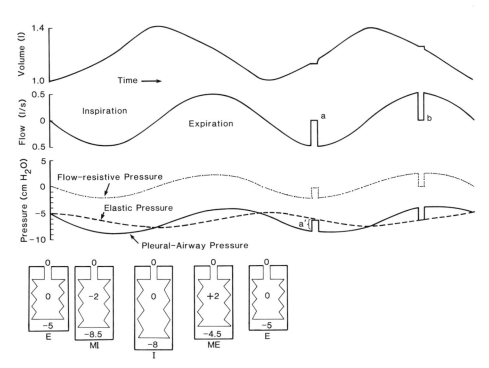

FIGURE 7–2. Lung volume, gas flow, and pleural minus airway pressure. The bellows box model corresponds to end-expiration (E), mid-inspiration (MI), end-inspiration (I), mid-expiration (ME), and end-expiration (E). The pressures shown in the bellows correspond to flow-resistive pressures (dashed-dotted line), and the pressure between the bellows and the box is the elastic pressure (dashed line). The flow resistance for the MI portion of the curve is:

$$\frac{\text{Flow-resistive pressure drop}}{\text{Flow}} = \frac{8.5 - 6.5 \text{ cmH}_2\text{O}}{0.5 \text{ l/s}} = 4 \text{ cmH}_2\text{O/l/s}$$

Another way to easily approximate the flow-resistive pressure drop is to interrupt breathing at some point in either the inspiratory (point a) or expiratory cycle (point b). The change in pleural minus airway pressure is equal to the flow-resistive pressure point (point a′). The resistance can be calculated by dividing this pressure drop by the flow that existed just prior to interruption of the flow.

flow is -8 cmH$_2$O; this is the pressure required to maintain inflation of the elastic bellows at the new volume of 1.4 l. The change in pleural-minus-airway pressure from expiration to inspiration at the two 0 flow points is read from the pressure tracings and is equal to 3 cmH$_2$O (from -5 to -8 cmH$_2$O). The dynamic compliance (Cdyn) is therefore 0.4 l/3 cmH$_2$O, or 0.133 l/cmH$_2$O.

During inspiration and expiration, the volume of the bellows changes as gas flows through the airway. The airway offers resistance to flow, so part of the pressure applied to the model is necessary to overcome the airway resistance. To measure the resistance to flow, it is necessary to determine how much of the applied pressure actually produces gas flow. If the elastic component of pressure is subtracted from the pleural-minus-airway pressure during gas flow, the remainder will be the flow-resistive pressure drop.

The elastic pressure (as shown by the dashed line in Figure 7–2) can be predicted by assuming a constant compliance of the lung (0.133 l/cmH$_2$O). For example, at the time when one-half of the volume increase has occurred during inspiration (0.2 l), one-half of the total change in elastic pressure has also occurred (as shown by the arrow in the tracing of Figure 7–2 labeled elastic pressure). In this example, the elastic component of applied pressure at mid-inspiration (MI) would have increased from -5 to -6.5 cmH$_2$O (0.2 l/0.133 l/cmH$_2$O). Note that the total applied (pleural-minus-airway) pressure is -8.5 cmH$_2$O. Therefore, the difference between the total applied pressure and the elastic component of pressure is 2 cmH$_2$O (8.5 $-$ 6.5). This is the flow-resistive pressure drop. Using similar computations, the flow-resistive pressure drop can be computed at every point during the breath and is plotted just above the elastic pressure (dashed-dotted line). Thus, at mid-inspiration, the alveolar pressure is -2 cmH$_2$O. From the gas flow tracing, it can be seen that this pressure drop of 2 cmH$_2$O produces a gas flow of 0.5 l/sec. The resistance is, therefore, equal to $\Delta P/\dot{V} = 2/0.5 = 4$ cmH$_2$O/l/sec.

A simpler way to determine the flow-resistive pressure drop is demonstrated in the right-hand portion of Figure 7–2. First, during inspiration (point a), flow was suddenly stopped by occluding the airway. When flow goes to 0, the resistive pressure drop is also 0, and the pleural-minus-airway pressure drops to the value defined by the elastic recoil at that volume. The resistance at point a can be calculated by dividing the change in the pleural-minus-airway pressure (2 cmH$_2$O, a') by the flow that existed prior to the interruption (0.5 l/sec). The resistance can also be measured by interrupting expiration at point b and dividing the change in pleural-minus-airway pressure by the pre-existing flow.

In practice, the difference between pleural and airway pressure is frequently used to calculate pulmonary resistance to airflow (RL). Although RL largely reflects the resistance to gas flow in the airways, it also includes a component due to frictional resistance within lung tissue. In Figure 7–2, a constant lung compliance was assumed when computing the flow-resistive pressure. This pressure is equivalent to the alveolar gas pressure (Palv) during breathing. By measuring Palv directly, the resistance of the airways (Raw) can be measured.

In Figure 7–3, a body plethysmograph has been modified to measure alveolar pressure during breathing. The subject breathes in and out of the body box through a flowmeter ($\dot{V}$). The change in box volume during breathing is a function of airway resistance. If airway resistance were 0, then the box volume would not change during breathing. However, because there is gas flow resistance during expiration, alveolar gas pressure will exceed the pressure at the mouth (i.e., the pressure in the box). As alveolar gas is compressed, the spirometer will move to the left. The converse occurs during inspiration. These changes in box volume that occur during breathing are direct reflections of alveolar gas pressures. To measure Raw, the subject breathes in and out of the box through the flowmeter, and gas flow ($\dot{V}$) and volume changes in the box (ΔVbox) are measured to obtain the ratio ΔVbox/$\dot{V}$. Next, the airway is occluded and the subject attempts to inhale and exhale against the occluded airway, yielding a measure of changes in alveolar gas pressure as a function of changes in box volume (Palv/ΔVbox). By utilizing these data, airway resistance (Raw) can be calculated as:

$$\text{Raw} = \frac{\Delta \text{Vbox}}{\dot{V}} \times \frac{\text{Palv}}{\Delta \text{Vbox}} = \frac{\text{Palv}}{\dot{V}} \qquad (7\text{–}6)$$

Generally, airway resistance is measured during panting, since small breaths minimize thermal changes in the box. However, it is possible with appropriate modifications to measure Raw during quiet breathing.

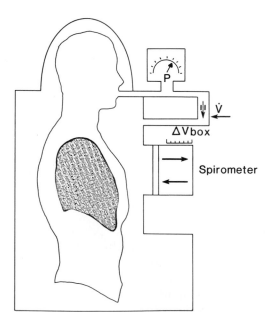

FIGURE 7–3. Body plethysmograph modified to measure airway resistance (Raw). The subject breathes through a circuit that contains a flowmeter ($\dot{V}$) and a pressure gauge (P). The box volume change, ΔV, is measured by a spirometer attached to the box. The subject breathes back and forth to obtain ΔVbox/$\dot{V}$ and inhales and exhales against an occlusion to obtain Palv/ΔVbox. From this, Raw is calculated as their product, which equals Palv/$\dot{V}$.

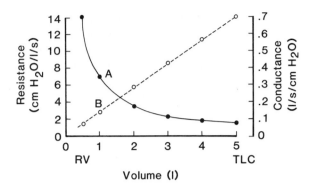

FIGURE 7–4. Plot of resistance (solid line-closed circles) and conductance (dashed line-open circles) as a function of lung volume. For a lung volume of 1 l, the resistance is 7 cmH₂O/l/s (A). The corresponding conductance is 0.14 l/s/cmH₂O (B).

Factors Affecting Resistance

Figure 7–4 shows that flow resistance (solid line, closed circles) steadily increases as lung volume decreases. This occurs because the elastic recoil pressure, acting on the outside of the airways, decreases as lung volume decreases (see Fig. 6–2) until the airways finally collapse.

Conductance (G) is also used to describe the relationship between flow and pressure. Conductance is the reciprocal of resistance, i.e., $G = 1/R$, and varies linearly with lung volume. In Figure 7–4, the conductance-volume relationship has also been plotted (dashed line, open circles). In this example resistance varied as $7/V$. When resistance is 7 cmH₂O/l/s (point A), the conductance is 0.14 l/s/cmH₂O (point B).

Upper Airway Resistance

Measurements of airway resistance include the resistance of not only the intrathoracic airways but also the extrathoracic (or upper) airways, including the nose, mouth, and larynx. Since the resistance of the intrathoracic airways is an important determinant of lung function, it is useful to determine what percentage of the total airway resistance is due to the upper airways. In normal subjects, upper airway resistance during mouth breathing is 45 to 50 per cent of the total resistance at functional residual capacity (FRC). During nasal breathing, upper airway resistance constitutes 66 per cent of the total airway resistance at FRC. With obstructive lung disease, intrathoracic airway resistance increases greatly above upper airway resistance, and, therefore, upper airway resistance becomes less important.

Distribution of Airway Resistance

Based on the total cross-sectional area of the airways at each generation illustrated in Figure 1–6, it is possible to predict the airway resistance of each generation (Fig. 7–5). The highest resistance is found in the central airways (generations 5 through 8), with a steady decrease in resistance in the more peripheral airways. The central airways are larger but fewer in number. Therefore, the total cross-sectional area of the central airways is small relative to that of the peripheral airways, which have a tremendous number of small branches and a correspondingly huge cumulative cross-sectional area.

Clinicians are often faced with the difficult problem of detecting disease in the peripheral airways, although peripheral airways contribute only a small portion of overall resistance (20 to 30 per cent). The problem is depicted by the electrical analog of a branching airway system (Fig. 7–6). The circuit is a combination of a single resistance (R_1, which is analogous to the central airways) in series with four parallel resistances (R_2, which represent peripheral airways). To find the total resistance of the system, the resistance of the parallel system is first computed. Assume that each resistor is equal to 1. The parallel circuit has a conductance of: $1/R_2 = 1/1 + 1/1 + 1/1 + 1/1 = 4$, or $R_2 = 1/4 = 0.25$. The series resistor (R_1) is 1, and the total resistance is $R_1 + R_2$, or 1.25. The lower half of the figure shows what occurs if two of the parallel resistances are increased four-fold. The parallel resistance only increases from 0.25 to 0.4, and the total resistance becomes 1.4, a change of 12 per cent. Therefore, even a large change in peripheral airway resistance is extremely hard to detect using currently available methods owing to the parallel arrangements of the small airways.

MAXIMAL EXPIRATORY FLOW

Up to this point, lung mechanics have been described during quiet breathing. However, procedures that stress a system to its maximum often provide information not obtained from measurements made under normal conditions. *Maximal expiratory flow* is an example of a pulmonary test performed under

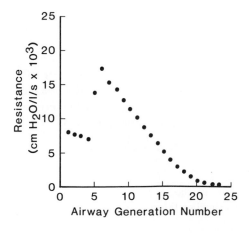

FIGURE 7–5. Resistance calculated at each airway generation. Note that the resistance is higher in the more central airways (generations 5 to 8) and less in the smaller airways.

Combination of Series and Parallel Resistances:

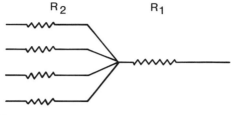

$R_{total} = R_2 + R_1$

if each R = 1,

$$\frac{1}{R_2} = \frac{1}{1} + \frac{1}{1} + \frac{1}{1} + \frac{1}{1} = 4$$

and $R_2 = 0.25$

since $R_1 = 1.0$

$R_{total} = 1.25$

Effect of four-fold increase in half of the R_2 elements:

$$\frac{1}{R_2} = \frac{1}{4} + \frac{1}{4} + \frac{1}{1} + \frac{1}{1}$$

$$= 0.25 + 0.25 + 2 = 2.5$$

$$R_2 = 1/2.5 = 0.4$$

$$R_{total} = 1 + 0.4 = 1.4$$

FIGURE 7–6. Diagrammatic representation illustrating the difficulty in measuring changes in small airway resistance. The small airways are represented here as four parallel resistances (R_2) connected to a large airway represented as R_1. When the resistance of each element is equal to 1, the resistance of the total circuit is $R_1 + R_2 = 1.25$. Increasing two of the peripheral resistances four-fold will only alter total resistance by 0.15, i.e., 12%. Therefore, a large change must occur in peripheral resistance before a change in total resistance can be measured, even with very accurate techniques.

stress. It is a useful clinical measurement of lung mechanics because of its reproducibility, ease of measurement, and sensitivity to changes in the lung's mechanical properties. The basic procedure is called the forced expiratory vital capacity (FVC) test and is performed as follows. The subject inhales to total lung capacity (TLC) and then exhales as completely and with as much force as possible. The data are collected using a spirometer as shown in Figure 7–7A. More recent techniques measure instantaneous expiratory flow and volume and directly produce the maximal expiratory flow-volume (MEFV) plot as shown in Figure 7–7B. If the slopes from the spirogram are calculated, the lower curve can be obtained from the upper. From either figure, it is seen that the flows are very high early in expiration but gradually decrease as expiration continues, approaching 0 near residual volume (RV). An important parameter obtained by the FVC test is the FEV_1 (see Fig. 7–7A). FEV_1 is the volume of

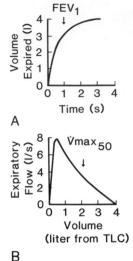

A

FIGURE 7-7. Plot of volume expired as a function of time *(A)* and expiratory flow as a function of volume *(B)* during a forced expiratory vital capacity maneuver.

B

gas expired in the first second of forced expiration. In addition, $\dot{V}max_{50}$, which is the expiratory flow at 50 per cent of vital capacity, can be obtained as shown in Figure 7-7B.

Expiratory Flow Limitation

The value of the FVC test resides in the fact that there is an upper limit to expiratory flow at any lung volume. The concept of expiratory flow limitation is demonstrated in Figure 7-8B. Shown are three isovolume pressure flow (IVPF) curves. Curve A was measured at a high lung volume, about 1 liter from total lung capacity, whereas curves B and C were measured at lower lung volumes. To generate the IVPF curves, the pleural-minus-airway pressure is plotted against flow at a fixed volume. This is done by having the subject breathe in and out through the volume of interest; pressure is plotted against flow *only* when the subject breathes through the volume of interest. Note that at high lung volumes (curve A), flow continues to increase as pressure increases, and there is no well-defined limit to expiratory flow. However, at volumes below curve A, flow increases with increasing pressure, reaches a maximum, and plateaus. Flow will not increase further despite large increases in pressure or expiratory effort. Note that the pressure at which the plateau occurs depends on the volume at which the curve is measured, i.e., curve B plateaus at a higher pressure than does curve C, which is measured at a lower volume. The plateau flow also depends on volume. Once maximal flow is reached, any further increase in applied pressure is matched by an increase in resistance such that flow remains constant. Therefore, there is a limit to expiratory flow over at least the lower 80 per cent of the vital capacity. Furthermore, excessively high pressures are not required to reach this limit. These are the reasons that the

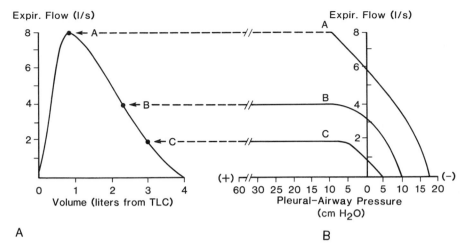

FIGURE 7–8. *A,* Maximal expiratory flow volume (MEFV) curve. *B,* Three isovolume pressure flow (IVPF) curves. The maximal flow from each isovolume pressure flow curve is plotted at its corresponding volume (points A, B, and C). Note that expiratory flow depicted in curves B and C, which were measured in submaximal lung volumes, plateau even though transpulmonary pressure increases.

maximal expiratory flow-volume (MEFV) curve, or the forced vital capacity (FVC) maneuver, is very reproducible and valuable.

In Figure 7–8A, maximal flow at each lung volume is plotted on the flow-volume graph to the left. Curve C, which has a maximal flow of 2 l/sec, is plotted at the volume of its measurement, 3 l from total lung capacity. If a large number of IVPF curves are measured, the full MEFV curve can be generated as shown in Figure 7–8A. In practice, MEFV curves are not constructed from IVPF curves. Instead, expiratory flow is plotted directly against volume during the FVC maneuver to obtain the curve.

The concept of expiratory flow limitation is further illustrated in Figure 7–9 using flow-volume (FV) curves. Figure 7–9B shows the expiratory pressure as a function of lung volume for four expirations of increasing effort, 4 to 1, where 1 is a maximum expiratory effort. Figure 7–9A demonstrates the corresponding FV curves for each expiratory effort. At high lung volumes near TLC, the expiratory flow (Fig. 7–9A) is effort dependent. That is, greater expiratory effort leads to increased flow until the maximum expiratory flow is achieved. As the volume of gas remaining in the lungs approaches RV, expiratory flow becomes less dependent on effort. Near RV, where the downslope of the FV curve is identical for all four efforts, flow has become independent of effort. At intermediate lung volumes, the expiratory flow is limited by the MEFV curve obtained with maximum expiratory effort (curve 1); increases in effort at these lower volumes cannot produce expiratory flows that exceed those of the maximum effort at that lung volume.

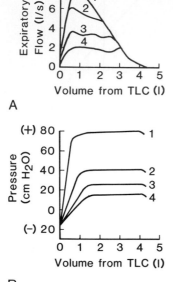

A

FIGURE 7–9. *A,* Plot of expiratory flow versus volume expired from TLC. Note that all four curves representing expirations of increasing effort have the same down slope. *B,* Pressure (pleural minus airway) as a function of volume from total lung capacity for the four different expiratory efforts in *A.*

B

Dynamic Compression

Dynamic compression of the elastic airways is the mechanism responsible for the expiratory flow limitation seen during forced expiration. An elastic airway responds to the pressure acting across its wall, the transmural pressure (Ptm = Paw − Ppl). When the pressure inside the airway (Paw) is less than that acting on its outer wall (Ppl), the airway will be narrowed or compressed. Figure 7–10 shows how airway compression causes limitation of the maximum expiratory flow, using a slight modification of the basic elastic bellows with its elastic resistance tube in a rigid chamber. The rigid chamber is the analog of the chest wall. In Figure 7–10A, flow is 0 and the pressure within the airway (Paw) is equal to atmospheric pressure (0 cmH$_2$O). The pressure in the pleural cavity (Ppl) surrounding the lung and the airway is − 16 cmH$_2$O, which, at that volume, is the elastic recoil pressure of the lung that distends the airway. Keeping lung volume constant, pleural pressure is increased to +1 cmH$_2$O (Fig. 7–10B). Alveolar pressure rises to +17 cmH$_2$O, so that the alveolar-pleural pressure difference (due to elastic recoil) is still 16 cmH$_2$O. Expiratory flow rises to 3 l/s, and airway pressure falls gradually to 0 at the outlet. Some narrowing of the airway tube occurs because the pressure across the airway (Ptm) becomes less as the airway pressure drops owing to flow. However, the pressure inside the airway is still greater than that outside, so the tube is not maximally narrowed. Figure 7–10C shows what happens when pleural pressure is increased to +20 cmH$_2$O and alveolar pressure rises to +36 cmH$_2$O. Near the outlet of the chamber, the pressure inside the tube equals that outside the

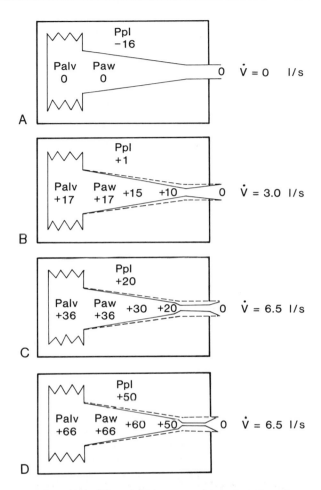

FIGURE 7–10. Illustration of four different driving pressures and gas flows in a model consisting of a bellows connected to a collapsible outflow tube. In A, the original surrounding pleural pressure (Ppl) is exactly equal to the recoil pressure of the bellows (16 cmH$_2$O). As Ppl increases in B, Palv and flow velocity increase and the diameter of the outflow tube decreases. In C, for a Ppl of 20, the airway pressure (Paw) at the distal end falls to 20 cmH$_2$O and is equal to the pleural pressure. This is the equal pressure point, and beyond this point the outflow tube is narrowed. At D (Ppl of 50 cmH$_2$O), the flow is identical to that in C. Thus, flow has plateaued, and a further increase in expiratory pressure does not increase flow.

tube, the equal pressure point. Beyond the point where airway pressure equals pleural pressure, the airway is compressed, since the airway pressure is now below pleural pressure. That flow limitation has been achieved is shown in Figure 7–10D. If pleural pressure rises to +50 cmH$_2$O, alveolar pressure increases to +66 cmH$_2$O, but flow does not increase above 6.5 l/s (which is the same as that seen in Figure 7–10C), because more narrowing of the downstream compressed airway segment has occurred. There is no change in the pressure distribution along the airway upstream of the narrowed portion, and the radius of the tube up to that point remains the same. Thus, the example in Figure 7–10 illustrates that outlet or downstream pressure can be lowered below alveolar pressure without increasing flow; the outlet pressure is actually uncoupled from the pressure that is driving the flow. This uncoupling of driving pressure from flow has been termed the "waterfall" effect, since the height of a waterfall (or sluice) has no influence on the flow over the fall. A similar phenomenon occurs in the pulmonary circulation (see Fig. 5–8).

Determinants of Maximal Expiratory Flow (MEF)

The maximal expiratory flow that can be achieved at a given lung volume depends on several factors. MEF is dependent on the elastic recoil pressure of the lungs. When flow limitation is attained, the pressure drop from alveolus to the point of airway compression, where intra- and extramural pressures are equal, is the value of the recoil pressure at that lung volume.

Airway size is another important determinant of MEF and is a function of elastic recoil. Narrowing of the airways, as occurs in emphysema and asthma, decreases MEF. Airway stiffness or compliance is another important factor that determines MEF; stiffer airways allow higher maximum flow because they are less compressible. Resistance upstream from the compression site (i.e., toward the alveoli) influences MEF, since a higher upstream resistance causes a greater pressure drop, resulting in lower distending pressure at the compression site and, therefore, a more narrowed airway. Finally, the properties of the gas can alter MEF. Increasing the viscosity, such as in neon-oxygen mixtures, or increasing the density, as in a diving chamber, decreases maximal flow. An important fact to remember is that the FVC test is dependent on changes in the mechanical properties of the lungs and this is why it is useful for detecting and analyzing the type and severity of lung disease.

WORK OF BREATHING

Work (W) of the respiratory system in moving gas is defined as the product of pressure (P) times volume (V):

$$W = P \times V \qquad (7–7)$$

Work has units of g-cm when pressure is given as g/cm^2 and volume as cm^3. A pressure-volume (PV) loop is shown in Figure 7–11. During inspiration (line A), a large portion of the work is required to overcome the elastic properties of the lung. This work is defined by the area bound by the lines 0FDBC0. The remaining portion of the work is done to overcome flow resistance, defined by the area FABDF (crosshatched area). Total work done on the lung is a sum of

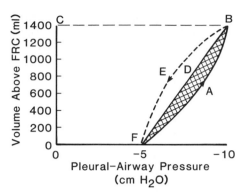

FIGURE 7–11. PV curve showing the work of breathing. 0FDBC0 is the inspiratory work done to overcome elastic forces (open area), whereas the airflow resistive work is FABDF (cross-hatched area).

these two, namely 0FABC0. During expiration, the potential energy stored in the elastic components of the lung is released; this normally overcomes any flow resistance as the lung deflates along the line BEF. The remaining stored elastic energy, defined by the area 0FEBC0, is dissipated as heat.

Two factors can increase the work of breathing: (1) increased flows will increase the resistive component of work, and (2) increased volume excursions will increase the elastic component of work. These considerations become important in certain diseases.

Consider the static deflation PV curves in Figure 7–12 for a normal subject, a subject with chronic obstructive pulmonary disease (COPD), and a subject with pulmonary fibrosis. Only a single inspiratory loop is shown for each condition. For simplicity, loops of the same volume, 1.5 l, are shown. Note that in the COPD subject, a large resistive component (crosshatched area) occurs in the work loop. This subject's strategy to decrease his work of breathing is to take slow deep breaths to minimize the resistive component (R) and maximize the elastic work (E), which is low owing to loss of lung recoil force. The converse occurs for a subject with pulmonary fibrosis, since this disease causes the elastic work (E) to greatly increase, whereas the resistive work (R) remains fairly normal. This subject's strategy is to breathe shallowly but rapidly, thus minimizing the elastic work.

LUNG MECHANICS IN DISEASE

Additional details of tests used to quantify lung mechanics are discussed more fully in Chapter 9. Pulmonary function tests define functional impairment but rarely, if ever, provide a specific clinical diagnosis. However, they do provide important clues as to the severity and specific type of lung disease. Figure 7–13A shows a section of normal lung, whereas Figure 7–13B shows a section of lung with chronic obstructive lung disease and emphysema. The loss of functional lung tissue is easily seen on gross inspection and is responsible

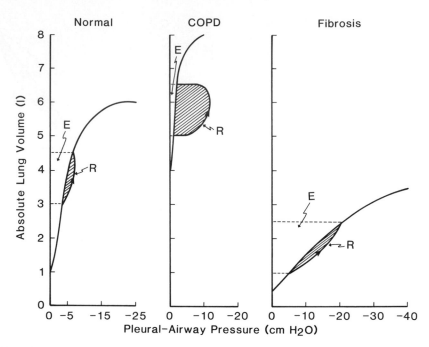

FIGURE 7–12. Plot of inspiratory loop for a normal subject and a subject with chronic obstructive pulmonary disease (COPD) and another subject with pulmonary fibrosis. The size of the inspiratory loop is determined by the resistive component of work (R), whereas distance from the lung volume axis determines the elastic component of work (E).

for the changes seen in the static pressure-volume curves of emphysematous subjects, i.e., a shift to the left due to loss of lung recoil.

Alterations in FRC

Recall from Figure 6–9 that FRC is determined by the balance between the elastic recoil pressures of the chest wall and the lung. Assume that the patient with COPD shown in Figure 7–12 has no change in his chest wall pressure-volume curve. This subject's chest wall and lung PV curves are shown in Figure 7–14. FRC increases considerably owing to the loss of lung recoil, which shifts the balance point between chest wall and lung recoil (FRC) to a higher value, i.e., to approximately 70 per cent of total lung capacity. Conversely, if a similar plot was constructed for the subject with pulmonary fibrosis, the FRC would be decreased, since the increased lung recoil pulls the chest down to lower volumes. In babies, the FRC is controlled by not only the recoil pressures of chest wall and lung but also inspiratory muscle tone and narrowing of the vocal cords (glottic throttling). Intubation of the trachea of these infants may reduce FRC and, therefore, impair gas exchange.

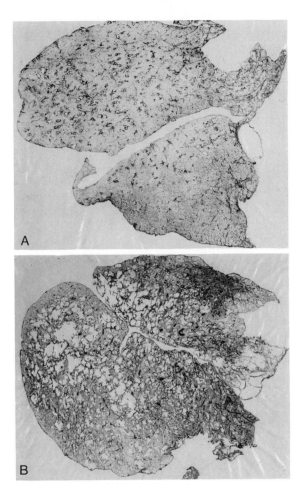

FIGURE 7–13. Whole lung section from a normal individual *(A)* and a patient with COPD and emphysema *(B)*.

Frequency Dependence of Compliance

In discussing Figure 7–6, the difficulty in detecting disease in the small peripheral airways was presented. One way to detect early peripheral airway disease is to determine the dynamic compliance when breathing rate is increased. The normal bellows, shown in Figure 7–15A, each have a compliance of 0.133 l/cmH$_2$O. A combination of two normal bellows as in Figure 7–15A has a compliance of 0.266 l/cmH$_2$O. Static and dynamic compliances are assumed to be equal. When this lung is ventilated at gradually increasing rates, the dynamic compliance does not change from its static value even for breathing rates as high as 60 breaths/min. Therefore, compliance is not frequency dependent for units with equal time constants.

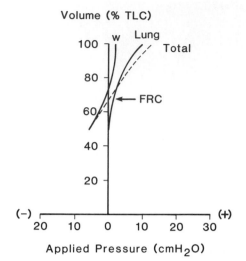

FIGURE 7–14. Plot of PV curves for the chest wall (w) and lung for the subject in Figure 7–12 with COPD. Even with normal chest mechanics, FRC will be increased from its normal value of 50 to almost 70% of TLC.

Note what occurs in the two lungs in Figure 7–15B, one of which has a narrowed airway (increased resistance) similar to that seen in subjects with peripheral airway disease. Compliance at very low breathing rates is normal (graph, Fig. 7–15B); however, as the breathing rate increases, compliance falls, and less and less volume is delivered to the lung with the narrowed airway. Finally, at high ventilation rates, gas only enters and leaves the normal bellows,

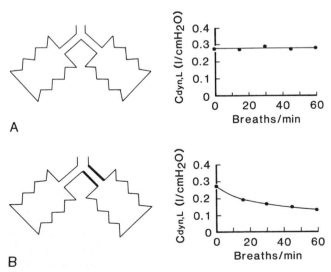

FIGURE 7–15. Influence of breathing frequency on lung dynamic compliance (C dyn, L). *A* shows two lung units with equal time constants, demonstrating that dynamic compliance is independent of breathing frequency. *B* shows two lung units with different time constants owing to increased airway resistance in one unit; note that the dynamic compliance is very frequency dependent under these conditions.

i.e., the abnormal lung is not ventilated. The compliance of the system is now equal to that of a single bellows, 0.133 l/cmH$_2$O. Thus, early airway disease causes compliance to become frequency dependent. In this indirect manner, diseases of the peripheral airways can be detected.

Maximal Respiratory Pressures

In Figure 6–1, the normal maximal respiratory pressures were discussed. In chronic obstructive pulmonary disease, muscle strength is usually well preserved despite hyperinflation of the chest wall. However, toward the end of the disease course, there is often a decrease in muscle strength due to muscle fatigue, which may contribute to the onset of respiratory failure. Moderate loss of muscle strength has little effect on lung volumes, since fairly low pressures are required to inflate and deflate the lung. There is also very little effect on the FVC test, because muscle strength is still sufficient to reach maximal flows. However, the cough mechanism will always be weakened. Interestingly, patients with neuromuscular diseases of various sorts often develop dyspnea (shortness of breath) well before pulmonary function tests become abnormal. Patients have been described whose pulmonary function tests were still normal despite a 50 per cent reduction in maximal pressures. It is only by measuring maximal muscle strength in these individuals that their complaints can be evaluated and the cause of the dyspnea understood.

SUGGESTED READING

Hyatt, R.E.: Expiratory flow limitation. *J. Appl. Physiol.*, 55:1–8, 1983.
Hyatt, R.E., and Black, L.F.: The flow-volume curve. A current perspective. *Am. Rev. Resp. Dis.*, 107:191–199, 1973.
Mead, J., Turner, J.M., Macklem, P.T., and Little, J.B.: Significance of the relationship between lung recoil and maximal expiratory flow. *J. Appl. Physiol.*, 22:95–108, 1967.

QUESTIONS

1. A subject is exercising in a chamber in which the surrounding pressure is 10 atmospheres. The subject experiences dyspnea, which is relieved by breathing an 80% helium:20% oxygen mixture. Why does dyspnea occur, and why does the He:O$_2$ mixture relieve it?
2. In a given subject, airway conductance is decreased when the subject breathes near TLC. True or false?
3. During a forced expiration (when the airways are dynamically compressed), the subject increases expiratory effort. Maximal expiratory flow will do which of the following? a. increase; b. decrease; c. not change.

PHYSIOLOGIC DEAD SPACE

RIGHT-TO-LEFT INTRAPULMONARY SHUNTING

THE ALVEOLAR GAS EQUATION

THE O_2–CO_2 DIAGRAM
  The Gas R Lines
  The Blood R Lines

REGIONAL $\dot{V}_A/\dot{Q}$ INEQUALITIES

MEASUREMENT OF ALVEOLAR VENTILATION-PERFUSION INEQUALITIES

8

ALVEOLAR VENTILATION-PERFUSION ($\dot{V}_A/\dot{Q}$)

The efficiency of gas exchange in the lungs is critically dependent on the appropriate balance between alveolar ventilation and blood flow. For the normal subject, the regions of the lungs that are best ventilated also receive the most pulmonary blood flow, and, as a result, the lungs function as nearly optimal gas exchangers. In diseased lungs, the distribution of alveolar ventilation and blood perfusion may change, impairing the oxygenation of the blood in the lung as well as CO_2 elimination.

PHYSIOLOGIC DEAD SPACE

Gas exchange in the lungs cannot occur efficiently unless there is a proper balance between perfusion and ventilation. For instance, if a portion of a lung was ventilated but not perfused, O_2 and CO_2 could not be exchanged between alveolar gas and the pulmonary circulation. Hence, the gas ventilating the unperfused region would have a composition similar to that of the inspired gas. The volume of gas ventilating unperfused alveoli is referred to as the *alveolar dead space volume*. In normal lungs, the alveolar dead space is virtually zero, but in diseased lungs or during anesthesia the alveolar dead space may increase.

The alveolar dead space must be differentiated from the anatomic dead space, which is determined by Fowler's single-breath nitrogen clearance test (see Chap. 2). The anatomic dead space is the volume of the conducting (non–gas exchanging) airways, whereas the physiologic dead space is the sum of all dead spaces (anatomic and alveolar). The physiologic dead space (VD) cannot be measured directly but can be calculated in the following fashion (Fig. 8–1). At end-inspiration, gas residing in the conducting airways has the composition of inhaled gas; that is, it contains essentially no CO_2. This gas is exhaled first. On further exhalation, the gas comes from the alveoli, which contain CO_2. As a result, the partial pressure of CO_2 in mixed expired gas ($P\overline{E}CO_2$) is lower than that of alveolar gas ($PACO_2$). When the volume of the dead space increases relative to the volume of gas that participates in alveolar gas exchange, the mixed expired gas will have an even lower CO_2 partial pressure. Therefore, the difference between $P\overline{E}CO_2$ and $PACO_2$ indicates the magnitude of physiologic dead space relative to alveolar ventilation. This intuitive conclusion is expressed quantitatively by the *Bohr equation*. Assume that the lung consists of an alveolar volume (VA) and a physiologic dead space volume (VD) and that the lung is ventilated with a tidal volume (VT) (see Fig. 8–1). The volume of CO_2 exhaled per breath from this hypothetical lung ($VT \times F\overline{E}CO_2$) equals the sum of the volume of CO_2 exhaled from the alveolar volume ($VA \times FACO_2$) plus the volume of CO_2 eliminated from the dead space ($VD \times FICO_2$), or:

$$VT \times F\overline{E}CO_2 = (VA \times FACO_2) + (VD \times FICO_2) \qquad (8-1)$$

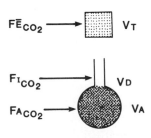

$$VT \times F\overline{E}CO_2 = (VT-VD) \times FACO_2 + (VD \times FICO_2)$$

FIGURE 8–1. Diagrammatic representation of alveolar volume (VA) and dead space volume (VD). The volume of CO_2 exhaled per breath from this hypothetical lung equals the fractional concentration of CO_2 in mixed expired gas ($F\overline{E}CO_2$) times the exhaled volume (VT). The volume of CO_2 exhaled per breath from this lung also equals the volume of CO_2 eliminated from the alveolar volume ($VA \times FACO_2$) plus the CO_2 exhaled from the dead space volume ($VD \times FICO_2$), which is 0 if inspired CO_2 concentration is 0, i.e., $FICO_2 = 0$.

Since the inspired air usually does not contain CO_2, $F_{ICO_2} = 0$, and since V_A = $V_T - V_D$, Equation 8–1 reduces to:

$$V_T \times F_{\bar{E}CO_2} = (V_T - V_D) \times F_{ACO_2} \qquad (8\text{–}2)$$

Solving for V_D/V_T and replacing fractional CO_2 concentrations with CO_2 partial pressures, Equation 8–2 can be rewritten as:

$$V_D/V_T = \frac{P_{ACO_2} - P_{\bar{E}CO_2}}{P_{ACO_2}} \qquad (8\text{–}3)$$

Equation 8–3 is the classic Bohr equation. If P_{ACO_2} is replaced by arterial CO_2 tension (Pa_{CO_2}), Equation 3 is written as the Enghoff modification:

$$V_D/V_T = \frac{Pa_{CO_2} - P_{\bar{E}CO_2}}{Pa_{CO_2}} \qquad (8\text{–}4)$$

To evaluate V_D/V_T, the arterial and mean expired CO_2 tensions must be measured. Mean expired CO_2 tension is determined by the CO_2 concentration in the exhaled gas, and arterial CO_2 tension is measured by blood gas analysis or estimated by end-tidal P_{CO_2}. To obtain the alveolar dead space, the anatomic dead space, as measured by the N_2 washout method, is subtracted from the physiologic dead space.

The value of V_D/V_T for healthy subjects is approximately 0.30, meaning that one-third of the inspired gas does not participate in gas exchange. However, in diseased lungs, the alveolar dead space can greatly increase, and V_D/V_T values as large as 0.85 are observed in clinical practice. Although V_D/V_T is a reliable indicator of physiologic dead space, it is affected by large right-to-left shunts; this is particularly true if the difference between venous and arterial CO_2 content is large, as occurs with low cardiac output. Small right-to-left shunts have little effect on V_D/V_T if the CO_2 content of the shunted blood is near normal.

RIGHT-TO-LEFT INTRAPULMONARY SHUNTING

As previously mentioned, efficient gas exchange in the lungs cannot occur without appropriate matching of alveolar ventilation and perfusion. If a lung segment is perfused but not ventilated, the gas tensions in this lung segment will approach those of mixed venous P_{CO_2} and P_{O_2}, and the blood flowing through the nonventilated lung segment will not be oxygenated. This shunted blood is added to the properly oxygenated blood leaving the lung and therefore will decrease the P_{O_2} of arterial blood.

Two major sources of right-to-left shunting have been identified: (1) blood perfusing poorly ventilated lung regions, and (2) blood bypassing the pulmonary alveolar capillary bed through anatomic connections between the right and left

TABLE 8–1. Anatomic Right-to-Left Shunts

Anterior cardiac veins
Thebesian veins
Giant pleural capillaries
Bronchial veins

circulations. The O_2 content of the shunted blood from these two sources is slightly different, but most calculations assume that shunted blood has the same composition as mixed venous blood.

Mixed venous blood enters the lungs by way of the pulmonary artery. Some of the blood in the pulmonary artery perfuses poorly ventilated lung regions and is not adequately oxygenated. Although most venous blood from the coronary and bronchial circulations drains into the right side of the circulation, a small fraction enters the left side of the circulation. Blood flow through the thebesian veins (venae cordis minimae), bronchial veins, and other sources also contributes to this *anatomic right-to-left shunt* (Table 8–1). The poorly oxygenated blood from these sources reduces the O_2 content and the O_2 tension of arterial blood. Normally, less than 2 to 3 per cent of the total cardiac output passes through these anatomic shunts. However, blood flow through these channels can increase considerably in patients with emphysema, bronchiectasis, coarctation of the aorta, bronchial diseases, and some congenital heart diseases, particularly when an obstruction to the right-sided outflow exists.

Using the O_2 concentrations defined in Figure 8–2, the quantity of blood passing through right-to-left shunts can be mathematically defined. The volume of blood flowing into the lungs per unit time is $\dot{Q}$, and the O_2 content of this

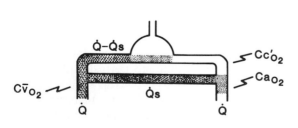

FIGURE 8–2. Diagrammatic representation of the distribution of pulmonary blood flow. Blood flow into the lungs ($\dot{Q}$) has an O_2 content equal to that of mixed venous blood ($C\bar{v}_{O_2}$). The blood flow divides into two pathways, one perfusing the lung regions that do not participate in oxygenation ($\dot{Q}s$), and the other perfusing the ventilated regions ($\dot{Q} - \dot{Q}s$). The amount of O_2 carried per unit time in the arterial blood leaving the lungs equals the product of blood flow times the arterial O_2 content ($\dot{Q} \times Ca_{O_2}$), which, in turn, equals the volume of O_2 carried in the blood that perfuses the ventilated regions [($\dot{Q} - \dot{Q}s) \times Cc'_{O_2}$] plus the volume of oxygen in the blood that perfuses the regions not participating in oxygenation ($\dot{Q}s \times C\bar{v}_{O_2}$).

blood equals the O_2 content of mixed venous blood ($C\bar{v}_{O_2}$). Assume that this blood flow follows two different pathways, one bypassing the regions that participate in oxygenation, i.e., shunted blood ($\dot{Q}s$), and another perfusing regions participating in oxygenation ($\dot{Q} - \dot{Q}s$). The volume of O_2 entering the arterial blood per unit time equals the product of blood flow and arterial O_2 content ($\dot{Q} \times Ca_{O_2}$). In a steady state, this volume equals the sum of the volume of O_2 carried in the shunted blood, which has the O_2 content of mixed venous blood ($\dot{Q}s \times C\bar{v}_{O_2}$), plus the volume of O_2 carried in the blood that perfuses the ventilated regions [($\dot{Q} - \dot{Q}s$) $\times$ Cc'$_{O_2}$], where Cc'$_{O_2}$ is the O_2 content of end-capillary blood. This relationship is expressed mathematically as:

$$\dot{Q} \times Ca_{O_2} = Cc'_{O_2}(\dot{Q} - \dot{Q}s) + (\dot{Q}s \times C\bar{v}_{O_2}) \tag{8–5}$$

Equation 8–5 can be rearranged to yield:

$$\frac{\dot{Q}s}{\dot{Q}} = \frac{Cc'_{O_2} - Ca_{O_2}}{Cc'_{O_2} - C\bar{v}_{O_2}} \tag{8–6}$$

This equation expresses the fraction of the cardiac output that perfuses lung regions that do not participate in oxygenation of the blood. When using this equation, remember that all shunted blood was assumed to have the composition of mixed venous blood. The disadvantage of Equation 8–6 is that end-capillary O_2 content cannot be determined and must, therefore, be estimated. Since hemoglobin in end-capillary blood is completely saturated with O_2 during 100% oxygen breathing, end capillary O_2 content can be estimated as:

$$Cc'_{O_2} = (Hb \times 1.38) + P_{A_{O_2}} \times \frac{\alpha}{760} \tag{8–7}$$

Substituting Cc'$_{O_2}$ and Ca$_{O_2}$ into Equation 8–6 yields:

$$\frac{\dot{Q}s}{\dot{Q}} = \frac{(P_{A_{O_2}} - Pa_{O_2}) \times 0.0031}{(P_{A_{O_2}} - Pa_{O_2}) \times 0.0031 + (Ca_{O_2} - C\bar{v}_{O_2})} \tag{8–8}$$

Equation 8–8 indicates that both the alveolar-arterial O_2 tension difference ($P_{A_{O_2}} - Pa_{O_2}$) and the arteriovenous O_2 content difference ($Ca_{O_2} - C\bar{v}_{O_2}$) are important determinants of the fraction of right-to-left shunt. Figure 8–3 depicts the relationship between arterial O_2 tension (Pa_{O_2}) and arteriovenous O_2 content difference ($Ca_{O_2} - C\bar{v}_{O_2}$) for 0, 11 and 20 per cent shunts in subjects breathing 100% O_2 at sea level. From Figure 8–3 it can be seen that the same Pa_{O_2} can be achieved with two different shunt flows (11 or 20 per cent). Note that for any arteriovenous O_2 content difference, the 11 per cent shunt (point A) has a higher Pa_{O_2} than the 20 per cent shunt (point B). Why is the same Pa_{O_2} obtained with different shunts? This is shown in Equation 8–8, where it can be seen that changes in arteriovenous oxygen content difference can compensate for changes in shunt fraction to produce the same Pa_{O_2}. These examples clearly

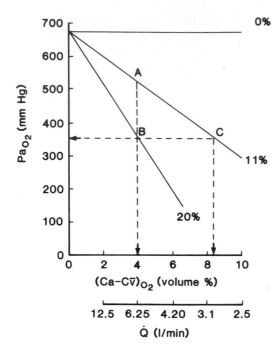

FIGURE 8–3. Relationship between arterial O_2 tension (Pa_{O_2}) and arteriovenous O_2 content difference (Ca − $C\bar{v})_{O_2}$ or cardiac output $\dot{Q}$. In this example, a subject is breathing 100% O_2 at sea level. The subject's arterial CO_2 tension is 40 mmHg, the alveolar water vapor tension at a body temperature of 37°C is 47 mmHg, and the oxygen uptake is 250 ml/min. The alveolar O_2 tension is therefore 673 mmHg (760 − 40 − 47). If there is no right-to-left shunting (shunt = 0 per cent), alveolar O_2 tension is equal to arterial O_2 tension regardless of the arteriovenous O_2 content difference. This figure shows that, with a given right-to-left shunt, arterial O_2 tension depends on the arteriovenous O_2 content difference. Note that at the same (Ca − $C\bar{v})_{O_2}$ or $\dot{Q}$, the Pa_{O_2} decreases as shunting increases (points A and B). The same Pa_{O_2} can be obtained at different degrees of shunting when (Ca − $C\bar{v})_{O_2}$ increases or $\dot{Q}$ decreases (points B and C).

illustrate that, in the presence of a right-to-left shunt, arterial O_2 tension depends critically on the arteriovenous O_2 content difference.

The Fick equation can be arranged to:

$$\frac{\dot{V}_{O_2}}{\dot{Q}} = (Ca_{O_2} - C\bar{v}_{O_2}) \tag{8–9}$$

Equation 8–9 shows that the magnitude of the arteriovenous O_2 content difference is inversely related to cardiac output ($\dot{Q}$) and directly related to O_2 consumption ($\dot{V}_{O_2}$). Therefore, for a given shunt, the arterial O_2 tension is affected by changes in cardiac output, $\dot{V}_{O_2}$, or both. For a constant $\dot{V}_{O_2}$, cardiac output is inversely related to arteriovenous oxygen content difference (see Fig. 8–3). Since the arteriovenous oxygen content difference is in the denominator of the shunt equation (see Eq. 8–8), an increase in arteriovenous oxygen content difference reduces the shunt fraction ($\dot{Q}s/\dot{Q}$) for a given arterial oxygen tension (point B → point C). Clinically, any improvement in Pa_{O_2} could be due to decreased shunt, increased cardiac output, decreased $\dot{V}_{O_2}$, or a combination thereof. To determine the underlying mechanism for the improved Pa_{O_2}, (Ca − $C\bar{v})_{O_2}$ must be measured.

THE ALVEOLAR GAS EQUATION

The alveolar gas equation relates the alveolar partial pressure of O_2 (PA_{O_2}) to the partial pressure of O_2 in the inspired gas (PI_{O_2}) and to the alveolar partial pressure of CO_2 (PA_{CO_2}). This equation also indicates that the alveolar partial pressure of O_2 decreases as the alveolar partial pressure of CO_2 increases.

The alveolar gas equation is derived in Appendix A and is defined as:

$$PA_{O_2} = PI_{O_2} + \left[FI_{O_2} \frac{(1 - R)}{R} - \frac{1}{R} \right] PA_{CO_2} \qquad (8\text{--}10)$$

where R is the respiratory exchange ratio. The student should note that Equation 8–10 indicates a linear relationship between PA_{O_2} and PA_{CO_2}. The slope of the line is $\left(FI_{O_2} \dfrac{(1 - R)}{R} - \dfrac{1}{R} \right)$ and the x-intercept is PI_{O_2}, i.e., when PA_{CO_2} = 0, $PA_{O_2} = PI_{O_2}$.

The alveolar gas equation is used to compute the alveolar O_2 tension when gas mixtures other than 100% O_2 are breathed. When 100% O_2 is breathed, the alveolar gas equation is simplified. Since FI_{O_2} = 1, the bracketed term in Equation 8–10 reduces to -1, yielding Equation 8–11:

$$PA_{O_2} = PI_{O_2} - PA_{CO_2} \qquad (8\text{--}11)$$

When breathing 100% O_2, PI_{O_2} = 760 $-$ 47 mmHg, and Equation 8–11 becomes:

$$PA_{O_2} = 713 \text{ mmHg} - PA_{CO_2}$$

In a patient breathing room air with an R of 0.8, the alveolar gas equation reduces to:

$$PA_{O_2} = 150 \text{ mmHg} - (1.2)PA_{CO_2}$$

Assuming that $PA_{CO_2} = Pa_{CO_2}$, one can quickly obtain an estimate of PA_{O_2} by measuring Pa_{CO_2}. Comparison of this estimate of PA_{O_2} to the measured Pa_{O_2} indicates the degree of respiratory insufficiency, i.e., the greater the difference between PA_{O_2} and Pa_{O_2}, the more severe the respiratory insufficiency.

THE O_2–CO_2 DIAGRAM

The Gas R Lines

So far, the two extremes of ventilation and perfusion have been considered: (1) right-to-left shunting ($\dot{V}A/\dot{Q}$ = 0), and (2) alveolar dead space ($\dot{V}A/\dot{Q}$ = ∞).

The slope of the alveolar gas equation (Eq. 8–10) is equal to:

$$FI_{O_2} \frac{(1 - R)}{R} - \frac{1}{R}$$

that is, the alveolar gas equation predicts a negative slope relating PA_{O_2} to PA_{CO_2}. Figure 8–4 shows three examples of the relationship between PA_{O_2} and PA_{CO_2} at three different R values. These examples demonstrate a negative linear relationship between PA_{O_2} and PA_{CO_2} for a given R value, i.e., when PA_{O_2} decreases, PA_{CO_2} will increase. The student may be surprised that R can be greater than 1, but since R = $\dot{V}_{CO_2}/\dot{V}_{O_2}$, R can be greater than 1 when the rate of CO_2 elimination exceeds the rate of oxygen uptake. This can occur, for instance, during hyperventilation.

The Blood R Lines

In a steady state, O_2 uptake in the lungs from alveolar gas ($\dot{V}_{O_2}$) equals the volume of O_2 taken up by the blood in the lungs [$\dot{Q} \times (Ca_{O_2} - C\bar{v}_{O_2})$]. Similarly, the volume of CO_2 eliminated from the blood into the lungs [$\dot{Q} \times C\bar{v}_{CO_2} - Ca_{CO_2})$] equals CO_2 elimination from the lungs into the environment ($\dot{V}_{CO_2}$). The following equation expresses this relationship quantitatively:

$$R = \frac{\dot{V}_{CO_2}}{\dot{V}_{O_2}} = \frac{\dot{Q}(C\bar{v}_{CO_2} - Ca_{CO_2})}{\dot{Q}(Ca_{O_2} - C\bar{v}_{O_2})} \tag{8–12}$$

Figure 8–5 shows the relationship between P_{O_2} and P_{CO_2} in blood. In contrast to the linear relationship between PA_{O_2} and PA_{CO_2} in alveolar gas, the relationship between P_{O_2} and P_{CO_2} in blood is curvilinear. This curvilinearity is caused by the nonlinear oxyhemoglobin and CO_2 dissociation curves. All possible combinations of P_{O_2} and P_{CO_2} in blood are defined by the line labelled R = 1.0, as long as R = 1.0 and the mixed venous blood has the composition defined by point $\bar{v}$ in Figure 8–5. Because the slope of the CO_2 dissociation curve is steeper than that of the oxyhemoglobin curve (see Fig. 4–6B), a given change in CO_2 blood tension is associated with a larger change in the blood O_2 tension, i.e., the blood R lines are nearly horizontal.

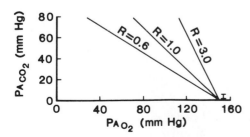

FIGURE 8–4. Graphic solution of the alveolar gas equation. The alveolar gas equation predicts that the relationship between alveolar O_2 and CO_2 tensions is linear. If the inspired O_2 and CO_2 tensions are known (in this example, PI_{O_2} = 150 mmHg and PI_{CO_2} = 0 mmHg), only one point needs to be calculated for a given R value to characterize the unique relationship between PA_{O_2} and PA_{CO_2}. Three examples, R = 0.6, R = 1.0, and R = 3.0, are given.

FIGURE 8–5. Graphic solution of Equation 8–12. In contrast to the relationship between P_{AO_2} and P_{ACO_2}, the relationship between P_{O_2} and P_{CO_2} in blood is curvilinear. The shape of this curve is due to the curvilinear oxyhemoglobin and CO_2 dissociation curves. Point $\bar{v}$ represents the partial pressures of oxygen and carbon dioxide in mixed venous blood.

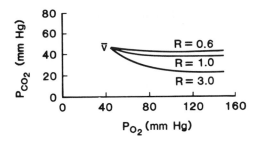

Figure 8–6 combines the gas and blood R lines from Figures 8–4 and 8–5. If the inspiratory gas (I) and the mixed venous blood ($\bar{v}$) have the compositions shown in Figure 8–6, the intercepts of the gas and blood R lines indicate, for a given R value, the unique P_{O_2} and P_{CO_2} relationships in alveolar gas and pulmonary end-capillary blood that must exist in a uniform lung. For instance, the intercept of the blood and gas R lines of 1.0 describes the only gas tensions that can exist in a uniform lung where O_2 uptake and CO_2 elimination are equal (R = 1), ventilation is with a gas mixture described by point I ($P_{O_2} = 150$ mmHg), and blood with a $P\bar{v}_{O_2}$ and $P\bar{v}_{CO_2}$ defined by point $\bar{v}$ ($P_{O_2} = 40$ mmHg and $P_{CO_2} = 45$ mmHg) perfuses the lung.

To convert the R values to $\dot{V}A/\dot{Q}$ values, the ventilation-perfusion equation is derived as:

$$\dot{V}A = \frac{\dot{V}_{CO_2}}{P_{ACO_2}} \qquad (8\text{–}13)$$

when $F_{ICO_2} = 0$.

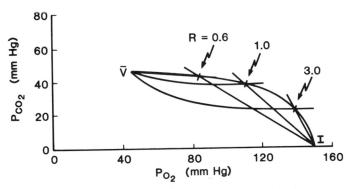

FIGURE 8–6. Blood and gas R lines plotted together. For a given R value, the intercepts of the blood and gas R lines define the gas tensions that exist in the alveolar gas and the pulmonary end-capillary blood of a lung or a lung region if a subject breathes gas of the composition defined by point I and if the lung is perfused with mixed venous blood of the composition defined by point $\bar{v}$.

Rearranging Equation 8–9 yields:

$$\dot{Q} = \frac{\dot{V}_{O_2}}{(Ca_{O_2} - C\bar{v}_{O_2})} \qquad (8\text{–}14)$$

Dividing Equation 8–13 by Equation 8–14 and inserting R for $\dot{V}_{CO_2}/\dot{V}_{O_2}$ yields the alveolar ventilation-to-perfusion equation:

$$\frac{\dot{V}_A}{\dot{Q}} = \frac{R \times (Ca_{O_2} - C\bar{v}_{O_2})}{Pa_{CO_2}} \times K \qquad (8\text{–}15)$$

where K is a constant needed to transform fractional concentrations to partial pressures and to express $\dot{V}_{CO_2}$ in BTPS (body temperature and pressure, saturated) rather than STPD (standard temperature and pressure, dry). K = 8.63 mmHg when O_2 contents are expressed in volume %.

Using Equation 8–15, the R values shown in Figure 8–6 can be converted to $\dot{V}_A/\dot{Q}$ values, as shown in Figure 8–7. The line connecting the mixed venous point ($\bar{v}$), the intercepts of the blood and gas R lines, and the inspiratory point (I) defines the P_{O_2}'s and P_{CO_2}'s that may exist in a hypothetical lung perfused with mixed venous blood of the composition defined by point $\bar{v}$ and ventilated with an inspired gas mixture defined by point I. When $\dot{V}_A/\dot{Q} = 0.44$, P_{O_2} values are lower and P_{CO_2} values higher than when $\dot{V}_A/\dot{Q} = 0.89$. It is also apparent from Figure 8–7 that reducing $\dot{V}_A/\dot{Q}$ below 0.89 results in a dramatic decrease in P_{O_2} with only a slight change in P_{CO_2}. Conversely, increasing the value of $\dot{V}_A/\dot{Q}$ over a value of 1 has a progressively larger effect on P_{CO_2} and a progressively smaller effect on P_{O_2}.

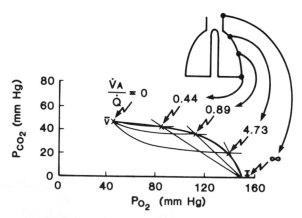

FIGURE 8–7. The R values from Figure 8–6 have been converted to $\dot{V}_A/\dot{Q}$ values by solving Equation 8–15. Note that low $\dot{V}_A/\dot{Q}$ values are associated with low O_2 tensions and high CO_2 tensions. Reducing the $\dot{V}_A/\dot{Q}$ from 0.89 to 0 reduces P_{O_2} drastically, while having only a minimal effect on P_{CO_2}. Conversely, increasing the $\dot{V}_A/\dot{Q}$ from 0.89 to infinity has a progressively smaller effect on P_{O_2} and a progressively larger effect on P_{CO_2}. The lung insert shows appropriate $\dot{V}_A/\dot{Q}$ ratios for various lung heights and for the trachea ($\dot{V}_A/\dot{Q} = \infty$).

REGIONAL $\dot{V}$A/$\dot{Q}$ INEQUALITIES

Chapters 5, 6, and 7 discussed the distribution of ventilation and pulmonary blood flow and stressed that neither ventilation nor perfusion is uniform in a normal lung. In a seated or standing subject, ventilation and perfusion progressively increase from apex to base. The increase in perfusion per unit lung volume from the top to the bottom is larger than the increase in ventilation. At the apex, alveolar ventilation is large relative to perfusion, whereas the reverse is true at the base. It follows that $\dot{V}$A/$\dot{Q}$ is larger than 1 at the apex and less than 1 at the base as shown by the schematic lung in the upper part of Figure 8–7.

The following example demonstrates the effect of mixing blood from three lung regions with different $\dot{V}$A/$\dot{Q}$ values on arterial O_2 and CO_2 contents. Assume that a lung consists of three regions, each with a uniform $\dot{V}$A/$\dot{Q}$ value. One region has a $\dot{V}$A/$\dot{Q}$ value of 0.44, the second of 0.89, and the third of 4.73. Assume also that the inspired gas has the composition defined by point I (see Fig. 8–7) and that the mixed venous blood has the composition defined by point $\bar{v}$. Alveolar ventilation and cardiac output are assumed to be 5.1 and 7.62 l/min, respectively. Ventilation and blood flow are distributed to the three regions as shown in Table 8–2. The overall alveolar O_2 and CO_2 tensions can be calculated from the weighted average of the P_{AO_2} and P_{ACO_2} in the three lung regions (overall P_{ACO_2} and P_{AO_2}, see Table 8–2). In contrast, the overall

TABLE 8–2. Effects of $\dot{V}$A/$\dot{Q}$ Inequality on Efficiency of Pulmonary Gas Exchange

	Region 1	Region 2	Region 3	Overall
$\dot{V}$A/$\dot{Q}$	0.44	0.89	4.73	0.67*
Gas phase:				
VA, l/min	2.04	2.55	0.51	5.10
$\dot{V}$A, % of overall	(40%)	(50%)	(10%)	(100%)
P_{ACO_2}, mmHg	44	39	23	39.4
P_{AO_2}, mmHg	84	111	139	103.1
Blood phase:				
$\dot{Q}$, l/min	4.64	2.87	0.11	7.62
$\dot{Q}$, % of overall	(61%)	(38%)	(1%)	(100%)
P_{aCO_2}, mmHg	44	39	23	41.5*
C_{aCO_2}, vol %	50.3	48.0	38.2	49.3
P_{aO_2}, mmHg	84	111	139	92*
C_{aO_2}, vol %	19.4	19.7	19.9	19.52

*Cannot be calculated directly as weighted average.
Example for gas phase calculation of overall P_{ACO_2}: $(44 \times 0.40) + (39 \times 0.50) + (23 \times 0.10) = 39.4$.
Example for blood phase for C_{aO_2}: $(19.4 \times 0.61) + (19.7 \times 0.38) + (19.9 \times 0.01) = 19.52$.
Refer to the oxyhemoglobin dissociation curve (see Fig. 4–1) to arrive at the overall P_{aO_2} of 92 mmHg for a C_{aO_2} of 19.52 vol %.
    (A − a)D_{O_2} is $(103.1 − 92) = 11.1$ mmHg
    (a − A)D_{CO_2} is $(41.5 − 39.4) = 2.1$ mmHg

mixed arterial O_2 and CO_2 tensions (overall $PaCO_2$ and PaO_2, see Table 8–2) cannot be calculated from the weighted average of the end-capillary O_2 and CO_2 tensions in the three regions because of the nonlinear oxyhemoglobin and CO_2 dissociation curves. One must first determine from the $\dot{V}A/\dot{Q}$ line (see Fig. 8–7) the appropriate PO_2 and PCO_2 values in the end-capillary blood of each of the three lung regions and then determine the gas contents of the capillary blood in each of the three regions from the oxyhemoglobin and CO_2 dissociation curves, respectively (see Fig. 4–6B). The O_2 and CO_2 contents of the arterial blood (overall CaO_2 and $CaCO_2$, see Table 8–2) are then calculated from the weighted average, and the arterial PO_2 and PCO_2 values are determined from the appropriate dissociation curves.

It is apparent from Table 8–2 that the nonuniform distribution of $\dot{V}A/\dot{Q}$ in this hypothetical lung results in an impairment of gas exchange. The calculated PaO_2 is lower than the calculated PAO_2, and $PaCO_2$ is larger than $PACO_2$. The high PO_2 in the blood from the lung regions with a high $\dot{V}A/\dot{Q}$ value raises the O_2 content of this blood only minimally owing to the nearly horizontal shape of the oxyhemoglobin dissociation curve in this range. In contrast, the low PO_2 in the blood from the lung regions with a low $\dot{V}A/\dot{Q}$ value results in a low O_2 content because of the steeper slope of the oxyhemoglobin dissociation curve in this range. Hence, lung regions with high $\dot{V}A/\dot{Q}$ values cannot compensate in terms of O_2 content for lung regions with low $\dot{V}A/\dot{Q}$ values. This phenomenon is further aggravated because, by definition, the major portion of blood perfusing the lung comes from regions with a low $\dot{V}A/\dot{Q}$ value. Thus, the functional effect of $\dot{V}A/\dot{Q}$ mismatching is an impairment of oxygenation. In other words, it is similar to a right-to-left shunt; therefore, $\dot{V}A/\dot{Q}$ mismatch is referred to as a "shunt-like" effect. The sum of the shunt-like effect and right-to-left shunting is called the venous admixture.

Of course, $\dot{V}A/\dot{Q}$ mismatching also interferes with CO_2 elimination from the lung. However, when the chemoreceptors sense an elevated $PaCO_2$, overall ventilation is increased. Because the CO_2 dissociation curve is nearly linear, lung regions with a high $\dot{V}A/\dot{Q}$ value can nearly compensate for the lower CO_2 elimination for lung regions with a low $\dot{V}A/\dot{Q}$ value, thus keeping the $PaCO_2$ within the normal range. In the presence of very large $\dot{V}A/\dot{Q}$ mismatching, this compensatory mechanism fails, resulting in an elevated $PaCO_2$.

That the lung is not a perfect gas exchanger is illustrated in Figure 8–8. The intercept of the gas and blood R lines determines the "ideal" gas tensions for O_2 and CO_2 in a uniform lung with a given R; this is point i in Figure 8–8. Point a on the blood R line represents the true PaO_2 and $PaCO_2$ values, and point A on the gas R line represents the true PAO_2 and $PACO_2$ values. The horizontal distance from point A to point a equals the difference in alveolar and arterial O_2 tensions [$(A - a)DO_2$]. Assuming no diffusion limitation, this is a measure of the nonuniformity of $\dot{V}A/\dot{Q}$ distribution. The vertical distance from point a to point A is the difference between $PaCO_2$ and $PACO_2$ [$(a - A)DCO_2$] and is also a measure of the nonuniformity of $\dot{V}A/\dot{Q}$.

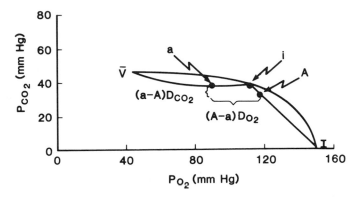

FIGURE 8–8. Point i indicates the "ideal" gas tension of alveolar gas and pulmonary end-capillary blood if lung function were completely uniform and if the relationship between O_2 uptake and CO_2 elimination were defined by the gas and blood R lines as shown in this figure. In a nonuniform lung, arterial and alveolar gas tensions differ from the ideal. The true arterial gas tension must lie on the blood R line (point a), and gas tensions in the gas phase must lie on the gas R line (point A). The vertical distance between points a and A is $(a - A)D_{CO_2}$, and the horizontal distance between points A and a is $(A - a)D_{O_2}$.

The alveolar to arterial P_{O_2} difference is small in young healthy humans breathing room air at sea level. In these subjects, both right-to-left shunting and $\dot{V}_A/\dot{Q}$ contribute equally to this small P_{O_2} difference, whereas the diffusion barrier to O_2 at the alveolar-capillary membrane does not contribute at all (Fig. 8–9, $P_{AO_2} = 100$). Increased alveolar O_2 tensions will decrease the relative contribution of $\dot{V}_A/\dot{Q}$ so that right-to-left shunting constitutes the major cause of the $(A - a)D_{O_2}$. In contrast, at low alveolar O_2 tensions ($P_{AO_2} < 100$), the $(A - a)D_{O_2}$ becomes much more dependent on the diffusional impedance for O_2.

Hypoxemia resulting from right-to-left shunting cannot be corrected by increasing the inspired O_2 concentration. By contrast, hypoxemia resulting from $\dot{V}_A/\dot{Q}$ mismatching is greatly improved by increasing the inspired O_2 concentration. This improvement is illustrated in Figure 8–10, which depicts the relationship between arterial O_2 tension (Pa_{O_2}) and fractional inspired O_2 concentration (F_{IO_2}) in an individual with a constant Pa_{CO_2}, pH, and hemoglobin level and $\dot{V}_A/\dot{Q}$ mismatches equivalent to right-to-left shunting of 10 to 70 per cent of cardiac output. For a mild $\dot{V}_A/\dot{Q}$ mismatch, which is equivalent to a 10 per cent right-to-left shunting (upper curve, see Fig. 8–10), Pa_{O_2} increases greatly as F_{IO_2} increases. In contrast, if the $\dot{V}_A/\dot{Q}$ mismatch is equivalent to a 70 per cent right-to-left shunting (lower curve, see Fig. 8–10), only a small increase in Pa_{O_2} can be expected even with an F_{IO_2} of 100 per cent. For intermediate shunts (i.e., 30 per cent), very high F_{IO_2}'s will increase Pa_{O_2}.

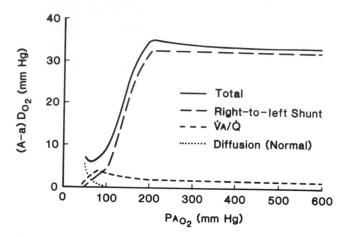

FIGURE 8–9. Relationship between $(A - a)D_{O_2}$ and $P_{A_{O_2}}$, assuming a right-to-left shunt of 2 per cent, normal $\dot{V}_A/\dot{Q}$ mismatching, and normal diffusing capacity. At high $P_{A_{O_2}}$, the $(A - a)D_{O_2}$ is predominantly due to right-to-left shunt, whereas at low $P_{A_{O_2}}$, impaired diffusion is a major contributor. (Modified from Farhi, L.E., and Rahn, H.: A theoretical analysis of the alveolar-arterial O_2 difference with special reference to the distribution effect. J. Appl. Physiol., 7:699–703, 1955.)

MEASUREMENT OF ALVEOLAR VENTILATION-PERFUSION INEQUALITIES

The whole lung is usually modeled as consisting of three compartments: (1) a shunt compartment, (2) a $\dot{V}_A/\dot{Q}$ compartment, and (3) a dead space compartment (Fig. 8–11A). The shunt and dead space can be calculated as previously discussed, and radioactive tracers have been used to study the topographic distributions of ventilation and perfusion throughout the lung. However, the radiographic technique has a poor spatial resolution, which severely limits its

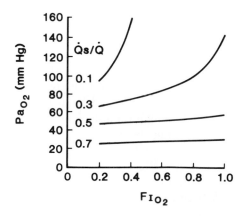

FIGURE 8–10. Relationship between arterial O_2 tension (Pa_{O_2}) and fractional inspired O_2 concentration ($F_{I_{O_2}}$) at different shunt values ($\dot{Q}s/\dot{Q}$).

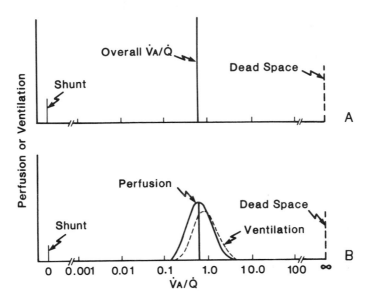

FIGURE 8–11. *A,* Three compartment model. One compartment has a $\dot{V}A/\dot{Q}$ of 0 (shunt), one is represented by the overall $\dot{V}A/\dot{Q}$, and the third is represented by a $\dot{V}A/\dot{Q}$ of infinity (dead space). *B,* The inert gas elimination technique allows the determination of shunt and dead space as well as a virtually continuous description of the $\dot{V}A/\dot{Q}$ distribution.

value in quantitating the $\dot{V}A/\dot{Q}$ mismatch. More recently, a new method employing metabolically inert gases has become available. This technique defines a shunt compartment, a dead space compartment, and a compartment with a virtually continuous distribution of $\dot{V}A/\dot{Q}$ values (Fig. 8–11*B*). The resolution of this technique easily differentiates regions with low $\dot{V}A/\dot{Q}$ values from unventilated regions and also distinguishes regions with high $\dot{V}A/\dot{Q}$ values from unperfused regions.

To determine the virtually continuous distribution of $\dot{V}A/\dot{Q}$ values within the lung of intact man or animals, dextrose or saline solutions are equilibrated with traces of six inert gases and then intravenously infused in a continuous fashion. The inert gases are carried by the venous blood to the lung, where they are eliminated. After a steady state between uptake and elimination is achieved, the volume of each inert gas eliminated per unit time from the lung is equal to the volume of that inert gas added to the lung from the blood. Thus, the volume of an inert gas removed per unit time from the blood into the alveoli ($\dot{V}_{\text{inert gas}}$) can be defined as:

$$\dot{V}_{\text{inert gas}} = \dot{Q} \times \lambda \frac{(P\overline{v}_{\text{inert gas}} - Pa_{\text{inert gas}})}{760} \qquad (8\text{–}16)$$

where λ is the blood-gas partition coefficient (the greater the λ, the more soluble the gas). The volume of an inert gas exhaled from the lung per unit time ($\dot{V}_{inert\ gas}$) is:

$$\dot{V}_{inert\ gas} = \dot{V}A \times \frac{PA_{inert\ gas}}{760} \tag{8–17}$$

Assuming that $PA_{inert\ gas} = Pa_{inert\ gas}$, i.e., there is no diffusion barrier across the alveolar-capillary membrane for the inert gas, the retention (R) or excretion (E) of the gas can be obtained from Equations 8–16 and 8–17 as:

$$R = \frac{Pa_{inert\ gas}}{P\bar{v}_{inert\ gas}} = \frac{\lambda}{\lambda + \dot{V}A/\dot{Q}} \tag{8–18}$$

Equation 8–18 expresses the fractional retention (R) or fractional excretion (E) of an inert gas. This equation states that the retention or excretion of an inert gas depends on the gas solubility (λ) and the $\dot{V}A/\dot{Q}$. This relationship is used to determine a virtually continuous distribution of $\dot{V}A/\dot{Q}$ values, as depicted in Figure 8–11.

The relationship between retention and $\dot{V}A/\dot{Q}$ for inert gases with different values of λ is shown in Figure 8–12. This figure shows that substances that are relatively insoluble in blood (substances with a low λ, e.g., sulfur hexafluoride, $\lambda = 0.008$) are not retained if $\dot{V}A/\dot{Q}$ of the lung >1. Conversely, substances that are very soluble (e.g., acetone, $\lambda = 374$) are 100 per cent retained if $\dot{V}A/\dot{Q}$ <1. This dependence of gas retention on $\dot{V}A/\dot{Q}$ is used in the inert gas

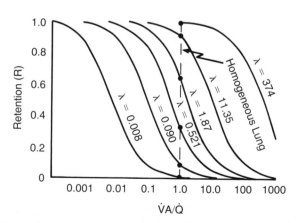

FIGURE 8–12. Relationship between retention and $\dot{V}A/\dot{Q}$ for six inert gases with Oswald partition coefficients (λ) ranging from 0.008 (sulfur hexafluoride) to 374 (acetone). The vertical dotted line predicts the retention for these six substances if the lung had a uniform $\dot{V}A/\dot{Q}$ of 1. Note that the retention of the substances with low solubility (e.g., sulfur hexafluoride) is primarily affected by low $\dot{V}A/\dot{Q}$ values; conversely, the retention of the more soluble substances is affected by high $\dot{V}A/\dot{Q}$ values. For example, at a $\dot{V}A/\dot{Q}$ ratio of 0.01, approximately 50 per cent of sulfur hexafluoride is retained and 50 per cent is eliminated via the lungs, whereas acetone is fully retained.

elimination technique to produce the virtually continuous distribution of $\dot{V}_A/\dot{Q}$ values within the lung.

The retentions, excretions, and blood gas partition coefficients of sulfur hexafluoride, ethane, cyclopropane, halothane, diethylether, and acetone are determined after a steady state has been attained in the subjects. From the relationship between λ and retention or excretion of these six gases, the distribution of ventilation and perfusion as a function of $\dot{V}_A/\dot{Q}$ can be computed for 50 lung compartments using special numeric analysis. The result of such an analysis is shown diagrammatically in Figure 8–13. If the lungs were completely homogeneous in terms of $\dot{V}_A/\dot{Q}$, the relationship between retention and λ shown by the dashed line would exist. But even in the normal lung, some $\dot{V}_A/\dot{Q}$ mismatching exists, which results in an increased retention of the less soluble gases; that is, the lower portion of the curve is shifted to the left (solid line). This relationship corresponds to a blood flow distribution as shown in Figure 8–13B and a ventilation distribution as shown in Figure 8–13C.

The inert gas elimination technique has been used as both a research and clinical tool. Figure 8–14 shows an example of its application. Figure 8–14A and B depicts the distributions of perfusion and ventilation in a healthy awake human in a supine position breathing 100% O_2. Induction of anesthesia and muscle paralysis with curare-like drugs plus mechanical ventilation of the lungs results in increased mismatching of $\dot{V}_A/\dot{Q}$ (as evidenced by a broadening of the ventilation-perfusion curves) and the development of a small right-to-left shunt of 4 per cent. Such an increased $\dot{V}_A/\dot{Q}$ mismatch is observed in nearly all normal subjects after induction of general anesthesia and is the basis for the impaired oxygenation and CO_2 elimination seen during general anesthesia. The $\dot{V}_A/\dot{Q}$ mismatching can be much worse in subjects with pre-existing lung disease, who may experience right-to-left shunts as high as 50 per cent.

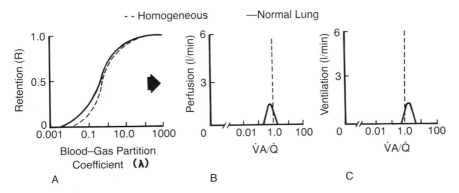

FIGURE 8–13. Using techniques of numerical analysis, the distribution of perfusion as a function of $\dot{V}_A/\dot{Q}$ (B) and the distribution of ventilation as a function of $\dot{V}_A/\dot{Q}$ (C) are determined from the relationship between excretion (not shown), retention, and blood-gas partition coefficient (A).

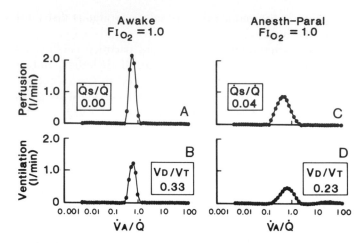

FIGURE 8–14. $\dot{V}A/\dot{Q}$ ratios and right-to-left shunt fractions ($\dot{Q}s/\dot{Q}$) observed in a healthy subject before *(A* and *B)* and after *(C* and *D)* induction of general anesthesia and muscle paralysis produced by curare-like drugs. The $\dot{Q}s/\dot{Q}$ of 0 in the awake state as measured with this technique differs from the normal $\dot{Q}s/\dot{Q}$ of approximately 0.03 because the inert gas technique cannot detect shunts associated with bronchial and thebesian circulations. VD/VT decreased because the anatomic dead space was reduced in the anesthetized-paralyzed state by endotracheal intubation. The reduction in anatomic dead space exceeded the increase in alveolar dead space, so that physiologic dead space was reduced.

SUGGESTED READING

Rahn, H., and Fenn, W.O.: *A Graphical Analysis of the Respiratory Gas Exchange:* The O_2-CO_2 Diagram. Washington, D.C.: The American Physiological Society, 1955.

Wagner, P.D., Saltzman, H.A., and West, J.B.: Measurement of continuous distributions of ventilation-perfusion ratios: Theory. *J. Appl. Physiol.,* 36:588–599, 1974.

West, J.B.: *Ventilation/Blood Flow and Gas Exchange.* London: Blackwell Scientific Publications, 1985.

QUESTIONS

1. What is the VD/VT ratio for a patient whose $PaCO_2$ is 60 mmHg and whose $P\overline{E}CO_2$ is 20 mmHg?
2. A patient has a cardiac output of 6.0 l/min and an oxygen consumption of 240 ml/min. A. What is the arteriovenous O_2 content difference? B. How much of the cardiac output is shunted from right-to-left if the alveolar-arterial oxygen tension difference is 180 mmHg?
3. Assuming a patient's lungs consist of two regions, each with a uniform $\dot{V}A/\dot{Q}$ and using the values given on the next page, fill in the missing values.

	Region 1	Region 2	Overall
V̇A/Q̇	0.20	2.0	0.99
Gas phase:			
V̇A, l/min	0.5	3.9	4.4
V̇A, % of overall			(100%)
PA_{CO_2}, mmHg	46	35	
PA_{O_2}, mmHg	53	129	
Blood phase:			
Q̇, l/min			
Q̇, % of overall			(100%)
Pa_{CO_2}, mmHg	46	35	41
Ca_{CO_2}, vol %	51.2	46	
Pa_{O_2}, mmHg	53	129	78
Ca_{O_2}, vol %	17.4	19.8	

$(A - a)D_{O_2}$

$(a - A)D_{CO_2}$

4. A patient is breathing 100% O_2 at sea level (barometric pressure 760 mmHg, body temperature 37°C). On admission, Pa_{O_2} = 100 mmHg and Pa_{CO_2} = 30 mmHg. The oxygen uptake is 250 ml/min, and the cardiac output is 3 l/min. What is the PA_{O_2}, the $(A - a)D_{O_2}$, the arteriovenous oxygen content difference, and the Q̇s?

5. Assume that the cardiac output of the patient in Question 4 increased on his second day of hospitalization to 6.0 l/min and the Pa_{O_2} is still 100 mmHg. What is his right-to-left shunt?

9

CLINICAL PULMONARY FUNCTION TESTS

Patients with respiratory abnormalities are often referred for pulmonary function testing. The greatest amount of information is obtained by testing lung mechanics. Specifically, the forced expiratory vital capacity is the most useful diagnostic test. In addition, certain patterns are suggestive of specific diseases (Table 9–1). Clearly, this testing does not provide specific diagnoses, but it does help to quantify the degree of physiologic abnormality. The specific diagnosis must be made by the clinician, who evaluates all available clinical information.

FORCED EXPIRATORY VITAL CAPACITY

Spirometry is used to measure the forced expiratory vital capacity (FVC). Although the measurement of FVC was discussed in Chapter 7, it will be briefly

TABLE 9–1.   Spirometry Values for Figure 9–1

	Normal	COPD	Fibrosis
FVC (l)	5	4	3
FEV$_1$ (l)	4	2	2.6
FEV$_1$%	80	50	87
Vmax$_{50}$ (l/sec)	3.5	0.6	3.5
FEF$_{25-75}$ (l/sec)	4.2	0.9	3.0

reviewed here. The subject inhales maximally, then exhales as forcefully and completely as possible. Recall from Chapter 7 (see Fig. 7–7) that the results of this maneuver are plotted as either expired volume as a function of time (a classic spirogram) or expiratory flow versus volume [the maximal expiratory flow-volume (MEFV) curve]. In Figure 9–1, both types of plots are presented. The results fall into one of several patterns. The subject may be normal, or the pattern may be consistent with either airway obstruction or pulmonary restrictive disease (e.g., pulmonary fibrosis). In certain instances, a combined obstructive-restrictive pattern is present.

Obstructive Pattern

In obstructive pulmonary disease, which is associated with an increased airway resistance, maximal expiratory flows are decreased. Figure 9–1B and E presents typical tracings from a subject with chronic obstructive pulmonary disease (COPD). It is quite apparent from the MEFV curve (Fig. 9–1B) that flows are markedly reduced relative to normal. There are several ways of evaluating decreases in expiratory flow. One is to measure the volume of gas expired during the first second of the FVC maneuver, the FEV$_1$. The greater the obstruction, the lower the FEV$_1$ and the lower the FEV$_1$ relative to the FVC. This FEV$_1$/FVC ratio (times 100) is designated as the FEV$_1$%. Another commonly used method requires measurement of the average flow over the middle 50 per cent of FVC, the FEF$_{25-75}$. The FEF$_{25-75}$, as shown in Figure 9–1D through F, is calculated by taking the middle 50 per cent of the FVC, i.e., the difference in volume expired at 25 and 75 per cent VC, (a), divided by the time required to exhale this volume (b). In the normal subject, this volume is 2.5 l, which, divided by the time (0.6 sec), gives an FEF$_{25-75}$ of 4.2 l/sec. Another important variable of expiratory flow is the Vmax$_{50}$, which is the maximum expiratory flow at one-half of vital capacity and is shown in Figure 9–1A, B, and C.

From Table 9–1 it can be seen that the FEV$_1$ is one-half of normal in the COPD patient and that only 50 per cent of the vital capacity is expired in 1 second (FEV$_1$% = 50%). Significant reductions are also seen in the Vmax$_{50}$ and the FEF$_{25-75}$. In COPD, there is a slight reduction in the vital capacity, but, as shown in Table 9–2, the vital capacity is not always reduced, particularly in the early stages of obstructive disease. The subject shown in Figure 9–1B

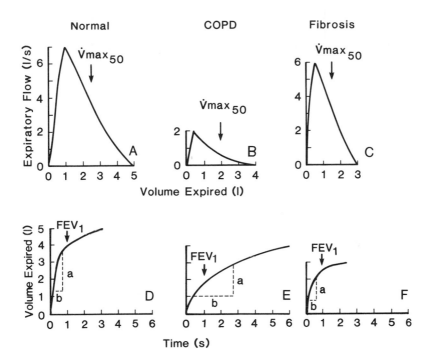

FIGURE 9–1. Plots of data obtained from a forced expiratory vital capacity test. *A, B,* and *C* are plots of the expiratory flow as a function of expired volume, and *D, E,* and *F* represent volume expired as a function of time. *A, B,* and *C* are the slopes of the bottom curves ($\Delta V/\Delta t$), or a direct measurement of flow. Curves are shown for normal subjects and for subjects with chronic obstructive pulmonary disease (COPD) or pulmonary fibrosis. FEV_1 is the volume of air expired during the first second, and FEF_{25-75} is the average flow over the middle 50 per cent of the forced expiratory vital capacity and is calculated as *a* divided by *b*. $\dot{V}max_{50}$ is shown in *A, B,* and *C* and represents the maximum expiratory flow at 50 per cent vital capacity.

and *E* clearly has airway obstruction. Other ways of quantifying this obstruction, to distinguish its possible cause, will be presented in a more detailed fashion later. However, for the majority of clinical situations, the data obtained by simple spirometry are adequate.

Restrictive Pattern

As its name implies, there is a decrease in all lung volumes in restrictive lung disease. Pulmonary fibrosis is a frequent cause of a restrictive pattern as seen from the curves in Figure 9–1*C* and *F*. Clearly, even with a reduced vital capacity, the flows are well preserved. Table 9–1 shows that the flows can be

TABLE 9–2. Typical Patterns of Abnormal Function

	Obstructive			Restrictive	
	Emphysema	*Chronic Bronchitis*	*Asthma*	*Parenchymal*	*Extraparenchymal Skeletal/ Neuromuscular*
VC	N or ↓	N or ↓	N or ↓	↓	↓
TLC	↑	N or ↑	N or ↑	↓	N or ↓
FRC	↑	N or ↑	↑	↓	N or ↓
RV	↑	↑	↑	↓	N or ↑
FEV$_1$	↓	↓	↓	↓	↓
FEF$_{25-75}$	↓	↓	↓	N or ↓	N or ↓
D$_{CO}$	N or ↓	N	N or ↑	↓	N
Pa$_{O_2}$	N or ↓	↓	↓	↓	N or ↓
Pa$_{CO_2}$	N or ↑	N or ↑	N or ↓	N or ↓	N or ↑
Pst,L$_{TLC}$	↓	N	N	↑	N
Cst,L	N or ↑	N	N	↓	N
Cdyn,L	↓	N or ↓	N or ↓	↓	N
R$_L$	↑	↑	↑	N	N
Phase III	↑	↑	↑	N	N

mildly reduced, associated with a reduction in volume, but the $FEV_1\%$ is normal. The descending limb of the FV curve frequently shows a steep slope in restrictive disease. Often these data are sufficient to describe restrictive disease, i.e., the characteristic pattern is a decrease in the vital capacity with a normal $FEV_1\%$. However, to be quite certain that a subject has a restrictive disease, the total lung capacity should be measured.

Mixed Pattern

Occasionally, subjects have pulmonary diseases with both restrictive and obstructive components. Pulmonary sarcoidosis or cancer, developing in a smoker with COPD, can produce mixed types of disease. In this mixed pattern of disease, the decrease in vital capacity is accompanied by a decrease in airflow, particularly the $FEV_1\%$. To prove that this is not simple obstructive disease, total lung capacity (TLC) should be measured and would be decreased in the mixed type of disease. Mixed obstructive-restrictive patterns occur fairly infrequently.

In summary, in most cases spirometry provides at least 80 per cent of the important information in pulmonary function testing. However, if the defect is to be further characterized, or if the physical examination or roentgenogram is not consistent with the pulmonary function tests, then further tests are warranted. The various types of obstructive and restrictive patterns are described in Table 9–2, with the different possible lung measurements shown on the left.

OBSTRUCTIVE PATTERN

The causes of obstructive patterns can be subdivided into (1) emphysema, (2) chronic bronchitis, and (3) asthma, as shown in Table 9–2, although mixtures of these conditions are often encountered clinically. The general term chronic obstructive pulmonary disease (COPD) may refer to pure emphysema, pure bronchitis, or a mixture of the two. Remember that the results of pulmonary function testing must always be considered with the patient's history, chest roentgenograms, and other available clinical data.

Emphysema

Emphysema is actually an anatomic diagnosis with the destruction of lung tissue documented by anatomic examination. True emphysema implies normal airways, i.e., airways without bronchitis. Patterns consistent with emphysema are listed in Table 9–2. As a consequence of lung tissue destruction, there is a loss of lung elasticity, and the static pressure-volume (PV) curve of the lung is shifted to the left (see Fig. 7–12). The data in Figure 7–12 for the COPD patient are typical of a patient with emphysema. The recoil pressure at total lung capacity, Pst,L_{TLC}, which is equal to pleural pressure at TLC, is changed from the normal value of -25 to -10 cmH$_2$O. An associated increase in static compliance has occurred, since the slope of the static PV curve is increased. However, the dynamic compliance is normal or decreased owing to the non-uniformity of time constants, as discussed in Chapter 7.

With the loss of lung tissue in emphysema, radial traction on the airways is decreased and the airways are narrowed, resulting in increased resistance to gas flow. In addition, an increase in residual volume occurs because the airways collapse more readily as the person exhales. Maximal flows are greatly reduced, even though the airways are anatomically normal. The importance of the lung's elastic recoil in determining maximal expiratory flows (V̇max) is graphically demonstrated in Figure 9–2, where V̇max is plotted against static lung recoil pressure, Pst,L, producing maximal flow-static recoil (MFSR) curves. The MFSR curves are generated by measuring V̇max and Pst,L at various lung volumes as explained in the figure legend. Note in bronchitis that for a given recoil pressure, the flows are lower (open circles). In contrast, in emphysema with a recoil pressure <2 cmH$_2$O, the flow is normal but higher flows cannot be obtained because maximal recoil is reduced (closed dots).

Figure 9–3 shows the MEFV curves as a function of absolute lung volume. The subject with COPD, in this case emphysema, functions with very high lung volumes, yet flows are markedly reduced as compared with the normal. The larger volumes are necessary to raise lung recoil pressure and drive flow through the obstructed airways. In contrast, the pulmonary fibrosis subject has low lung volumes but normal flow.

Associated with the loss of lung tissue in COPD is loss of pulmonary capillaries. This reduction in diffusing area causes a decreased diffusing capacity. Such subjects frequently show mild chronic increases in minute ventilation and often maintain a normal Pa$_{CO_2}$ with only a normal or slightly reduced Pa$_{O_2}$. Only late in the course of the disease do hypoxemia and CO$_2$ retention develop. The hypoxemia results from a ventilation-perfusion mismatch combined with a decreased diffusing capacity.

Single-breath nitrogen washout curves from a normal subject and a patient with COPD are presented in Figure 9–4. The slope of phase III is abnormally steep in the COPD patient owing to prolonged, nonuniform time constants. In addition, the phase IV (closing volume) has become obscured. These changes in the single-breath nitrogen washout curve also occur in chronic bronchitis, making the closing volume test of little value in evaluating advanced disease.

In summary, there are four alterations in pulmonary function tests (besides the decreased expiratory flows) that strongly suggest the diagnosis of emphysema: (1) an increased TLC, seen as hyperinflation on chest roentgenogram, (2) loss of peripheral vascular elements on chest roentgenogram, reflecting loss of tissue, (3) a decrease in static recoil of the lung, and (4) a decrease in diffusing capacity.

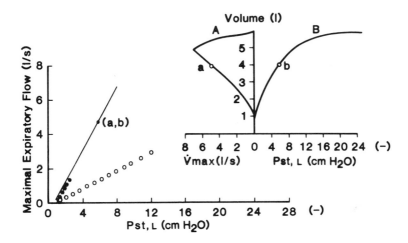

FIGURE 9–2. Maximal expiratory flow versus lung recoil (MFSR) curves for normal subjects (solid line) and subjects with emphysema (solid circles) or bronchitis (open circles). These curves are constructed by measuring V̇max from maximal MEFV curves and lung recoil pressures (Pst,L) from static pressure-volume curves. The insert is composed of the normal maximal expiratory flow volume (MEFV) curves (left axis, A) and the normal static deflation curve of the lungs (right axis, B). The normal MFSR curve (solid line, point a,b) was constructed by finding, at a given volume, the maximum expiratory flow (point a) and the appropriate recoil pressure (point b). At each lung volume this measurement provides points that allow construction of the MFSR curve as shown by the solid line and the indicated point (a, b). The flow volume curves and static pressure-volume curves for subjects with emphysema or bronchitis used to construct the MFSR curves indicated by solid and open circles are not shown. For emphysema, V̇max is normal for the recoil pressure (closed dots), but the curve is very short over the entire forced expiration. For bronchitis, the curve is shifted down (open dots).

Chronic Bronchitis

Bronchitis in its pure form is limited to the airways. Therefore TLC is often normal (see Table 9–2). The diseased airways are narrowed, however, causing increased airway resistance, increased residual volume, and a decreased vital capacity. The FEV_1 and FEF_{25-75} are reduced. The functional residual capacity (FRC) is often increased, even though the pressure-volume curve of the lung is normal. The FRC is increased dynamically in an attempt to compensate for the high airway resistance, since resistance decreases as lung volume increases (see Fig. 7–4).

Since the lung parenchyma is normal, the static compliance and recoil pressure at total lung capacity are normal. Despite the normal PV curve, the

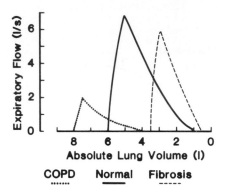

FIGURE 9–3. Forced expiratory flow as a function of total lung volume is shown for normal subjects (solid line) and for subjects with COPD (dotted line) and pulmonary fibrosis (dashed line). Note that for COPD, the total lung volume is high, whereas expiratory flow is decreased. In fibrotic disease, flows are near normal, but total lung volume is much smaller.

maximum flow-static recoil curve (open circles, see Fig. 9–2) is greatly abnormal owing to airway disease, indicating how emphysema and bronchitis can be separated using this type of analysis. Dynamic compliance is generally not normal owing to differences in the regional time constants of the lung. These changes in time constants are also responsible for the increased slope of phase III (see Fig. 9–4). The diffusing capacity is frequently normal in the early

FIGURE 9–4. Single-breath nitrogen washout curve for a normal subject and a patient with COPD. Remember that after inhaling pure O_2, the expired gas contains no oxygen as the dead space is cleared (phase I), but then the gas rapidly approaches the concentration in the alveoli (phase II) (see Fig. 6–11). However, the phase III portion of these washout curves is not flat, since different areas of the lung have different time constants of emptying and filling. For COPD, the time constants for the various lung elements are greatly different, and the slope of phase III N_2 is much higher (7 per cent N_2 per liter of volume expired) than the normal slope of 1.5 per cent N_2 per liter volume expired. The onset of phase IV (closing volume) occurs at 20 per cent of vital capacity (1 liter) in the normal subject but is absent in the COPD subject.

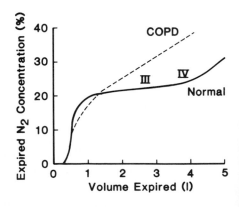

stages, but owing to severe mismatching of ventilation and perfusion, Pa_{O_2} is reduced and CO_2 is retained.

In summary, the major characteristics of bronchitis are (1) reduction in Pa_{O_2}, (2) CO_2 retention, (3) decreased dynamic compliance, and (4) near normal TLC.

Asthma

If the subject is experiencing symptoms of asthma, such as cough, wheezing, and mild dyspnea at the time of testing, and if there is a long history of episodic attacks of wheezing (bronchospasm), a diagnosis of asthma is fairly certain. But some asthmatics have symptom-free periods during which their pulmonary function tests are normal.

In the symptomatic subject with severe narrowing of the airways, the FEV_1 and maximum expiratory flows are decreased. The respiratory system attempts to compensate for this increased airway resistance with an acute increase in TLC and an increased FRC. Residual volume is increased secondary to the high airway resistance. Consequently, the vital capacity is reduced. Since there is no basic abnormality in the lung parenchyma, the static lung PV curve and static lung compliance are normal. However, dynamic compliance is decreased owing to the abnormality in time constants; this will produce an abnormal distribution of inspired gas and an increase in the slope of phase III during exhalation (see Fig. 9–4). The diffusing capacity is typically normal. In some cases, however, it is increased, owing to increased pulmonary blood volume. Owing to abnormalities in ventilation-perfusion matching, the Pa_{O_2} is decreased, but typically these individuals increase their minute ventilation and maintain a normal Pa_{CO_2}.

The airway constriction in asthma is reversible to varying degrees. Hence it is most useful to perform spirometry before and after the administration of an inhaled bronchodilator drug, since significant increases in airway flows and vital capacity after administration of the drug are consistent with a diagnosis of asthma. In asymptomatic subjects, a bronchoprovocation study with inhaled histamine or methacholine is used to provoke an asthmatic episode. Sometimes an antigen for which the subject has tested positive is used to provoke an asthmatic attack.

In summary, the characteristic findings in asthma are (1) decrease in FEV_1, (2) decrease in FEF_{25-75}, (3) lowered Pa_{O_2}, (4) normal Pa_{CO_2} associated with an increased respiratory frequency, and (5) increased TLC and FRC.

RESTRICTIVE PATTERN

A decreased vital capacity with normal flows, i.e., a normal $FEV_1\%$, is consistent with restrictive lung disease. The clinician can be totally confident of this diagnosis if a decreased TLC is present. Two classes of defects lead to a restrictive pattern: (1) alterations in lung parenchyma, and (2) extraparenchymal changes.

Parenchymal Changes

Alterations in the lung tissue caused by conditions such as idiopathic pulmonary fibrosis or diffuse carcinomatosis fall into this category of restrictive lung disease. The roentgenogram is abnormal. The effect of this type of abnormality on lung volumes is depicted in Figure 9–3. Total lung capacity, vital capacity, and residual volume are decreased. FRC is also decreased owing to a decreased static lung compliance (as discussed for Fig. 7–14).

In restrictive disease due to parenchymal changes, maximal expiratory flows are generally normal or slightly decreased and $FEV_1\%$ is normal, as shown in Figure 9–1 and Table 9–1. Increased radial traction on the airways due to increased lung recoil may actually promote increased airflow, as evidenced by the steep slope seen in the MEFV curve. Airway resistance is normal.

The shift to the right of the PV curve shown in Figure 7–12 causes an increased lung recoil at TLC, in this case to -40 cmH$_2$O. Both static and dynamic compliances are reduced. Invariably, the diffusing capacity for carbon monoxide (DL_{CO}) is decreased. This is due to increased thickness of the alveolar-capillary membrane and alterations in ventilation-perfusion matching. This results in a decreased Pa_{O_2}. Arterial P_{CO_2} may be maintained at normal levels, but some subjects chronically hyperventilate and decrease their Pa_{CO_2}.

In summary, the hallmarks of parenchymal restrictive lung disease are as follows: (1) $FEV_1\%$ is normal, (2) TLC, VC, and RV are decreased, (3) DL_{CO} is decreased, (4) Pa_{O_2} is decreased, (5) Pa_{CO_2} is usually normal, (6) Pst,L is increased, and (7) dynamic and static compliances are decreased.

Extraparenchymal Changes

In extraparenchymal disease, the lung is essentially normal. The restriction may be due to a variety of conditions such as thoracic tumors, obesity, accumulation of pleural fluid, or skeletal deformities such as kyphoscoliosis. Restriction has also been seen in conditions that produce weakness of the respiratory muscles; for example, the chest cage cannot be expanded adequately with poliomyelitis or with neurologic conditions such as amyotrophic lateral sclerosis (Lou Gehrig's disease) or myasthenia gravis. In these neurologic conditions, respiratory muscle strength must be measured. The important details of making this measurement were discussed in Chapter 6. Although the normal expiratory pressure exerted at total lung capacity is approximately 230 cmH$_2$O, it is not uncommon to find reductions to as low as 80 cmH$_2$O in various forms of neuromuscular disease. Similarly, maximal inspiratory pressures at residual volume may change from -125 to -30 cmH$_2$O. Early in the disease course, these subjects often experience dyspnea, with little or no change in the standard pulmonary function tests. The first overt abnormality is a decrease in respiratory muscle strength.

Table 9–2 indicates that the patterns due to parenchymal and extraparenchymal causes are very similar. Vital capacity, total lung capacity, and FRC are decreased. However, the residual volume may be increased in the extraparenchymal conditions, because the respiratory muscles are not strong enough to compress the chest. The $FEV_1\%$ is normal or slightly increased. Since the lung (and hence the pressure-volume curve) is normal, near normal recoil pressures at total lung capacity, normal compliances, and a normal phase III are seen. Moreover, the diffusing capacity and gas exchange are normal, but arterial blood gases may be abnormal.

In summary, the major findings in extraparenchymal restrictive disease are (1) decreased VC, TLC, and FRC with a possible increase in RV, (2) decreased Pa_{O_2}, (3) increased Pa_{CO_2}, (4) normal D_{LCO}, and (5) normal or decreased Pst,L. Note that the major difference between parenchymal and extraparenchymal restrictive disease is that lung compliance and D_{LCO} are decreased in parenchymal disease, whereas both are normal in extraparenchymal disease.

ABNORMAL BLOOD GASES

Causes of Hypoxemia

HYPOVENTILATION (DECREASE IN ALVEOLAR VENTILATION)

The importance of decreased alveolar ventilation is clear from the modified Equation 2–8:

$$\dot{V}_A = \dot{V}_{CO_2}/Pa_{CO_2}$$

When CO_2 production remains constant, a decreased alveolar ventilation causes an increased Pa_{CO_2}. When the respiratory exchange ratio (R) and the fractional inspired oxygen concentration are unchanged, for every increase in arterial CO_2 there is a decrease in alveolar O_2 tension leading to a decreased arterial O_2 tension. Hypoventilation itself, however, does not produce severe hypoxemia; this form of hypoxemia is readily corrected by increasing the inspired oxygen concentration. Common causes of hypoventilation include decreases in central neurologic drive (idiopathic or secondary to depressant drugs); diseases that weaken the respiratory muscles, such as poliomyelitis or myasthenia gravis; and abnormal loads placed on the thoracic cage, such as extreme obesity.

SHUNT

Right-to-left shunting of blood commonly occurs in congenital heart disease but is also seen with arteriovenous malformations within the lung. *Hypoxemia secondary to shunting is the one case that cannot be corrected with 100% oxygen.* With shunting, there is usually no increase in the arterial CO_2 tension, except in severe cases.

DIFFUSION DEFECT

Hypoxemia due to diffusion defects can be reversed with 100% oxygen, which increases the diffusion gradient for oxygen. The exact contribution of the diffusion defect to the hypoxemia is difficult to assess. Generally, there is an associated ventilation-perfusion mismatch that also contributes to the hypoxemia. Usually, arterial P_{CO_2} does not increase with diffusion defects.

VENTILATION-PERFUSION ($\dot{V}A/\dot{Q}$) MISMATCH

This is the most common cause of both hypoxemia and CO_2 retention. One generally arrives at a diagnosis of $\dot{V}A/\dot{Q}$ mismatching by excluding the previously mentioned causes. However, an increased difference between alveolar and arterial O_2 tension [$(A - a)D_{O_2}$] is a good indicator of a $\dot{V}A/\dot{Q}$ abnormality. In contrast to right-to-left shunts, the hypoxemia due to $\dot{V}A/\dot{Q}$ mismatch is abolished by breathing pure oxygen. Of course, a combination of the conditions discussed previously may cause hypoxemia, i.e., hypoventilation caused by muscle weakness in subjects with chronic obstructive lung disease who already have $\dot{V}A/\dot{Q}$ abnormalities.

Causes of Hypercapnia

The major causes of hypercapnia have been previously discussed; these are *hypoventilation* and $\dot{V}A/\dot{Q}$ *mismatch*. The $\dot{V}A/\dot{Q}$ mismatch is generally seen in subjects with chronic obstructive pulmonary disease who have not increased their alveolar ventilation, resulting in a rise in Pa_{CO_2} tension.

UPPER AIRWAY LESIONS

This is an interesting but rare group of lesions that affect the upper airways, primarily the trachea. A very high-pitched noisy inspiration or an atypical history of asthma suggests the presence of an upper airway lesion. Routine pulmonary function tests may be normal, with the most obvious abnormality being an unexplained decrease in the maximum expiratory flow or maximum breathing capacity. Obviously, the final diagnosis depends on a direct visualization of the lesion by bronchoscopy. However, flow-volume loops, such as those shown in Figure 9–5, can be very helpful in characterizing such abnormalities. The maximal inspiratory flow and the maximal expiratory flow are measured to produce the flow-volume loops as shown in Figure 9–5. For the

FIGURE 9–5. Plot of maximal expiratory flow (curve above zero-flow axis) and maximal inspiratory flow (curve below zero-flow axis). Shown are flow volume loops for a normal subject and for subjects with fixed, variable extrathoracic, and variable intrathoracic tracheal lesions.

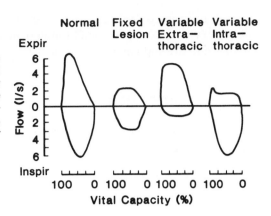

normal loop, peak flows during inspiration and expiration and the flows at 50 per cent of the vital capacity are very similar.

For the *fixed lesion,* both inspiratory and expiratory flows are markedly decreased and both exhibit a plateau in flow. This type of flow-volume loop is usually caused by a tumor of the trachea, which produces a fixed airway narrowing during both inspiration and expiration. The tumor can be either intrathoracic or extrathoracic. A fractured larynx, which causes fixed narrowing of the vocal cords, can also produce this pattern. The flow-volume loop associated with a fixed tracheal lesion can be mimicked easily in the laboratory by measuring forced inspiratory and expiratory flows through a small orifice.

Some loop patterns are called variable, since their shapes depend on lesion location. A variable loop indicates that flow is reduced during either inspiration or expiration but not both, as seen in the fixed lesion. The *variable extrathoracic* pattern predominantly shows a reduction in inspiratory flow, with a fairly normal expiratory flow. This pattern is commonly seen when the vocal cord muscles are paralyzed or when the extrathoracic trachea has been damaged because of prolonged tracheal intubation. The flow dynamics associated with these abnormalities primarily affect inspiratory flow. During forced inspiration, the subatmospheric intratracheal pressure causes the lesion to be pulled inward, which narrows the airway and reduces inspiratory flow. During expiration, however, the positive intratracheal pressure holds the airway open so that expiratory flow is not greatly affected.

For a *variable intrathoracic* lesion, the extramural pressure acting on the airway is not atmospheric but pleural pressure. During forced inspiration, the subatmospheric pleural pressure holds the airway open, and the inspiratory flow is little affected. However, during expiration, the high positive pleural pressure causes partial collapse in the lesion area and a substantial reduction in airflow. This produces the typical intrathoracic pattern showing a reduction in peak expiratory flow, an expiratory plateau, but almost no change in the inspiratory flow. Note the small initial overshoot in expiratory flow. This overshoot is due to a sudden compression of the airways, which expel their contents.

OTHER PROCEDURES

Maximum Breathing Capacity (MBC), or Maximum Voluntary Ventilation (MVV)

This was one of the first pulmonary function measurements developed. In this test, the subject breathes as rapidly and forcefully as possible for 15 seconds, and the volume of expired gas is measured in liters and multiplied by 4 to obtain l/min. The test has two disadvantages: (1) it is a tiring procedure, and (2) it depends on patient effort. Of all pulmonary function tests presented in this book, however, the MBC is best correlated with the patient's subjective evaluation of dyspnea, regardless of the causative factor. The MBC is abnormal in many conditions and does not indicate specific abnormalities, but it is quite sensitive and may be the first test to become abnormal with upper airway lesions. In addition, it is generally the first routine pulmonary function test to indicate neuromuscular disease. Therefore, many laboratories still use the MBC.

Detection of Early Airway Disease

Many investigators feel that airway disease associated with chronic bronchitis begins in the peripheral airways. This belief has led to the development of a large number of pulmonary function tests designed to detect early small airway disease. The first of these tests involved measuring the frequency dependence of compliance, which was discussed in Chapter 7. This procedure is very demanding and requires prior training, since the subjects must increase their respiratory frequency but maintain constant tidal volume and FRC. For many subjects, even those with little airway obstruction, this is very difficult. The test is also not specific for small airway disease, since nonuniform alterations in compliance, which lead to abnormal time constants, result in a fall in compliance with increasing frequency of ventilation.

Another test highly proclaimed as a measure of early small airway disease was the onset of phase IV, or the closing volume, of the single-breath nitrogen washout curve. There are now many published reports indicating that closing volume does not correlate with peripheral airway disease, in part because of problems associated with reproducibility.

More recently, pulmonary clinicians have begun to use the effects of inspired gas density on maximal expiratory flow as a means of detecting small airway disease. At low lung volumes, i.e., near residual volume, flow is limited in the periphery of the lung where laminar flow predominates. Recall that laminar flow decreases with increased viscosity but is not affected by changes in gas density. At high lung volumes, gas flow is limited by the larger airways, where turbulent flow predominates. Under these circumstances, flow is inversely related to the gas density. Because gas flow is markedly density dependent in the larger airways but density independent in the small airways, changing the inspired gas to a mixture of 80% helium and 20% oxygen (which is only 35 per cent as dense as air) produces an approximate 50 per cent increase in flow at 50 per cent of the vital capacity owing to reductions in turbulence. If early airway disease begins in the peripheral airways, then they would be more important in determining maximal flow. MEFV curves obtained after breathing a helium-oxygen mixture would show a less than normal increase in maximal flow at 50 per cent vital capacity in subjects with small airway disease. The change in $\dot{V}max_{50}$ while breathing a He:O_2 mixture is mathematically defined as:

$$\Delta\dot{V}max_{50} = \frac{\dot{V}max_{50,He} - \dot{V}max_{50,air}}{\dot{V}max_{50,air}} \tag{9–1}$$

where $\dot{V}max_{50,He}$ is the maximal flow at 50 per cent VC when the subject breathes a He:O_2 mixture, and $\dot{V}max_{50,air}$ is the maximal flow at 50 per cent VC when the subject breathes air.

$\Delta\dot{V}max_{50}$ of 20 per cent or less was originally thought to indicate small airway disease. However, this test has limited usefulness, since some individuals with severe airway disease have a $\Delta\dot{V}max_{50}$ well within the normal range. Another problem arises because of the poor reproducibility of the measurement. Two MEFV curves must be made, one using air and the other using helium:oxygen, and the variability associated with each measurement reduces the reliability of the test. Thus, the density-dependence measurements appear to have no advantage over conventional spirometry in detecting small airway disease.

In summary, there is no test presently used that accurately detects small airway disease. Indeed, there is little conclusive evidence that early airway disease begins in the peripheral airways.

NORMAL VALUES

Table 9–3 lists normal values for all tests discussed in this chapter. Relevant regression equations are given, as are references for the normal values. Mean values are for an average male [age 40, height 5'10" (178 cm)] or an average female [age 40, height 5'5" (165 cm)]. Note that sex, height, and age are important determinants of normal values. It is important that normal values be obtained from subjects who have never smoked. Many published values

TABLE 9–3. List of Normal Respiratory Values

Test (Units)	Normal Male (M)	Normal Female (F)	Prediction Equation*	LLN†	Reference
TLC (l)	6.8	5.2	(M) 0.076H − 6.69 (F) 0.0646H − 5.44	− 1.37 − 1.10	1
FVC (l)	5.0	3.5	(M) 0.0844H − 0.0298A − 8.78 (F) 0.0444H − 0.0169A − 3.19	× 0.78 × 0.752	2
RV (l)	1.8	1.7	TLC − FVC		
FRC (l)	3.4	2.6	50% pred TLC		
FEV$_1$ (l)	4.1	2.9	(M) 0.0665H − 0.0292A − 6.51 (F) 0.0332H − 0.0190A − 1.82	× 0.791 × 0.779	2
FEV$_1$% (%)	82	83	(M) −0.105A + 86.7 (F) −0.1852H − 0.1896A + 121.7	× 0.869 × 0.859	2
FEF$_{25-75}$ (l/sec)	4.3	3.3	(M) 0.0579H − 0.0363A − 4.52 (F) 0.0300H − 0.0309A − 0.41	× 0.553 × 0.448	2
Vmax$_{50}$ (l/sec)	5.2	3.9	(M) 0.0684H − 0.0366A − 5.54 (F) 0.0321H − 0.0240A − 0.44	× 0.651 × 0.542	2
MVV (l/min)	168	112	(M) 1.15H − 1.27A + 14 (F) 0.55H − 0.72A + 50	−33 −33	3
Resistance (cmH$_2$O/l/sec)	1–2.5	1–2.5			
Pst,L$_{TLC}$ (cmH$_2$O)	−30	−30		− 20	6
Cst,L‡ (l/cmH$_2$O)	0.260	0.230		− 0.06	7

Test			Prediction formula	± value	Ref.
Cdyn,L§ (l/cmH$_2$O)	0.190	0.150		-0.04	4
Phase III (% N$_2$/l)	2.9	2.8	(M&F) $-$ 0.007H $-$ 0.0002A $+$ 1.7	1.96	5
MEP‖ (cmH$_2$O)	233	152		(M) ±84 (F) ±54	5
MIP# (cmH$_2$O)	124	87		(M) ±44 (F) +32	1
DL$_{CO}$ (ml/min/mmHg)	33	24	(M) 0.1646H $-$ 0.2290A $+$ 12.9 (F) 0.1602H $-$ 0.1111A $+$ 2.2	-8.0 -6.5	
Pao$_2$ (mmHg)	85	85	[(P$_B$ $-$ 47) × 0.2093 $-$ (Paco$_2$ × 1.17)] × 0.58 $+$ 42.7 $-$ (A × 0.24)		
Paco$_2$ (mmHg)	40±5	40±5			

*H = height in centimeters; A = age in years; P$_B$ = barometric pressure.
†Add or subtract number shown or multiply the predicted value by the factor shown.
‡Static compliance from deflation limb of static pressure-volume curve.
§Dynamic compliance, measured during inspiration.
‖Maximal static expiratory pressure measured at TLC.
#Maximal static inspiratory pressure measured at RV.

References

1. Miller, R.D., et al., Am. Rev. Resp. Dis., 127:270, 1983.
2. Knudson, R.J., et al., Am. Rev. Resp. Dis., 127:725, 1983.
3. Composite of several studies.
4. Knudson, R.J., et al., Am. Rev. Resp. Dis., 115:423, 1977.
5. Black, L.F., and Hyatt, R.E.: Am. Rev. Resp. Dis., 99:696, 1969.
6. Turner, J.M., et al., J. Appl. Physiol., 25:664, 1968.
7. Permutt, S., & Martin, H.B., J. Appl. Physiol., 15:819, 1960.

include smokers and nonsmokers in their groups and hence are not reliable as baseline values. One should also be extremely careful when making predictions outside the range of age or height included in the original sample from which the regression equations were developed. There are also racial effects; the best documented racial effect is for blacks, for whom it is necessary to reduce all the predicted volumes and flows by 12 per cent.

One must be cautious in applying these equations to an individual who has a thoracic deformity such as kyphoscoliosis, the abnormality seen in the hunchback of Notre Dame. In this case, using height would underestimate lung volumes. For example, assume the male in this table with a predicted FVC of 5 l developed a spinal deformity that reduced his height to 5 ft (152.4 cm). Using the latter height measurement, one would predict his normal FVC to be only 2.89 l. This prediction value would severely underestimate his FVC. To circumvent this type of problem, the individual's arm span is substituted for height in the prediction equations, since arm span is little affected by such thoracic deformities.

Finally, Table 9–3 lists the lower limit of normal (LLN). Approximately 95 per cent of normals lie either above this value, as with the FVC, or below this value, as with phase III.

SUGGESTED READING

Black, L.F., Hyatt, R.E., and Stubbs, S.E.: Mechanism of expiratory airflow limitation in chronic obstructive pulmonary disease associated with alpha-1-antitrypsin deficiency. *Am. Rev. Resp. Dis.*, 105:891–899, 1972.

Hyatt, R.E., and Rodarte, J.R.: Closing volume, one man's noise—other men's experiment. *Mayo Clin. Proc.*, 50:17–27, 1975.

Miller, R.D., and Hyatt, R.E.: Evaluation of obstructing lesions of the trachea and larynx by flow-volume loops. *Am. Rev. Resp. Dis.*, 108:475–481, 1973.

QUESTIONS

1. The patient is a 45-year-old nonsmoking female who has noted progressive dyspnea on exertion for 5 years. Her father and a brother died of lung disease. Pertinent test results are:

Test	Predicted	Observed	Bronchodilator Rx
TLC (l)	5.6	7.0	7.0
FVC (l)	4.0	3.0	3.0
FEV_1 (l)	3.0	1.5	1.5
D_{LCO} (ml/min/mmHg)	25	10	

a. Is this a restrictive or obstructive pattern?
b. What are the major features consistent with your answer?
c. Can you further subclassify the pattern and on what basis?
d. What additional finding would help you most in your further classifications?

2. A husky 20-year-old male complains of periodic cough, which on close questioning appears to occur during exertion, especially jogging on cold days. He is a nonsmoker. Otherwise, the history is negative.

Test	Predicted	Observed	Bronchodilator Rx
TLC (l)	8.0	8.4	8.4
FVC (l)	6.0	5.0	6.0
FEV_1 (l)	4.8	3.0	4.5
D_{LCO} (ml/min/mmHg)	30	35	

a. Is this a restrictive or obstructive pattern?
b. What are the major features consistent with your answer?
c. Can you further subclassify the pattern and on what basis?
d. What additional finding would help you most in your further classifications?

3. The patient is a 40-year old white female who has noted progressive dyspnea on exertion since age 35. She also has a persistent dry cough and notes that her fingernails often look blue and puffy. She is a non-smoker, and there is no history of unusual exposure to environmental or industrial irritants.

Test	Predicted	Observed
TLC (l)	6.0	4.0
FVC (l)	4.2	2.2
FEV_1 (l)	3.4	2.0
D_{LCO} (ml/min/mmHg)	25	7

a. Is this a restrictive or obstructive pattern?
b. What are the major features consistent with your answer?
c. Can you further subclassify the pattern and on what basis?
d. What additional finding would help you most in your further classifications?

4. The patient is a 56-year-old male who has noted progressive dyspnea on exertion for 5 years. He has smoked two packs of cigarettes for 40 years (80 pack-years). For the past 10 years, he has noted a morning "smoker's" cough productive of phlegm. He has averaged three respiratory infections per winter for 5 years. Pertinent test results are:

Test	Predicted	Observed	Bronchodilator Rx
TLC (l)	6.5	6.8	
FVC (l)	5.0	3.5	3.5
FEV$_1$ (l)	4.0	1.8	1.8
D$_{LCO}$ (ml/min/mmHg)	30	25	

    a. Is this a restrictive or obstructive pattern?
    b. What are the major features consistent with your answer?
    c. Can you further subclassify the pattern and on what basis?
    d. What additional finding would help you most in your further classi-
       fications?
5. During his annual physical exam, this 45-year-old white male admitted
to the recent onset of mild to moderate dyspnea on exertion and difficulty
in raising secretions during a recent respiratory infection. He had quit
smoking 15 years ago.

Test	Predicted	Observed
TLC (l)	7.0	5.0
FVC (l)	5.0	3.0
FEV$_1$ (l)	3.8	2.7
D$_{LCO}$ (ml/min/mmHg)	26	24

    a. Is this a restrictive or obstructive pattern?
    b. What are the major features consistent with your answer?
    c. Can you further subclassify the pattern and on what basis?
    d. What additional finding would help you most in your further classi-
       fications?
6. A 21-year-old male complained of dyspnea on exertion of 2 months
duration. He was a nonsmoker and had been well until five months
prior, when he was injured in a home furnace explosion and received
serious burns to his chest, head and neck, and upper airway. Owing to
initial respiratory distress, a tracheostomy was performed. He recovered
nicely, and the tracheostomy tube was removed in 1 week. One month
later he had no symptoms, and chest examination and chest roentgenogram were normal. He returned to college and did well until his present
symptoms began.

Test	Predicted	Observed	Bronchodilator Rx
TLC (l)	7.2	7.6	7.6
FVC (l)	5.4	5.5	5.5
FEV$_1$ (l)	4.3	3.3	3.3
D$_{LCO}$ (ml/min/mmHg)	35	35	

a. Is this a restrictive or obstructive pattern?
b. What are the major features consistent with your answer?
c. Can you further subclassify the pattern and on what basis?
d. What additional finding would help you most in your further classifications?

FLUID EXCHANGE IN THE LUNG
Pulmonary Microcirculation
Capillary Pressure (Ppc)
Interstitial Hydrostatic Fluid Pressure (P$_T$)
Plasma Colloid Osmotic Pressure (ΠP)
Tissue Colloid Osmotic Pressure (ΠT)
Solvent Permeability of the Capillary Wall (Kfc)
Solute Selectivity of the Capillary Wall (σd)
Starling's Law of the Capillaries
Pulmonary Lymphatic System
Volume Overload
Clearance of Particulate Matter from Airways
Pleural Fluid Exchange
Airway Fluid Exchange and Alveolar Epithelial Transport

PULMONARY EDEMA

TISSUE EDEMA SAFETY FACTORS
Hydrostatic Edema
Damaged Endothelium

CLINICAL PROBLEMS ASSOCIATED WITH PULMONARY EDEMA

FACTORS THAT DAMAGE LUNGS
Detection of Edema Fluid

10

PULMONARY FLUID EXCHANGE

Fluid is normally exchanged between the pulmonary circulation and interstitium, between the interstitium and the pleural spaces, and between the airway interstitium and epithelial surfaces. These fluid exchanges are well regulated so that excessive fluid does not accumulate in the pulmonary interstitium or pleural spaces. The accumulation of excess fluid is also prevented by the extensive lymphatic system that drains these areas. In normal lungs, fluid formation always equals fluid removal so that excess fluid cannot enter the lung interstitium, alveoli, or airways to interfere with function. A major portion of this chapter is devoted to describing the mechanisms responsible for transcapillary fluid exchange, since each of the fluid exchange processes listed previously requires fluid to leave the capillaries serving the particular lung region. Normally, transcapillary fluid exchange is controlled within very narrow limits, but in many pathologic conditions, fluid may accumulate in alveoli and limit gas exchange. Fluid may also enter the pleural spaces, altering the mechanics of the lungs and chest wall. Alternatively, when inadequate amounts of fluid enter the airways the result is less compliant airways and dehydrated mucus, which cannot be properly removed from the airways by ciliary motion or cough. The remainder of this chapter deals with the role of transcapillary fluid exchange in various forms of lung pathology, providing the student with the necessary insight to apply these basic principles on the clinical level.

FLUID EXCHANGE IN THE LUNG

Pulmonary Microcirculation

It is important to remember the major differences between the pulmonary and systemic circulations. The pulmonary blood vessels are not as muscular as their systemic counterparts, and their intravascular hydrostatic pressures are lower. Thus, the pulmonary vascular system is a low-resistance, low-pressure, high-compliance circulation designed to accept changes in cardiac output with little change in intravascular pressure. In contrast to the peripheral circulation, the pulmonary vasculature does not autoregulate its blood flow. This lack of autoregulation in the lung's circulation plus its paucity of vascular smooth muscle makes it an ideal circulation to accept more blood flow without greatly elevating pulmonary vascular pressures. In fact, cardiac output has to increase to five times normal before pulmonary vascular pressure rises significantly.

The basic anatomy of the pulmonary blood vessels begins with the large muscular arteries that enter each lung lobe. These arteries then divide into numerous smaller arterioles (<100 μm), which contain little or no smooth muscle. These small arterioles branch into a system of 7-μm capillaries, which completely surround each alveolus. These capillaries coalesce to form the pulmonary venules, which combine into the large venous system, which empties its blood into the left atrium. Blood vessels in the lung have been further classified as alveolar or extra-alveolar, depending on whether the blood flow in these vessels is affected by changes in alveolar pressure (see Chap. 5).

It is generally thought that any pulmonary microvessel less than 100 μm in diameter is capable of exchanging fluid with the interstitium; the capillary density of the lung is so large that blood vessels larger than this cannot contribute greatly to fluid filtration. The exact location of transvascular fluid filtration is not known, but 60 per cent of the fluid filtration occurs in alveolar capillaries, whereas about 15 and 25 per cent occur in the extra-alveolar arterial and venous vessels, respectively. For the remainder of this chapter the term *pulmonary capillaries* will be used to refer to the entire fluid exchange portion of the pulmonary circulation.

Capillary Pressure (Ppc)

Figure 10–1 is a schematic representation of the pulmonary circulation indicating the large and small pulmonary arteries, pulmonary capillaries, and

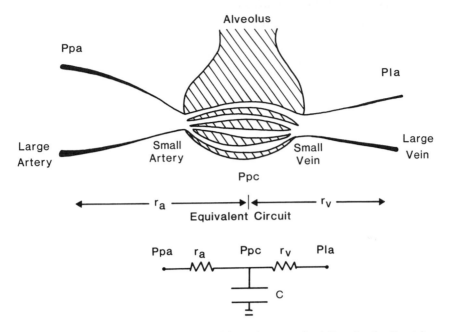

FIGURE 10–1. Schematic representation of the pulmonary circulation showing the pulmonary arterial pressure (Ppa), pulmonary capillary pressure (Ppc), and the left atrial pressure (Pla). Each alveolus is almost totally covered by capillaries. The lower portion of the figure shows an electrical analog of the pulmonary vascular circuit indicating precapillary (r_a) and postcapillary (r_v) resistances. The vascular compliance of the lung, where fluid is primarily exchanged, is denoted by the capacitor C.

small and large pulmonary veins. With most models used to analyze the pulmonary circulation, the large and small arteries are combined into a single resistance vessel and referred to as the precapillary (or upstream) resistance (r_a in Fig. 10–1). Similarly, the small and large veins are combined into a single postcapillary (or downstream) resistance vessel (r_v). Each segment of the pulmonary circulation has its own compliance characteristics. The region of the pulmonary circulation that primarily exchanges fluid with the lung tissue contains 75 to 80 per cent of the total vascular compliance of the lung. Therefore the pulmonary circulation can be represented as a simple resistance-capacitance electrical circuit in which the pulmonary arterial pressure (Ppa) is separated from the highly compliant capillary bed (represented by the capacitor, C) by the precapillary arterial resistance (r_a). The capillary pressure (Ppc) is located at the filtration midpoint of the pulmonary circulation and is separated from the left atrial pressure (Pla) by the postcapillary venous resistance (r_v). Using this simple electrical analog, the following equations describing the pulmonary circulation for a given cardiac output ($\dot{Q}B$) result:

$$Ppa - Pla = (r_a + r_v)\dot{Q}B \tag{10-1}$$

$$Ppa - Ppc = r_a\dot{Q}B \tag{10-2}$$

$$Ppc - Pla = r_v\dot{Q}B \tag{10-3}$$

and

$$r_a + r_v = r_t$$

where r_t is the total pulmonary vascular resistance.

Solving Equations 10–1 and 10–2 for Ppc yields the Gaar equation:

$$Ppc = Pla + (r_v/r_t)(Ppa - Pla) \tag{10-4}$$

Equation 10–4 states that Ppc is a function of Pla, the pressure gradient existing across the pulmonary circulation (Ppa − Pla), and the ratio of postcapillary resistance to the total vascular resistance r_v/r_t. Usually when Pla is elevated, 80 per cent of the pressure increase is reflected as an increased Ppa, which maintains blood flow in the lung.

The total pulmonary vascular resistance is normally equally divided between pre- and postcapillary resistances. Table 10–1 shows how capillary pressure changes when pulmonary arterial pressure changes and $r_a = r_v$, when $r_a > r_v$ (seen in alveolar hypoxia), or when $r_a < r_v$ (seen when histamine is released into the lung's circulation). The student should realize that the lung is basically a constant flow system as assumed in Table 10–1, because it must accept the cardiac output necessary to provide adequate oxygenation for the peripheral tissues. When total pulmonary vascular resistance increases while cardiac output remains constant and $r_a = r_v$, i.e., ΔP increases, capillary pressure increases

TABLE 10–1. Calculation of Capillary Pressure (Ppc) for
$r_a = r_v$, $r_a > r_v$, $r_a < r_v$ **at Normal, Increased, and Decreased r_t**
and Constant Cardiac Output (5 l/min)

		Ppa	Pla	ΔP	r_a	r_v	r_t	Ppc	Change in Ppc
A.	1.	20	5	15	1.5	1.5	3.0	12.5	Control
$r_a = r_v$	2.	35	5	30	3.0	3.0	6.0	20.0	↑
	3.	20	12.5	7.5	0.75	0.75	1.5	16.25	↑
B.	1.	20	5	15	2.0	1.0	3.0	10.0	↓
$r_a > r_v$	2.	35	5	30	4.0	2.0	6.0	15.0	↑
	3.	20	12.5	7.5	1.0	0.5	1.5	15.0	↑
C.	1.	20	5	15	1.0	2.0	3.0	15.0	↑
$r_a < r_v$	2.	35	5	30	2.0	4.0	6.0	25.0	↑
	3.	20	12.5	7.5	0.5	1.0	1.5	17.5	↑

Note: These numbers were calculated using Equation 10–4.

(see Table 10–1, A1 through A3). When $r_a > r_v$, Ppc is lower for any given total vascular resistance than when $r_a = r_v$ (compare A1 with B1), whereas Ppc is increased at both lower and higher vascular resistances but to a lesser extent than the increase occurring for $r_a = r_v$ (compare A2 and A3 with B2 and B3). When $r_a < r_v$, capillary pressure is elevated for normal, increased, and decreased pulmonary resistances and higher than when $r_a = r_v$ or $r_a > r_v$. Table 10–1 demonstrates that pulmonary capillary pressure is dependent on r_a, r_v, r_t, the pressure gradient existing across the pulmonary circulation, and the left atrial pressure. Many clinicians and physiologists calculate Ppc assuming it to be equivalent to Pla + 0.4 (Ppa − Pla), but this relationship will only predict Ppa when r_a/r_v is 60/40, i.e., r_v equals 40% of the total resistance.

INTERSTITIAL HYDROSTATIC FLUID PRESSURE (PT)

Interstitial hydrostatic fluid pressure acts to oppose the capillary pressure, since the difference between capillary pressure and interstitial hydrostatic pressure (Ppc − PT) is the net filtration pressure causing fluid movement out of the capillary into the interstitium. The pulmonary interstitial fluid pressure is subatmospheric, which results from lymphatic drainage and the recoil pressure of the lung. Some fluid always moves out of the alveolar capillaries into the perivascular spaces to be removed by the lymphatic vessels, as shown diagrammatically in Figure 10–2. The fluid exiting the alveolar capillaries is filtered through a dense basement membrane then percolates through the ground substance of the interstitium, which contains extracellular fluid, mucopolysaccharides, and collagen, before arriving in the larger perivascular spaces. The pressure surrounding the alveolar vessels is not known but is probably only 1 to 2 mmHg above the pressure in the perivascular spaces. The alveolar-capillary membrane swells only slightly when excess fluid enters the pulmonary interstitium because filtered fluid moves immediately into the more compliant perivascular spaces, which can accept large volumes of fluid with only small changes in pressure. Only after large amounts of fluid have entered the interstitium does fluid begin to enter the alveoli; that is, alveolar edema develops. The route that fluid uses to enter the alveoli is not known, but openings at the junction of alveolar ducts or at the alveolar epithelial membrane and/or leaks through large holes anywhere in the airways can serve as pathways for the fluid movements.

PLASMA COLLOID OSMOTIC PRESSURE (ΠP)

Proteins in plasma exert a colloid osmotic (or oncotic) pressure. This pressure tends to pull fluid from the tissues into the capillaries, i.e., colloid osmotic pressure acts as an absorptive force. Figure 10–3 shows the relationship between colloid osmotic pressure and plasma protein concentration. Albumin is the major protein in plasma (4 to 5 gm%), whereas α_2-, β-, and γ-globulins

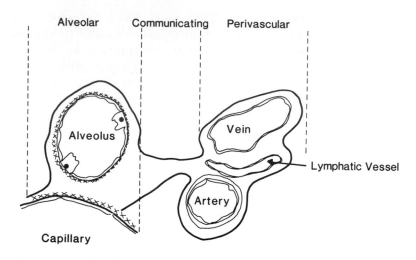

FIGURE 10–2. Schematic representation of the small alveolar tissue fluid spaces and the much larger perivascular fluid spaces and a communicating fluid space between the alveoli and perivascular spaces. The pressure is subatmospheric in all tissue spaces, but a pressure gradient exists between the alveolar and perivascular spaces since fluid moves in that direction to enter the lymphatic system.

together comprise approximately 3 gm% of the total proteins. Therefore, total plasma protein concentration is 7.5 gm%, which exerts an osmotic pressure of 28 mmHg (point A on dashed line in Fig. 10–3). Recall that the osmotic pressure of a solution is a function of the number of particles in solution. Since albumin is a smaller molecule than the globulins, it has more particles per gram weight and therefore exerts a greater colloid osmotic pressure per unit weight (upper curve labelled albumin).

The following equation can be used to approximate the colloid osmotic pressure of plasma:

$$\text{Colloid osmotic pressure } (\Pi_P) = 2.1 \; C_P + 0.16 \; C_P^2 \qquad (10\text{--}5)$$

The relationship between plasma colloid osmotic pressure and protein concentration (C_P) is not linear because plasma proteins are negatively charged particles holding a large number of cations. Since extracellular fluid is high in Na^+, proteins exist mostly as sodium salts. Of the 28 mmHg colloid osmotic pressure exerted by normal plasma proteins, about one-third is due to the Na^+ held by the negative charges on the plasma proteins (C_P^2 in Eq. 10–5), whereas the remaining two-thirds are due to the concentration of the total proteins in plasma ($2.1 \; C_P$ in Eq. 10–5). Whenever it is of clinical importance, Π_P should be measured rather than calculated because differences in the amount of albumin and globulins contained in plasma greatly affect the plasma colloid osmotic pressure, as shown in Figure 10–3.

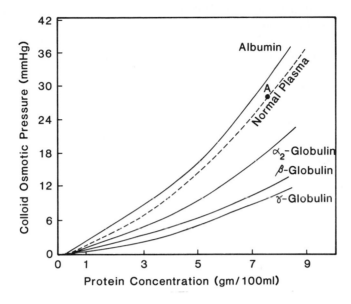

FIGURE 10–3. The effect of protein concentration on the colloid osmotic pressure for albumin, α_2-globulin, β-globulin, γ-globulin, and normal total plasma proteins (dashed line). The total plasma protein concentration is 7.5 gm/100 ml, which exerts 28 mmHg colloid osmotic pressure (point A). (Modified from Ott, H: Die Errechnung des kolloid osmotischen Serumdruckes aus dem Eiweiss-Spektrum und das mittlere Molekulargewicht der Serumeiweissfraktionen. *Klin. Wschr., 34:*1079–1083, 1956.)

The student should be aware that the colloid osmotic pressure of plasma is low relative to the crystalloid osmotic pressure of protein-free plasma, which is more than 200 times higher. However, crystalloids easily cross pulmonary capillary walls and enter the interstitium such that they exert no osmotic pressure difference between plasma and interstitial fluids. Therefore, only the plasma proteins are effective in promoting the movement of fluid across the pulmonary capillaries.

TISSUE COLLOID OSMOTIC PRESSURE (Π_T)

Since the walls of the capillaries are slightly permeable to plasma proteins, all plasma proteins are present in pulmonary interstitial fluid. Proteins leak continuously into the interstitium, where they exert an osmotic pressure tending to pull fluid from the capillaries into the interstitium. Fortunately, the lymphatic system of the lungs continuously removes these proteins from the interstitium and returns them to the systemic circulation. The plasma protein concentration in the pulmonary interstitium is about 4 to 5 gm% (i.e., a colloid osmotic pressure of 15 to 20 mmHg) and has a turnover rate of 30 hours in the normal functioning lung.

When the lung is diseased, the capillary endothelium may become abnormally leaky to plasma proteins so that the interstitial colloid osmotic pressure increases. Any abnormal protein accumulation in the interstitium decreases the colloid osmotic pressure gradient acting across the capillary wall (Π_P − Π_T) and thereby promotes capillary filtration leading to fluid accumulation in the pulmonary interstitium.

SOLVENT PERMEABILITY OF THE CAPILLARY WALL (Kfc)

The amount of fluid crossing the pulmonary capillary wall is a function of the total exchange surface area (about 100 m^2), the number of holes (or pores) contained within this area, and the radius to the fourth power of these holes. A membrane constant, called the filtration coefficient (Kfc), describes the filtration properties of the capillary wall. It defines the amount of fluid that crosses the capillary wall for a given difference in the filtrative and absorptive forces [(P_{pc} − P_T) − (Π_P − Π_T)]. The factors responsible for Kfc in lung tissue can best be appreciated by comparing them with Kfc's in other vascular beds. The Kfc for the lung is fairly high (0.2 ml/min/100 g/mmHg); the Kfc for the renal glomerular membrane is much larger (4.5 ml/min/100 g/mmHg); and the Kfc for skeletal muscle is markedly lower (0.015 ml/min/100 g/mmHg). The difference in the filtration properties of the capillaries between these tissues is due to either the number or size of the pores in the capillary walls. When Kfc values are expressed relative to the total exchange surface area, the Kfc values of lung and skeletal muscle, but not of the kidney, become similar. This indicates that the filtration properties of the pores are similar in lung and skeletal muscle but that the lung's microcirculation contains more pores. Because of its greater pore number and larger pore radius, the Kfc of the glomerular membrane is 10 to 100 times greater than that of the lung even when the Kfc value is expressed relative to total exchange surface area.

SOLUTE SELECTIVITY OF THE CAPILLARY WALL (σd)

Figure 10–4 shows the relationship between the ratio of protein concentration in the interstitium relative to plasma and the capillary filtration for normal pulmonary capillaries (solid line) and capillaries with damaged endothelium (dashed line). The concentration of protein in the tissues (C_T) relative to plasma (C_P) is defined as

$$\frac{C_T}{C_P} = \underbrace{\frac{(1 - \sigma d)J_v}{J_v}}_{\text{Convection}} + \underbrace{\frac{PS(C_P - C_T)}{J_v\,C_P}}_{\text{Diffusion}}, \qquad (10\text{–}6)$$

where σd is the osmotic reflection coefficient, C_P is the protein concentration

FIGURE 10–4. Effect of capillary filtration on the ratio of protein concentration in the interstitium (C_T) to plasma concentration (C_P) for normal pulmonary endothelium (solid line) and damaged endothelium (dashed line). The osmotic reflection coefficient can be calculated for both types of endothelia using $\sigma_d = (1 - C_T/C_P)$. Since π_T is directly proportional to C_T, the tissue colloid osmotic pressure changes in a similar fashion.

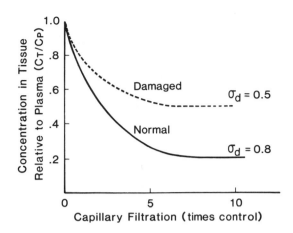

of plasma, J_V is the capillary filtration, and PS is the permeability coefficient times the surface area for exchange. The first term in Equation 10–6 represents the convective flux of solute, and the second term is diffusional flux. The osmotic reflection coefficient ranges from 0 to 1. If the membrane is freely permeable to protein, $\sigma_d = 0$. By contrast, if the membrane is impermeable to protein, $\sigma_d = 1$. When capillary filtration is small and diffusion of solute predominates, C_T approaches the concentration in plasma. Conversely, at high capillary filtration rates, when the diffusional component is small, C_T becomes a constant $[(1 - \sigma_d)C_P]$ because $PS(C_P - C_T)/J_V = 0$. The final C_T/C_P is directly related to the reflection coefficient, since $\sigma_d = (1 - C_T/C_P)$. Figure 10–4 shows that C_T/C_P approaches 0.5 for damaged endothelium and 0.2 for normal endothelium, indicating that $\sigma_d = 0.5$ and 0.8 for damaged and normal endothelium, respectively. In the following discussion, for simplicity it will be assumed that σ_d for total plasma proteins is unity for normal lung capillaries.

STARLING'S LAW OF THE CAPILLARIES (Fig. 10–5)

The forces discussed previously can now be used to describe quantitatively the fluid movement occurring across the pulmonary capillary using the Starling relationship:

$$
\begin{array}{cc}
\text{Filtration} & \text{Absorption} \\
\text{Pressure} & \text{Pressure}
\end{array} \qquad (10\text{–}7)
$$
$$
J_V = K_{fc}\,[(P_{pc} - P_T) - \sigma_d\,(\Pi_P - \Pi_T)]
$$

Pulmonary capillary pressure minus interstitial fluid pressure ($P_{pc} - P_T$) promotes fluid filtration from the capillaries into the interstitium and is therefore called the *net filtration pressure*. Plasma colloid osmotic pressure minus tissue

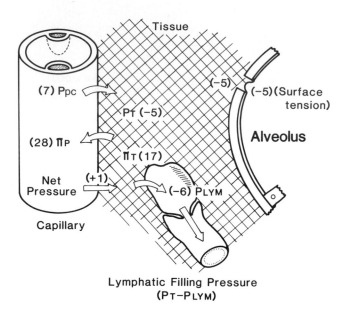

Lymphatic Filling Pressure
(P$_T$–P$_{LYM}$)

FIGURE 10–5. Schematic representation of the Starling forces operating between pulmonary capillaries and the interstitium. Note that the alveolar surface tension is exactly opposed by the subatmospheric interstitial fluid pressure (-5) and the lymphatic filling pressure (P$_T$ − P$_{LYM}$) [$-5-(-6)$] is positive, which promotes the filling of lymphatic vessels. (Redrawn from Guyton, *Textbook of Medical Physiology,* 7th edition, Saunders, 1986.)

colloid osmotic pressure times the osmotic reflection coefficient [σd (II$_P$ − II$_T$)] opposes the filtration pressure and is therefore called the *net absorption pressure.* The difference between the filtration and absorption pressures indicates the direction of fluid movement across the capillary, and the rapidity of the fluid movement is determined by Kfc.

A simple calculation will show how the Starling equation predicts the capillary filtration in both normal and damaged pulmonary capillary endothelium.

Normal Capillary Endothelium	**Damaged Capillary Endothelium**
Ppc = 7 mmHg	Ppc = 7 mmHg
P$_T$ = −5 mmHg	P$_T$ = −5 mmHg
II$_P$ = 28 mmHg	II$_P$ = 28 mmHg
II$_T$ = 17 mmHg	II$_T$ = 19 mmHg
Kfc = 0.2 ml/min/100 g/mmHg	Kfc = 0.4 ml/min/100 g/mmHg
σd = 1	σd = 0.5

$$Jv \text{ normal} = 0.2 \{[7-(-5)] - 1(28 - 17)\}$$
$$= 0.2 \ (12 - 11) = 0.2 \ \text{ml/min}$$

$$Jv \text{ abnormal} = 0.4 \{[7-(-5)] - 0.5 \ (28 - 19)\}$$
$$= 0.4 \ [(12 - 4.5)] = 3.0 \ \text{ml/min}$$

This calculation shows that the normal capillary filters a small amount of fluid that can be easily removed by the pulmonary lymphatic system (see Fig. 10–5). However, when the capillary endothelium becomes abnormally leaky to plasma proteins, σd is small and $(\Pi_P - \Pi_T)$ is reduced because Π_T is increased, resulting in the previous example in a 15-fold increase in capillary filtration. If the pulmonary lymphatic system cannot remove this increased fluid volume, excess fluid will accumulate in the tissues, resulting in *interstitial edema*. If fluid continues to accumulate in the interstitial spaces, the alveoli will fill with fluid, causing *alveolar edema*.

Pulmonary Lymphatic System

The pulmonary tissues have an extensive lymphatic drainage system. The smaller lymphatic vessels (called initial lymphatic vessels or lymphatic capillaries) are located in close approximation to the alveolar ducts (juxta-alveolar lymphatic system). These small lymphatic vessels coalesce and become more muscular and have valves to produce unidirectional flow. The lymph from these vessels empties into either the right lymphatic duct or the thoracic duct. Pulmonary lymphatic vessels can contract, producing lymphatic pressures of 25 to 30 cmH$_2$O. These contractions propel lymph from the tissues into the venous system. The lymph flow drops toward 0 at a lymph outflow pressure of about 15 cmH$_2$O rather than at 25 cmH$_2$O, which is the pressure generated in this example by the lymphatic pump (Fig. 10–6). This indicates that lymphatic drainage occurs easily at normal venous pressures but lymph flow decreases when the venous pressure is elevated, which occurs, for example, in heart failure. This reduction in lymph flow may be due to (1) incompetent valves within the lymph vessels and/or (2) a decrease in the effectiveness of the lymphatic pump. The lungs move with each respiratory cycle. This respiratory motion aids lymph propulsion, but the intrinsic lymphatic pump provides the major force to propel lymph from the interstitium of the lungs into the circulation.

VOLUME OVERLOAD

The major function of the lymphatic system is to remove proteins from the pulmonary interstitium. Without such removal of protein, the tissue protein

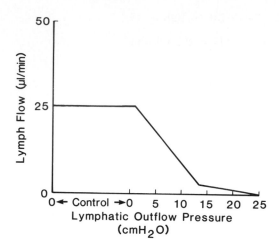

FIGURE 10–6. Diagrammatic plot of lymph flow as a function of lymphatic outflow pressure measured at the distal end of a lymphatic vessel. (Redrawn from Drake, R., Laine, G., Gable, J.: Effect of outflow pressure on lung lymph flow in unanesthetized sheep. *J. Appl. Physiol.*, 58:70–76, 1985.)

concentration would become equal to the plasma protein concentration, and gross edema would develop since the value of (P_{pc} − P_T) is always positive. The amount of fluid that can be removed by the pulmonary lymphatic system can increase about eight-fold when capillary pressure is increased to 20 mmHg (Fig. 10–7, points A to B, solid line). The lymphatic system eventually attains a maximum flow, and further increases in capillary filtration pressure will cause fluid accumulation in the tissues, which may result in alveolar edema, rather than a further increase in lymph flow.

Note that in Figure 10–7 lymph flow is higher when capillary endothelium is damaged. Under this condition, lymph flow increases 17 times above control (points A to C, dashed line). The underlying mechanisms responsible for this increased lymph flow are not known but may be related to a decreased tissue resistance to flow in addition to a greater initial lymphatic filling pressure, i.e., (P_T − P_{LYM}).

CLEARANCE OF PARTICULATE MATTER FROM AIRWAYS

Most particulate matter entering the lungs is trapped in the mucous layer of the airways and is expelled by coughing or propelled toward the mouth and swallowed (Fig. 10–8, arrow 1). Small particles that evade the mucous layer and are deposited in alveolar structures must be removed by other mechanisms. Alveolar macrophages may take up the particulate matter (arrow 2) and are then expelled up the airways (arrow 2a), or the particles may be phagocytized by alveolar type II cells (arrow 3) or type I cells (arrow 4). If the particles enter the tissues, they either enter the lymphatic vessels (arrow 6) or the pulmonary capillaries (arrow 5) or are phagocytized by interstitial macrophages (arrow 7), which can then enter the lymphatic vessels (arrow 7a). Many forms of particulate

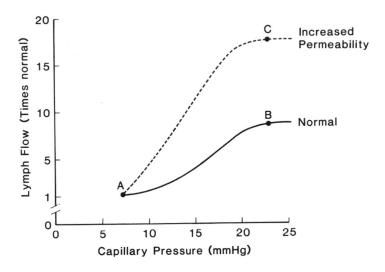

FIGURE 10–7. Lung lymph flow as a function of capillary pressure for normal capillaries (solid line) and capillaries with damaged endothelium (dashed line). Point A represents normal lymph flow and capillary pressures, whereas point B represents the increased lymph flow as seen with increased capillary pressure for normal endothelium and point C shows the response of damaged endothelium to increased capillary pressure.

matter are cleared from the lungs each day, but some, such as that found in smog and cigarette smoke, may remain in the lungs for several years.

Pleural Fluid Exchange

The fluid layer that separates the parietal and visceral pleura is formed by filtration, which occurs across both lung and chest wall pleural surfaces (Fig. 10–9). This fluid formation is a consequence of an imbalance in the Starling forces between the interstitial spaces of the lung and chest wall. The caudal chest wall, diaphragm, and inferior mediastinum have extensive lymphatic drainage systems through which pleural fluid can be readily removed (arrows pointing toward the chest wall). In an erect subject, the pleural fluid pressure (Ppl,f) at the cephalic level of the lung is more subatmospheric (-8 cmH$_2$O) than that at the caudal region of the lung (-1 cmH$_2$O). Therefore, the lymphatic filling pressure (Ppl,f $-$ PLYM) increases progressively toward the caudal region of the lung (progressively larger arrows in Fig. 10–9). Hence, the lymphatic drainage increases progressively from the top to the bottom. Thus, pleural fluid is predominantly formed at the top of the lung and mostly absorbed at the bottom of the lungs. The parietal pleura appears to both produce and remove pleural fluid, whereas the visceral pleura only forms pleural fluid when pulmonary edema is present.

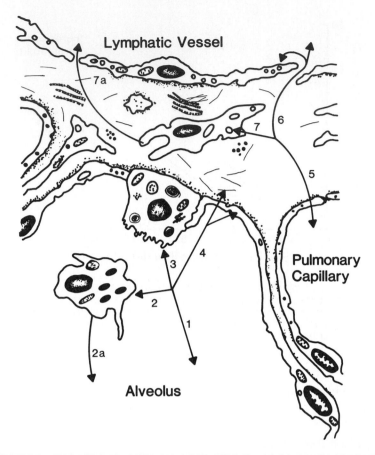

FIGURE 10–8. Schematic representation of alveolar clearance of particulate matter showing alveolar and tissue macrophages, alveoli, blood capillaries, and a lymphatic vessel. The arrows and numbers refer to possible pathways and mechanisms responsible for removing particulate matter deposited in the alveoli. (Modified from Lauweryns, J.M.: The juxta-alveolar lymphatics in the human adult lung. *Am. Rev. Resp. Dis., 102*:877–885, 1970.)

In many forms of lung pathology, pleural fluid volume increases, resulting in a collection of a pleural effusion. It is common for such an effusion to be associated with inflammation and infection (pleurisy), and the resulting cell debris may block the chest wall lymphatic drainage system of the parietal pleura. It is not known whether the fluid associated with pleural effusion is derived from the systemic blood vessels located in the parietal pleura or from the visceral pleura. Regardless of how the fluid is formed, it represents a failure of the lymphatic system to properly drain the pleural fluid.

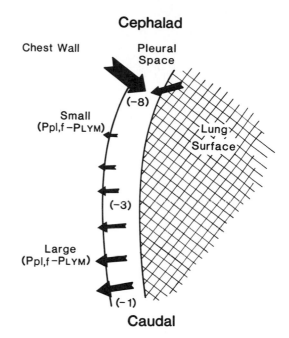

Cephalad

FIGURE 10–9. Schematic representation of pleural fluid dynamics in an upright lung. Pleural fluid is formed from the upper chest wall and lung surface. Because of the favorable hydrostatic pressure gradient, fluid flows toward the bottom of the lung. Since the lymphatic filling pressure becomes greater toward the bottom of the lung, the amount of pleural fluid removed by the chest wall lymphatic system increases progressively down the lung. (Drawn from Negrini, D., Capelli, C., Morini, M. and Miserocchi, G.: Gravity-dependent distribution of parietal subpleural interstitial pressure. *J. Appl. Physiol.*, 63:1912–1918, 1987.)

Airway Fluid Exchange and Alveolar Epithelial Transport

The large airways are normally covered by a thin layer of physiologic salt solution. This solution helps to maintain the mucosal barrier of the lung, to promote ciliary action, and to act as a low friction surface on which mucus is propelled toward the mouth. The salt solution is formed by at least four processes (Fig. 10–10): (1) secretion of an isotonic salt solution by submucosal glands, (2) delivery of surface liquid from more distal airways by ciliary motion (open arrows), (3) secretion of Cl^-, and (4) absorption of Na^+. In the fetus, Cl^- secretion is the dominant ion transport, resulting in net fluid secretion in the large airways. Conversely, Na^+ absorption is the major ion transport in the large airways in adults and net fluid absorption results. The manner in which the surface liquid is formed within small airways is not known, but a physiologic salt solution must be secreted to bathe the cilia. Clara cells may be responsible for this fluid secretion. At the alveolar level, alveolar type II epithelial cells actively transport Na^+ into the tissue, resulting in net removal of fluid from the airways. The observation that intra-alveolar fluid is removed by an active process in adults suggests that the alveoli may have a tendency to fill with fluid, which is counterbalanced by this active transport system. Alternatively, the system may have a low basal activity and only becomes stimulated when fluid accumulates in the airways. Interestingly, several compounds (e.g., β-adren-

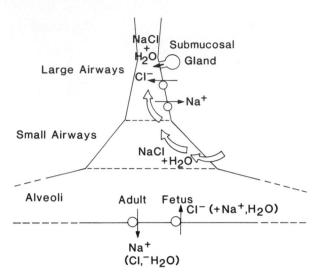

FIGURE 10–10. Transport processes in the large and small airways and alveoli of adult and fetal lungs. (Courtesy of Dr. J. Gatzy.)

ergic agonists) can accelerate alveolar fluid removal, and therefore these drugs may be useful in treating pulmonary edema. In contrast to adults, the fetus actually makes lung fluid by actively secreting Cl⁻ into the alveolar spaces.

PULMONARY EDEMA

Figure 10–11A shows the rate of edema formation in the lung following elevation of left atrial pressure for a normal endothelium (solid line) and a damaged endothelium (dashed line). An increase in left atrial pressure up to 23 mmHg, directly causing a rise in Ppc since Ppc = Pla + r_v/r_t(Ppa − Pla), causes essentially no tissue fluid accumulation in the lung with normal capillary endothelium. At higher left atrial pressures fluid rapidly accumulates in the pulmonary interstitium (Fig. 10–11A, 1), and at very high left atrial pressures the rate of edema formation is further accelerated (Fig. 10–11A, 2). The accelerated rate of edema formation is due to either an increased concentration of interstitial proteins or disruption of the alveolar-capillary membrane, or both. Once the interstitial space has expanded by approximately 50 per cent, alveolar edema begins to develop. The dashed line (Fig. 10–11A) shows the accumulation of edema fluid when the endothelium of the capillary wall is damaged. Note that the fluid begins to accumulate in the lung tissue at a much lower

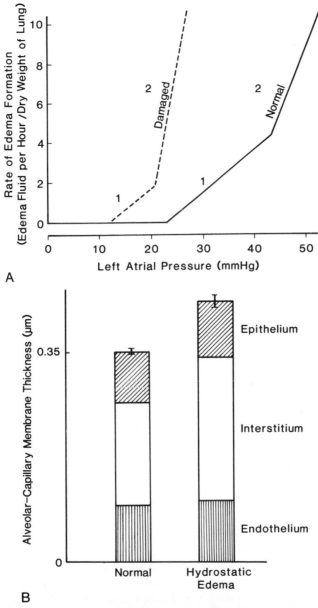

FIGURE 10–11. *A,* Rate of edema formation as a function of left atrial pressure. Solid line represents the behavior of normal endothelium, whereas the dashed line represents damaged endothelium. (Modified from Guyton, A.C., and Lindsey, A.W.: Effect of elevated left atrial pressure and decreased plasma protein concentration on the development of pulmonary edema. *Circ. Res., 7:*649–653, 1959.) Edema formation has two distinct components, a relatively slow rate of formation (1) and an accelerated rate of formation (2). Note that the rapid rate of edema formation occurs at low left atrial pressure when the endothelium is damaged. *B,* Thickness of the alveolar-capillary membrane for a normal lung and a lung with hydrostatic pulmonary edema. Note the minimal swelling of the alveolar-capillary membrane, which is confined to the interstitial space.

left atrial pressure and at a more rapid rate because of the damaged endothelium.

Figure 10–11*B* shows that edema formation increases the alveolar-capillary membrane thickness by only 15 to 20 per cent. This modest increase is due to an expanded interstitial space. This increase in the alveolar-capillary membrane thickness is so minimal that blood oxygenation is not significantly affected. The impairment in oxygenation is also minimal because the tissue fluid moves rapidly from the gas exchange sites into the more compliant perivascular spaces, providing a thin barrier for gas exchange during interstitial edema. Once the thickness of the interstitium has reached its maximum, fluid begins to fill the alveoli and blood oxygenation will be affected.

Why is there no detectable edema formation until left atrial pressure exceeds 23 mmHg? This question has led to the concept of *tissue edema safety factors*, which oppose the formation of pulmonary edema when capillary pressure is elevated.

TISSUE EDEMA SAFETY FACTORS

Hydrostatic Edema

The edema safety factor in normal lungs allows capillary pressure to increase from its normal value of 7 mmHg to about 23 mmHg. The forces that cause filtration across the pulmonary capillaries are the filtration pressure ($P_{pc} - P_T$) and the absorbing force [$\sigma d(\Pi_P - \Pi_T)$] as shown in Equation 10–7. When the left atrial pressure is increased and fluid filters into the lung interstitium, interstitial fluid pressure increases almost immediately because the pulmonary interstitium, in contrast to the vascular space, is very noncompliant. This increase in P_T decreases the net filtration pressure ($P_{pc} - P_T$) and opposes further edema formation. Furthermore, the protein concentration in the tissues is diluted (see Fig. 10–4), which increases the absorptive pressure [$\sigma d(\Pi_P - \Pi_T)$]. Finally, as excess fluid filters into the interstitium, the initial lymphatic vessels fill more easily and lymph flow increases five- to ten-fold (see Fig. 10–7), which provides an additional safety factor. The three tissue safety factors that oppose edema formation are shown in Figure 10–12 and represent (1) a decreased filtration pressure because tissue pressure increases, (2) an increased absorptive pressure because Π_T decreases, and (3) an increased lymph flow that carries away an additional amount of fluid. Because of these tissue safety factors, the tissues do not swell significantly until left atrial pressures are elevated above 23 mmHg in this example. Further increases in capillary filtration cause a rapid accumulation of tissue fluid because the tissue safety factors are exhausted and can no longer oppose even a small increase in the filtration pressure. It is interesting to note that patients with chronic heart failure and high left atrial pressure seem to have larger safety factors. Their left atrial

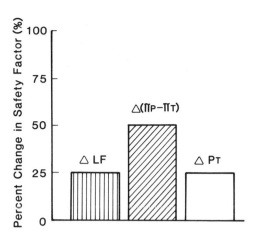

FIGURE 10–12. The per cent of the total tissue safety factor due to increased lymph flow (ΔLF), increase in the colloid osmotic pressure absorptive force $\Delta(\pi_P - \pi_T)$, and an increased tissue fluid pressure ΔP_T. (Redrawn from Taylor, A.E.: Capillary fluid filtration: Starling forces and lymph flow. *Circ. Res., 49*:557–575, 1981.)

pressures may rise above 40 mmHg without the development of pulmonary edema, indicating an increased lymph flow or absorption force factor.

Damaged Endothelium

Many conditions cause pulmonary capillary endothelial damage. Following such damage, edema develops at much lower capillary pressures as shown by the dashed line in Figure 10–11A. This occurs because (1) the lymphatic vessels are not as effective in fluid removal and (2) Π_T does not decrease as much because the capillary wall is leakier to plasma proteins (see Fig. 10–4). For example, Figure 10–4 shows how C_T (which determines Π_T) decreases less when filtration occurs across damaged endothelium as compared with normal endothelium: C_T decreases to only 50 per cent of C_P in leaky capillaries as compared with 20 per cent for normal capillaries. This form of edema has been termed the "leaky lung syndrome" or "low pressure edema" to differentiate it from the "high pressure edema" associated with left-sided heart failure. When the pulmonary capillary endothelium is damaged, alveolar edema can result even when capillary pressures are normal, as shown in Figure 10–11A. This form of pulmonary edema may constitute a severe threat to life because the lung's ability to properly oxygenate the hemoglobin may be severely limited.

CLINICAL PROBLEMS ASSOCIATED WITH PULMONARY EDEMA

Figure 10–13 shows the effects of increasing capillary pressure by volume expansion on extravascular lung water (edema formation, solid line) and arterial

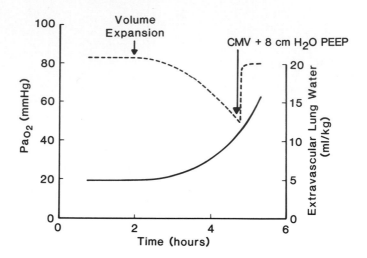

FIGURE 10–13. Effect of elevating capillary pressure on arterial oxygen tension (Pa$_{O_2}$, dashed line) and extravascular lung water (solid line). At the left arrow, capillary pressure was increased by volume expansion. Mechanical ventilation (CMV) at 8 cm PEEP was applied at the right arrow. Note the dramatic improvement of Pa$_{O_2}$ when mechanical ventilation (CMV) with PEEP was applied. (Modified from Noble, W.H.: Pulmonary oedema: A review. *Can. Anesth. Soc. J.,* 27:286–302, 1981.)

oxygen tension (Pa$_{O_2}$, dashed line). As capillary pressure is increased at the left arrow, the pulmonary blood vessels are dilated (congestion) and interstitial edema begins to develop. With further accumulation of extravascular lung water, alveolar edema begins to develop and Pa$_{O_2}$ drops dramatically. The figure shows that when mechanical ventilation with 8 cmH$_2$O positive end expiratory pressure is applied (PEEP, right arrow), Pa$_{O_2}$ increases dramatically even with additional increases in lung water. This improved Pa$_{O_2}$ is most likely due to recruitment of collapsed alveoli. When pulmonary edema is present, oxygenation can be improved by increasing the inspired oxygen concentration, positive end expiratory pressure, and diuretics. If the heart failure responds favorably to treatment, all signs of pulmonary edema usually disappear in one to three days.

Figure 10–14A shows the relationship between dynamic lung compliance and extravascular lung water in dogs. The initial sharp drop in dynamic lung compliance (points A to B) is associated with congestion of the pulmonary vasculature, and the drop from point B to point C is due to interstitial edema formation, whereas points C to D represent alveolar edema formation. The most likely cause of the decreased dynamic lung compliance is related to the reduced distensibility of the lungs because of the fluid within the interstitium

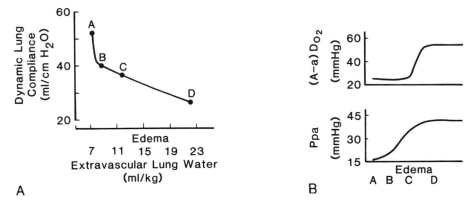

FIGURE 10–14. *A*, Change in dynamic lung compliance during edema formation in anesthetized dogs showing normal (point A), vascular congestion (point B), interstitial edema (point C), and alveolar edema (D). (Modified from Noble, W.H., Kay, J.C. and Obdrzalek, J.: Lung mechanics in hypervolemic pulmonary edema. *J. Appl. Physiol., 38*:681–687, 1975.) *B*, Change in $(A - a)Do_2$ and pulmonary arterial pressure (Ppa) during control (region A), vascular congestion (region B), interstitial edema (region C), and alveolar edema (region D).

and changes in surface properties related to the alveolar edema. Figure 10–14*B* shows the changes in the $(A - a)Do_2$ and pulmonary arterial pressure (Ppa) associated with edema formation. When alveolar edema forms, the $(A - a)Do_2$ increases owing to perfusion of poorly ventilated lung regions that are filled with edema fluid. During the vascular congestion (region B) and interstitial edema formation (region C), the vascular resistance increases and the pulmonary arterial pressure rises because cardiac output remains normal. Not shown is the fact that interstitial and alveolar edema may increase airway resistance because the blood vessel engorgement and fluid in the airways reduce the size of the airway lumen.

In summary, alveolar edema causes (1) an increased $(A - a)Do_2$; (2) an increased pulmonary vascular resistance and pulmonary arterial pressure; (3) a decreased dynamic lung compliance; and (4) an increased airway resistance.

FACTORS THAT DAMAGE LUNGS

Many factors can damage the alveolar-capillary membrane. The alveolar-capillary membrane can be damaged from the alveolar side, e.g., acid aspiration, or from the capillary side through processes that trigger an inflammatory response, e.g., sepsis syndrome. Many of the conditions associated with leaky lung capillaries also increase pulmonary capillary pressure because of increased pulmonary venous resistance resulting in a rapid formation of alveolar edema, even when the capillary endothelium is not severely damaged. The most important determinant of pulmonary edema is the capillary pressure; if the capillary endothelium is damaged, the rate of edema formation can be greatly accelerated in response to the increased capillary pressure.

The clinical syndrome associated with acute lung injury has been called the adult respiratory distress syndrome (ARDS). ARDS occurs in acid aspiration, fat and air emboli, near-drowning, trauma, oxygen toxicity, sepsis, hypovolemic shock, massive plasma volume expansion, and viral pneumonitis. On histologic examination of lungs from ARDS patients, one finds hyaline membranes covering the alveolar epithelium, type II alveolar cell proliferation, epithelial sloughing, and interstitial and alveolar edema.

The primary clinical finding in ARDS is the presence of hypoxemia that is refractory to oxygen therapy. The lung compliance is decreased, which increases the work of breathing, chest roentgenograms show bilateral diffuse infiltrates, and physiologic dead space is increased.

The exact cause of ARDS is not known, but it is thought to begin with capillary endothelial damage, resulting in a "low pressure" noncardiac type of interstitial edema accompanied by type I epithelial cell sloughing and impairment of surfactant production by the alveolar type II cells. It is interesting to contrast ARDS with the hydrostatic edema associated with heart failure. Edema associated with high vascular pressure does not damage endothelial or epithelial cells. Positive pressure ventilation is used successfully in both conditions to decrease the $(A - a)D_{O_2}$.

Detection of Edema Fluid

Edema fluid can be measured in patients by using the indicator dilution principle as developed in Appendix C. Heat is used as a measure of extracellular fluid volume plus vascular volume and Cardio-Green dye is used to measure the vascular volume. The edema fluid in the lung tissues is calculated as the difference between the space measured with heat and the space measured with the Cardio-Green dye. Also, interstitial edema fluid can be detected using roentgenograms, and alveolar edema is easily detected by listening to chest sounds. In addition, modern imaging techniques such as nuclear magnetic resonance and positron emission imaging are used to detect edema formation and endothelial damage in patients at risk for ARDS.

SUGGESTED READING

Fishman, A.P., and Renkin, E.M. (eds.): *Pulmonary Edema*. Clinical Physiology Series. Bethesda: APS, 1979.

Guyton, A.C., Taylor, A.E., Drake, R.E. and Parker, J.C.: Dynamics of subatmospheric pressures in the pulmonary interstitial fluid. In *Lung Liquid*. Ciba Symposium, Amsterdam: Elsevier, 1976, pp. 77–90.

Staub, N.C. (ed.): Lung water and solute exchange. In Lenfant, C. (ed.): *Lung Biology in Health and Disease*, Vol. 7. New York: Marcel Dekker, Inc., 1978.

Taylor, A.E., and Parker, J.C.: Pulmonary interstitial spaces and lymphatics. In Fishman, A.P. and Fisher, A.B. (eds.): *Handbook of Physiology, The Respiratory System, Circulation and Nonrespiratory Function*. Section 3, Volume I. Bethesda: APS, 1985, pp. 167–230.

QUESTIONS

Using the Starling equation:

$$\text{Capillary filtration} = \text{Kfc}\,[(\text{Ppc} - \text{P}_T) - \sigma\text{d}\,(\Pi_P - \Pi_T)]$$

1. Calculate the capillary filtration rate where Kfc = 1 ml/min/100 g/mmHg; Ppc = 7 mmHg; P_T = -7 mmHg; σd = 0.9; Π_P = 28 mmHg; and Π_T = 13 mmHg.

2. Calculate the capillary filtration rate after the capillaries have become very leaky to plasma proteins where Kfc = 3 ml/min/100 g/mmHg; Ppc = 7 mmHg; P_T = 0 mmHg; Π_P = 28 mmHg; Π_T = 20 mmHg; and σd = 0.5.

3. What are the safety factors operating in the lung that oppose the tendency for edema fluid to accumulate when pulmonary capillary pressure is elevated to 20 mmHg? Calculate the final capillary filtration rate using Kfc = 1 ml/min/100 g/mmHg and σd = 0.9. What would be the capillary filtration rate if the safety factors did not change, using the P_T, σd, Π_P, and Π_T values given in Problem 1; would edema develop?

MEDULLARY RESPIRATORY CENTERS
Dorsal Respiratory Group
Ventral Respiratory Group

PONTINE RESPIRATORY CENTERS

INSPIRATORY PATTERN GENERATION

CONTROL OF INSPIRATORY ACTIVITY

REFLEX CONTROL OF VENTILATION
Hering-Breuer Reflexes
Irritant Receptor Reflexes
J-Receptor Reflexes
Reflexes Mediated by Peripheral Receptors
Cortical Modulation

CHEMICAL CONTROL OF RESPIRATION
The Central Chemoreceptors
Mechanisms for Central Chemosensitivity
Adaptation of Central Chemoreceptors
Ventilatory Response to Carbon Dioxide and Hydrogen Ions
Peripheral Chemoreceptor Response to Arterial P_{O_2}
Mechanism of Peripheral Chemosensitivity

INTEGRATED CONTROL OF VENTILATION

DISORDERS OF VENTILATORY CONTROL
Sleep Apneas
Irregular Breathing Patterns

VENTILATORY RESPONSE TO EXERCISE

11

CONTROL OF VENTILATION

Hemostasis of blood pH and blood-gas tensions requires proper matching of ventilation to the body's oxygen consumption and CO_2 production. This matching is accomplished by a rhythmic pattern of ventilation, which can be interrupted by nonrespiratory functions such as mastication, speech, and cough.

MEDULLARY RESPIRATORY CENTERS

The search for a discrete respiratory center in the medulla that controls the rate and depth of ventilation has not been successful; indeed, several widely dispersed respiratory-related medullary groups of neurons have been identified. These groups of neurons have been divided into dorsal and ventral respiratory groups as shown in Figure 11–1; they are bilaterally symmetric and contain both inspiratory and expiratory neurons. Many of these neurons do not directly

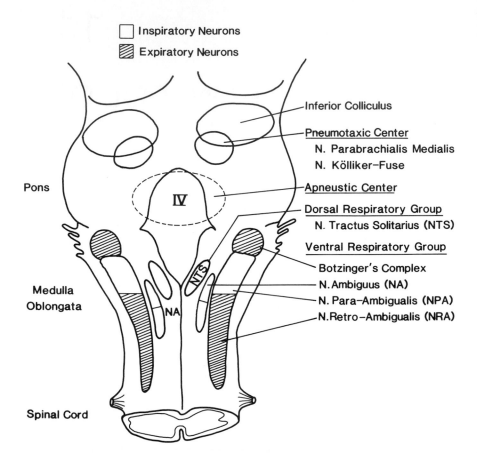

FIGURE 11–1. Dorsal view of the brainstem showing the major groups of respiratory-related neurons. IV refers to the fourth ventricle. Inspiratory and expiratory neurons are shown by open and hatched regions, respectively.

drive inspiratory or expiratory motor neurons but only serve to modulate the ventilatory pattern.

Dorsal Respiratory Group

Dorsal respiratory neurons are primarily inspiratory and are located bilaterally in the *nucleus tractus solitarius* (NTS). These neurons project contralaterally to the phrenic and external intercostal motor neurons in the spinal cord and provide the primary stimulus for *inspiration* (Fig. 11–2). Inputs from central and peripheral chemoreceptors, pulmonary stretch receptors, somatic pain receptors and mechanoreceptors, and cortical and pontine centers converge on the NTS to modulate the rate and depth of inspiration. Inhibitory

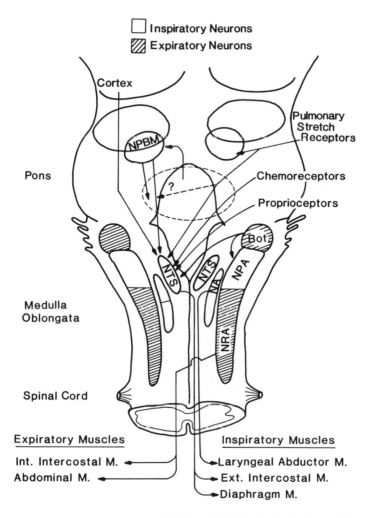

FIGURE 11–2. Dorsal view of the brainstem showing facilitory and inhibitory inputs to the nucleus tractus solitarius (NTS) and outflow pathways to inspiratory and expiratory muscle groups. Structures shown include the nucleus parabrachialis medialis (NPBM), nucleus ambiguus (NA), nucleus para-ambigualis (NPA), nucleus retro-ambigualis (NRA), and Botzinger's complex (Bot.).

fibers from the NTS to expiratory neurons of the ventral respiratory group have been identified, but only a few inhibitory fibers project from the ventral respiratory group to the NTS.

Ventral Respiratory Group

The ventral respiratory group is a bilateral collection of several nuclei containing both inspiratory and expiratory neurons. The *nucleus ambiguus* (NA) contains primarily *inspiratory neurons*, which project to muscles of the larynx, pharynx, and tongue, with the major output to the laryngeal abductor muscles. Stimulation of these neurons dilates the airways to minimize airway resistance during inspiration. The *nucleus retro-ambigualis* (NRA) is a long nucleus that is commonly divided into rostral and caudal areas. The *caudal portion* of the nucleus contains *expiratory neurons* that project contralaterally to motor neurons for the abdominal and internal intercostal muscles, but these expiratory neurons are activated only at high ventilatory rates. The rostral half of the NRA (often termed the *nucleus para-ambigualis*, NPA) contains *inspiratory neurons* whose discharge continuously increases during inspiration. The *Botzinger's complex* (Bot) is the most rostral nucleus of the ventral respiratory group and contains the only *expiratory neurons* shown to inhibit both the inspiratory NTS and phrenic motor neurons.

PONTINE RESPIRATORY CENTERS

Two major respiratory centers have been identified in the pons through brainstem transection experiments. Bilateral *pneumotaxic centers* in the rostral pons (see Fig. 11–1) consist of the nucleus *parabrachialis medialis* and the nucleus *Kölliker-Fuse*. Output of these nuclei stimulates the off-switch neurons, which terminate inspiration. Therefore, ablation of these nuclei or brainstem transection at the mid-pons results in prolonged inspiration. Furthermore, ablation of the nuclei combined with simultaneous section of the vagus nerves, which carry afferents from pulmonary stretch receptors that inhibit inspiration, results in sustained inspiration and produces apneustic breathing, a form of sustained inspiration punctuated by periodic expiratory gasps. The *apneustic center* is an ill-defined region in the caudal portion of the pons near the fourth ventricle (see Fig. 11–1) that may represent a switching station for pneumotaxic center inputs to the dorsal respiratory group.

INSPIRATORY PATTERN GENERATION

Phrenic nerve activity increases smoothly in both rate and amplitude during inspiration, then terminates abruptly and is very low during expiration.

Integration of inspiratory phrenic activity results in a smoothly increasing (ramp-like) signal, which produces a progressive increase in the number of diaphragmatic muscle units recruited during inspiration. The greater the number of muscle units recruited, the larger the tidal volume.

A complex mutual inhibition and facilitation between several types of respiratory neurons appears to shape the smoothly increasing discharge pattern of phrenic premotor neurons. These premotor neurons receive tonic facilitory activity from the reticular activating system. Inputs from chemoreceptors, peripheral afferents, and central afferents can enhance the reticular activating system's activity, increasing the rate and amplitude of inspiratory premotor neuronal discharge (tidal volume). Inhibitory neurons, whose activity peaks early in inspiration and then gradually decreases, cause the integrated inspiratory activity to become a smoothly increasing ramp function. Expiratory neurons inhibit the inspiratory neurons during the expiratory phase of the respiratory cycle, and they are also inhibited by inspiratory neurons during inspiration. Neurons whose activity builds rapidly only in late inspiration, as well as other neurons that exhibit a peak activity in early expiration, have a dramatic inhibitory effect on the inspiratory activity. These two neuron types serve as the off-switch for inspiratory activity and are under facilitatory control of the pneumotaxic center and the pulmonary stretch receptors. Feedback to the off-switch neurons limits the inspiratory time and influences both the rate and depth of respiration. A rhythmic pattern of inspiration and expiration results, with the rate and depth of respiration modulated by the activity of facilitory afferents and by off-switch neuron inhibition of inspiratory premotor neurons.

CONTROL OF INSPIRATORY ACTIVITY

Recall that activation of inhibitory neurons during late inspiration serves as an off-switch that limits the duration of inspiration. However, the underlying drive to the inspiratory neurons from chemoreceptor and other afferents has a marked influence on ventilatory frequency and tidal volume. Figure 11–3 shows integrated phrenic nerve activity as a function of time at different arterial P_{CO_2} values (A) and temperatures (B) in a cat in which the pneumotaxic center has been destroyed (i.e., an animal with sustained inspiratory activity). Since greater phrenic nerve activity recruits more diaphragmatic muscle units, the magnitude of the phrenic nerve activity is proportional to tidal volume. The time required to reach a plateau in tidal volume determines the time of inspiration and is inversely proportional to the respiratory frequency. The vertical dashed lines indicate the half-times to attain plateau activity. Figure 11–3A shows that increased arterial P_{CO_2} results in increased phrenic nerve activity (an increased tidal volume) at a constant respiratory frequency (dashed lines). This response serves to increase alveolar ventilation in response to an increased

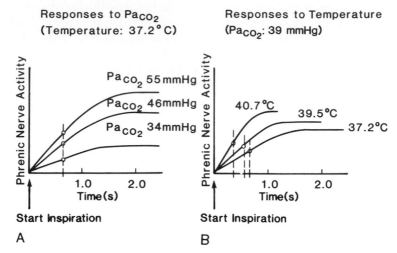

FIGURE 11–3. Rise of phrenic nerve activity with time after the start of inspiration in a cat with bilateral lesions in the pneumotaxic center. Open circles and dashed lines show the half-times for attaining plateau phrenic nerve activity. *A,* Increased Pa_{CO_2} causes the plateau (tidal volume) to increase. *B,* Increased temperature shortens the half-time for inspiratory activity to reach a plateau (increased respiratory frequency). (Redrawn from Euler, C.V., Marttila, I., Remmers, J.E., and Tippenbach, J.: Effects of lesions in the parabrachial nucleus on the mechanisms for central and reflex termination of inspiration in the cat. *Acta Physiol. Scand., 96*:324–337, 1976.)

P_{CO_2}. Stimulation by increased temperature results in a change in phrenic nerve activity but a more marked increase in breathing frequency (dashed lines). This phenomenon maintains alveolar ventilation at a constant level while increasing total ventilation for cooling purposes. This thermoregulatory function is important in animals that pant to decrease core temperature but has little importance in humans.

REFLEX CONTROL OF VENTILATION

Central ventilatory drive can be modulated by sensory information from a variety of peripheral inputs, including pain, temperature, and motion. In addition, a large number of reflexes originating in the lung serve protective and regulatory functions. These pulmonary reflexes are a result of sensory input from *unmyelinated C-fiber afferents* and naked nerve endings (*J-receptors*) as well as from *myelinated vagal afferents* derived from either slowly adapting stretch receptors in the airway smooth muscle or rapidly adapting receptors in the airway epithelium.

Hering-Breuer Reflexes

Slowly adapting pulmonary stretch receptors (SARs) are located in the smooth muscle of the bronchi and posterior trachea. The majority are present in intrapulmonary airways. These receptors send myelinated afferents through the vagus nerve to the dorsal respiratory neurons and the pneumotaxic center. Stimulation of these receptors by increased lung volume acts to shorten inspiration and limit the tidal volume. Figure 11–4 shows recordings of phrenic and inferior laryngeal nerve activities during a lung volume increase in the presence (1) or absence (2) of vagal nerve feedback. Inspiration is terminated earlier in the presence of vagal feedback but terminates spontaneously even in the absence of vagal nerve activity.

Brief stimulation of the slowly adapting stretch receptors only inhibits inspiration. Continued stimulation of these receptors by a sustained inflation of the lung during the expiratory phase causes excitation of the central expiratory neurons as well. Figure 11–5 illustrates the classic *Hering-Breuer* response and shows the inverse relationship between respiratory frequency (recorded from a phrenic nerve) and lung volume.

Although the Hering-Breuer inflation reflex is an important determinant of the respiratory frequency at rest in infants and most animals, it does not appear to be important in adult humans. Tidal volume must exceed 800 to 1000 ml before the slowly adapting stretch receptors influence the respiratory rate in humans. However, the Hering-Breuer reflex does contribute significantly to the regulation of respiratory frequency during moderate or strenuous exercise and may provide a protective mechanism for preventing overexpansion of the lungs.

The slowly adapting pulmonary stretch receptors may provide information to the respiratory center relative to alterations in small or large airway resistance. In addition, decreases in lung compliance stimulate the stretch receptors by augmenting the mechanical distending stresses acting on the airways, which causes an increased respiratory frequency. Thus, many types of chronic lung

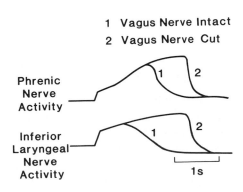

FIGURE 11–4. Effect of the presence (1) or absence (2) of vagal nerve feedback on phrenic nerve (diaphragm) and inferior laryngeal nerve (larynx) activities. Stretch receptor feedback transmitted through the vagus nerve shortens inspiratory drive to both the diaphragm and laryngeal abductor muscles (1). In the absence of vagal nerve feedback (2), inspiration ceases spontaneously. (Redrawn from Euler, C.V.: Brainstem mechanisms for generation and control of breathing pattern. In Cherniack, N.S., and Widdicombe, J.G. (eds.): *Handbook of Physiology:* Section 3, The Respiratory System, Volume II, Control of breathing, Part 2, Bethesda: APS 1986, pp. 529–593.)

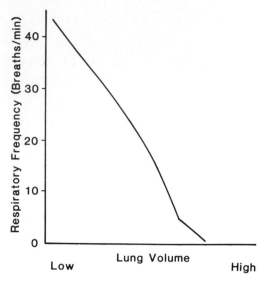

FIGURE 11–5. Respiratory frequency, measured from phrenic nerve activity, during static inflation of both lungs in an open-chested dog. A typical Hering-Breuer reflex was evoked, and frequency decreased linearly with increases in lung volume. (Redrawn from Nilsestuen, J.O., Coon, R.L., Woods, M., and Kampine, W.P.: Location of lung receptors mediating the breathing frequency response to pulmonary CO_2. *Resp. Physiol.*, 45:343–355, 1981.)

disease can influence ventilation through these receptors. Acute conditions such as vascular congestion, pulmonary edema, and pulmonary embolization also stimulate the slowly adapting pulmonary stretch receptors owing to a reduction in lung compliance.

An interesting feature of the stretch receptors is their ability to respond directly to changes in carbon dioxide tension in the airways. Receptor activity increases when airway P_{CO_2} falls below 10 mmHg during expiration, causing the expiratory neurons to reduce respiratory frequency. Stimulation of these receptors prevents hyperventilation.

Irritant Receptor Reflexes

Responses of the lung to irritants are mediated mainly by *rapidly adapting receptors* located in the epithelium of the carinal region. Mechanical or chemical irritation of the epithelium results in coughing, sneezing, tachypnea, bronchoconstriction, and increased secretions in the airways. Irritant receptors are also stimulated by various pollutants and endogenous compounds such as histamine and bradykinin.

J-Receptor Reflexes

Unmyelinated C-fiber nerve endings in the alveolar interstitium sense vascular distension and increases in interstitial fluid volume. These mechanoreceptors have been termed *pulmonary juxtacapillary receptors (J-receptors)* because of their location. Stimulation of these receptors may produce hyperpnea and/or dyspnea during pulmonary vascular congestion and edema. Figure 11–6 shows the activity of two such J-receptors when left atrial pressure is increased.

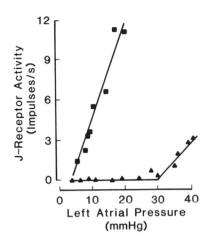

FIGURE 11–6. J-receptor activity measured in two J-receptor afferent nerve fibers as a function of left atrial pressure. Different pressure thresholds (left atrial axis intercept) and sensitivities (slopes) were observed for the two different J-receptor fibers. (Reproduced with permission from Coleridge, H.M., and Coleridge, J.C.G.: Afferent vagal C-fibers in the dog lung: Their discharge during spontaneous breathing, and their stimulation by alloxan and pulmonary congestion. In Paintal, A.S., and Gill-Kumar, P. (eds): *Respiratory Adaptations, Capillary Exchange and Reflex Mechanisms.* Delhi: Vallabhbhai Patel Chest Institute, pp. 396–405.)

One J-receptor responds at a low pressure, whereas the second J-receptor has a much higher threshold. In addition, the J-receptors also have different sensitivities (slopes of the line relating J-receptor impulses to left atrial pressure). J-receptors also respond to large increases in pulmonary blood flow, and this response may be due to the higher pulmonary vascular pressures and the associated vascular distention. In contrast, apnea associated with pulmonary embolism may be due to loss of J-receptor stimulation when vessels upstream from these receptors are blocked.

Reflexes Mediated by Peripheral Receptors

Proprioceptors in the muscles, tendons, and joints as well as pain receptors in the muscles and skin send afferent signals to the medulla. Stimulation of these receptors increases central inspiratory activity and produces hyperpnea. This is why somatic movements and painful stimuli, such as slapping and pinching, can stimulate ventilation in patients suffering from respiratory depression.

Reflex control of breathing effort is also mediated by stimulation of muscle spindles of the diaphragm and intercostal muscles when these muscles work against an increased load. This reflex response is more important in subjects with chronic lung disease who must work harder than normal subjects to achieve adequate ventilation because of increased airway resistance and decreased lung compliance.

Cortical Modulation

Voluntary control of ventilation rate can override the intrinsic neural rhythm of the respiratory centers and is essential for normal speech. Voluntary hyperventilation or hypoventilation (breath-holding) cannot continue indefinitely because the respiratory center's response to changes in Pa_{CO_2} and stretch receptor activity eventually overrides voluntary control.

CHEMICAL CONTROL OF RESPIRATION

Ventilation is controlled centrally by CO_2 and hydrogen ion concentrations in the cerebrospinal fluid and peripherally by the inputs from the carotid and aortic body receptors, which respond to changes in arterial pH, P_{CO_2}, and P_{O_2}. The principal controller of ventilation is the arterial P_{CO_2} acting at the central chemoreceptors. It may seem paradoxic that carbon dioxide should have a greater influence on alveolar ventilation than oxygen. However, CO_2 production by the tissues is directly related to oxidative metabolism as well as to pH through the bicarbonate buffer system. Thus, a CO_2-controlled system maintains a ventilation sufficient for adequate oxygen delivery, carbon dioxide removal, and optimal pH maintenance.

The Central Chemoreceptors

Cells located at or near the ventral surface of the medulla function as the central chemoreceptors (Fig. 11–7). These chemosensitive cells are concentrated into two major areas: a rostral area (RA) near the roots of cranial nerves VI through X, and a caudal area (CA) near the base of the hypoglossal nerve

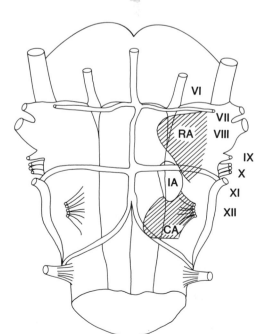

FIGURE 11–7. Central chemoreceptor areas on the ventral surface of the medulla. Rostral (RA) and caudal (CA) areas (hatched) are sensitive to CO_2 tension and hydrogen ion, whereas the intermediate area (IA) appears to relay chemoreceptor signals. (Roman numerals indicate nerves.) (Redrawn from Loeschcke, H.H.: Central chemoreceptors. In Pallot, D.J. (ed.): *Control of Respiration.* New York: Oxford University Press, 1983, p. 57.)

(XII). A small intermediate region (IA) appears to integrate activity of these surface receptors. Efferent fibers from the chemosensitive areas decussate to the contralateral brainstem and have a major input to the dorsal respiratory group. The *paragigantocellular nucleus* adjacent to the chemosensitive area also appears to mediate chemosensitivity.

Although the chemosensitive cells have no direct contact with arterial blood, they are bathed in cerebrospinal fluid. Wide interstitial spaces between the chemosensitive cells are continuous with the subarachnoid spaces. Therefore, even large molecules have ready access into the tissue. The ventral surface of the medulla is in close proximity to the choroid plexus. Since blood flow in the plexus is high and carbon dioxide equilibrates rapidly between blood and cerebrospinal fluid, the average cerebrospinal fluid and tissue P_{CO_2} approaches that of arterial blood.

MECHANISMS FOR CENTRAL CHEMOSENSITIVITY

The common pathway for the action of CO_2 and acidosis on the central chemoreceptors is the hydrogen ion concentration in the cerebrospinal fluid bathing the ventral surface of the medulla. Figure 11–8 shows the marked response of tidal volume to small changes in extracellular pH of the ventral surface of the medulla during inhalation of CO_2. This response to inhaled CO_2 occurs because CO_2 tension in the blood rapidly equilibrates with that in the cerebrospinal fluid. The CO_2 dissolved in the cerebrospinal fluid then combines with water to form carbonic acid, which dissociates into hydrogen and bicarbonate ions. The hydrogen ions enter the tissue and stimulate cholinergic synapses of the medullary chemoreceptor neurons to increase ventilation rate. Increased arterial hydrogen ion concentrations may also stimulate the chemoreceptors of the ventral medulla by increasing blood flow to the region. However, the effect of arterial hydrogen ion concentration is usually small because, unlike CO_2, hydrogen ion cannot easily cross the blood-brain barrier.

ADAPTATION OF CENTRAL CHEMORECEPTORS

Although ventilation rapidly responds to changes in arterial P_{CO_2}, the effects of P_{CO_2} tend to wane within hours to days. This adaptation is caused by the transport of bicarbonate ions across the endothelium of the blood-brain barrier. Bicarbonate then buffers the pH changes of the medullary extracellular fluid. Bicarbonate moves from plasma to cerebrospinal fluid during chronic hypercapnia and in the reverse direction during chronic hypocapnia. Exchange of bicarbonate for chloride ions between cerebrospinal fluid and plasma occurs through specific anion exchange channels and is mediated by a protein carrier. Return of the cerebrospinal fluid pH toward normal accounts for the decreased ventilatory drive in the presence of CO_2 retention associated with chronic obstructive lung disease. The P_{O_2} drive from peripheral chemoreceptors then

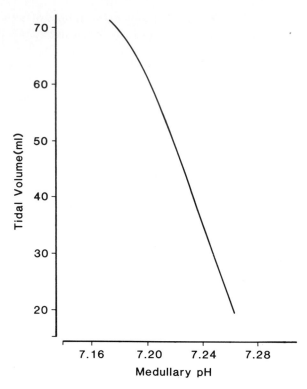

FIGURE 11–8. Relationship of tidal volume to medullary pH during progressive increases in inspired CO_2 concentrations. A decrease of 0.1 pH unit increased tidal volume by 3.5-fold. (Redrawn from Ahmad, H.R., and Loeschcke, H.H.: Transient and steady state responses of pulmonary ventilation to the medullary extracellular pH and approximately rectangular changes in alveolar P_{CO_2}. Pflugers Arch., 395:285–292, 1982.)

becomes the *only* means of maintaining sufficient ventilation, since cerebrospinal fluid pH approaches normal values.

VENTILATORY RESPONSE TO CARBON DIOXIDE AND HYDROGEN IONS

The ventilatory response to changes in arterial P_{CO_2} is shown in Figure 11–9. At a Pa_{CO_2} of 40 mmHg, the pH is 7.4 and alveolar ventilation is one unit. At a Pa_{CO_2} of 70 mmHg, alveolar ventilation has increased eight-fold. This is due to a direct stimulation of the central chemoreceptors by CO_2. The CO_2 effect can be altered by central depressant drugs that reduce the response of these receptors to CO_2 such that there is less of an increase in alveolar ventilation for a given increase in arterial CO_2 tension.

Metabolic acidosis also stimulates ventilation, but the ventilatory drive that can be achieved in response to decreases in arterial pH is less than one-half that observed in the presence of an increased Pa_{CO_2}. Increased arterial

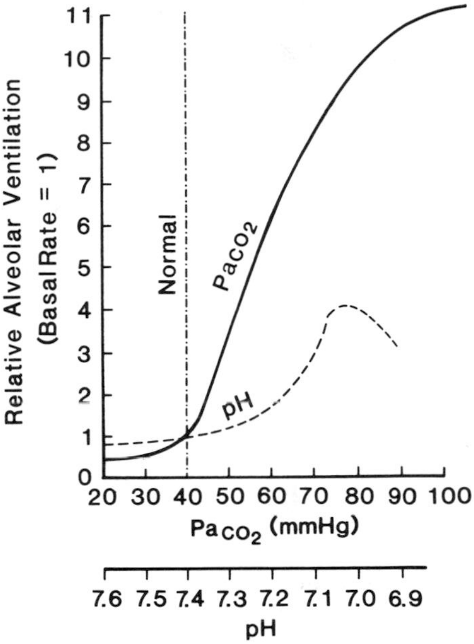

FIGURE 11–9. Stimulation of alveolar ventilation by decreased arterial pH or increased Pa_{CO_2}. (Redrawn from Guyton, A.C.: *Textbook of Medical Physiology.* 4th ed. Philadelphia: W.B. Saunders, 1971, p. 500.)

H^+ concentration stimulates peripheral chemoreceptors and, therefore, increases alveolar ventilation. However, this hyperventilation causes a decrease in arterial and cerebrospinal fluid CO_2 tensions. Since CO_2 leaves the cerebrospinal fluid much faster than H^+ enters, the pH of the cerebrospinal fluid close to the central chemoreceptor areas increases, opposing the hyperventilation.

Peripheral Chemoreceptor Response to Arterial Po_2

In addition to the central chemoreceptors in the medulla, the peripheral chemoreceptors in both the carotid and aortic bodies also modulate ventilation. Carotid bodies are small bilateral organs, only 2 to 3 mm in diameter, located at the bifurcation of the common carotid arteries (Fig. 11–10). The aortic bodies are found between the ascending aorta and pulmonary artery. These organs sense both arterial Po_2 and Pco_2, but only the carotid body responds to decreasing pH in humans. The carotid bodies send afferent inputs into the brainstem's respiratory centers through a branch of the glossopharyngeal nerve (Hering's nerve), whereas the aortic bodies transmit impulses through the vagus nerve.

Blood flow to the carotid bodies per gram organ weight is one of the highest in the body, approximately 2 l/min/100 g of tissue. Although the oxygen utilization (8 ml O_2/min/100 g) is actually higher than that of working muscle, only an insignificant net arteriovenous oxygen difference results across the carotid

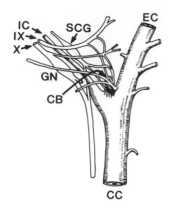

FIGURE 11–10. Anatomic location of the carotid body (CB) at the bifurcation of the common carotid artery (CC) into external (EC) and internal carotid arteries (IC). Adjacent structures are the ganglion nodosum (GN), superior cervical ganglion (SCG), and branches of the glossopharyngeal (IX) and vagus (X) nerves. (Redrawn from Adams, W.E.: *Comparative Morphology of the Carotid Body and Carotid Sinus.* Springfield, IL: Charles C Thomas, 1958.)

body (0.4 vol %). This allows the entire organ to sense a P_{O_2} that is nearly equivalent to that of arterial blood.

Aortic bodies show a weaker response to decreases in arterial P_{O_2} and a much lower sensitivity to changes in arterial P_{CO_2} than that noted for carotid bodies. Because of a higher arteriovenous oxygen difference, the aortic bodies respond to changes in either oxygen content or partial pressure. Thus, aortic bodies, but not carotid bodies, are stimulated by conditions in which arterial P_{O_2} is normal but arterial oxygen content is decreased, e.g., anemia and carbon monoxide poisoning. A rapid decrease in systemic arterial pressure from 160 to 60 mmHg can also transiently excite the carotid bodies, but this excitation persists only at pressures below 60 mmHg. Aortic bodies are somewhat more sensitive to arterial hypotension than are the carotid bodies.

The carotid bodies normally provide about 20 per cent of the total ventilatory drive. This can increase to 40 per cent or more during hypoxia or anesthesia, since the peripheral chemoreceptors are the only receptors that detect changes in arterial P_{O_2}. As shown in Figure 11–11, at a normal pH and Pa_{CO_2}, the carotid body receptors discharge at a low frequency until arterial P_{O_2} decreases to about 75 to 80 mmHg; then nerve activity sharply increases (middle curve). Note that the carotid body response begins at a relatively high Pa_{O_2} in normal conditions (7.4 pH and 40 mmHg Pa_{CO_2}), but maximum activity requires a large change in P_{O_2}. A considerable degree of interaction occurs between stimuli in the carotid body at normal O_2 tensions. In the presence of hypercapnea and acidosis, the firing rate is increased to 20 per cent of maximum (upper curve) even at normal oxygen tensions. Conversely, hypocapnia and alkalosis (lower curve) markedly depress nerve activity at normal oxygen tensions and lower the threshold P_{O_2} necessary to produce significant activity. Frequently hypercapnia and hypoxia occur concurrently, and their mutiplicative interaction causes a stronger ventilatory drive than would occur with only a lowered Pa_{O_2}.

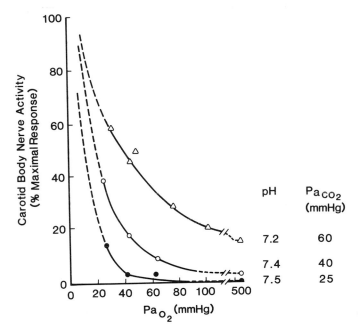

FIGURE 11–11. Carotid body nerve activity (per cent of maximal) as a function of Pa_{O_2}. The enhanced response to hypoxia as arterial pH decreases from 7.5 to 7.2 and P_{CO_2} increases from 25 to 60 is shown. (Redrawn from Hornbein, T.P.: The relation between stimulus to chemoreceptors and their response. In: Torrance, R.W. (ed.): *The Proceedings of the Wates Foundation Symposium on Arterial Chemoreceptors.* Oxford: Blackwell, 1968, pp. 65–76.)

MECHANISM OF PERIPHERAL CHEMOSENSITIVITY

Carotid and aortic bodies consist of two major cell types: spherical glomus cells (type I) and elongated sustentacular cells (type II). These cells are surrounded by numerous capillaries and vascular sinusoids. The glomus cells contain catecholamine granules and many mitochondria. Sensory axons from the glossopharyngeal or vagus nerves synapse on the glomus cells, as do sympathetic fibers from the stellate ganglion. The exact mechanism of signal transduction in response to changes in Pa_{O_2} is not known, but the glomus cells or the nerve endings are believed to be essential components.

INTEGRATED CONTROL OF VENTILATION

Integration of neural and humoral ventilatory stimuli occurs both within and between central and peripheral chemoreceptors. This complex interaction is illustrated in Figure 11–12, which shows the ventilatory response to changes in alveolar P_{CO_2} at different levels of alveolar P_{O_2} in humans. For a Pa_{O_2} of

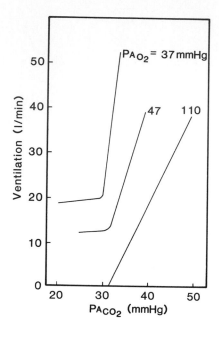

FIGURE 11–12. Ventilatory response to changes in $P_{A_{CO_2}}$ at various fixed $P_{A_{O_2}}$ values. The slopes progressively increased as $P_{A_{O_2}}$ was decreased, but the slope of the curve was unchanged when $P_{A_{O_2}}$ exceeded 110 mmHg. (Redrawn from Nielson, M., and Smith, H.: Studies on the regulation of respiration in acute hypoxia with an appendix on respiratory control during prolonged hypoxia. *Acta. Physiol. Scand.,* 24:293–313, 1952.)

110 mmHg, ventilation increases by only 2 l/min for each mmHg increase in $P_{A_{CO_2}}$. This response is enhanced at lower alveolar P_{O_2} values. For instance, when alveolar $P_{A_{O_2}}$ is reduced to 47 or 37 mmHg, the slopes relating ventilation to $P_{A_{CO_2}}$ become much steeper. The ventilation plateau seen at low $P_{A_{O_2}}$ values and $P_{A_{CO_2}}$ values results from the hypoxic stimulation of peripheral chemoreceptors. Acidemia enhances both $P_{A_{CO_2}}$ and $P_{A_{O_2}}$ effects, i.e., the curves are shifted to the left without significantly altering their slopes.

Figure 11–13 diagrammatically summarizes the major components of ventilatory control. These include phasic inputs from the reticular activating system to inspiratory neurons and reciprocal inhibition of inspiratory and expiratory neurons. Inspiratory neurons deliver an efferent drive to phrenic motor neurons, which stimulates diaphragmatic muscle. The intensity of this response is related to tidal volume and is a function of $P_{a_{CO_2}}$, arterial pH, and $P_{a_{O_2}}$ stimulation of central and peripheral chemoreceptors. The off-switch neurons are inhibited during most of the inspiratory cycle, but this inhibition decreases with time. These neurons can be stimulated by the pneumotaxic center or by feedback from pulmonary stretch receptors to discharge more quickly during inspiration and terminate inspiratory neuron activity. Although the duration of inspiration can be limited by vagal afferent feedback, ventilatory rate is closely regulated to maintain blood gas and pH homeostasis.

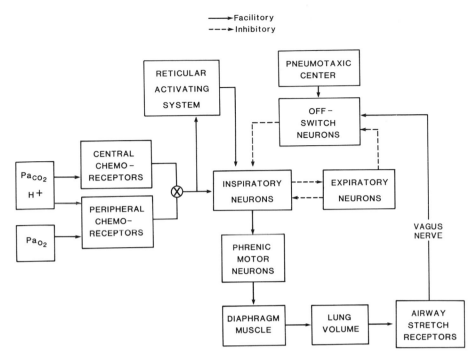

FIGURE 11–13. Block diagram showing major components of ventilatory control. Inspiratory neurons are facilitated by the reticular activating system and chemoreceptor output but inhibited by expiratory neurons throughout expiration and off-switch neurons late in inspiration. These off-switch neurons are facilitated by the pneumotaxic center and the vagal stretch receptor input. Note that the effects of the central and peripheral chemoreceptors are multiplicative ($\times$), not additive.

DISORDERS OF VENTILATORY CONTROL

Sleep Apneas

Sleep apneas are classified as either *central*, resulting from a failure of central inspiratory drive; or *obstructive*, which results from closure of the glottis, larynx, or pharynx without loss of inspiratory muscle effort; or some combination of the two. Figure 11–14 shows the three different patterns of sleep apneas. Shown on the figure are gas flow, esophageal pressure, and arterial O_2 saturation. For the central type (Fig. 11–14A), there is no respiratory drive as indicated by the lack of respiratory pressure changes (as measured with esophageal pressures) during the period of apnea. This indicates that the central receptors are not responding in a normal fashion. In obstructive and mixed types (Fig. 11–14B and C), gas flow ceases in spite of very strong, progressively increasing inspiratory efforts as indicated by the large esophageal pressure changes. The clinical characteristics associated with these types of apnea are shown in Table 11–1. Sleep apnea is much more common in older men than

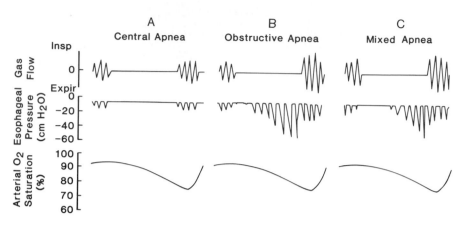

FIGURE 11–14. Patterns of gas flow, esophageal (pleural) pressure, and arterial oxygen saturation during *(A)* central, *(B)* obstructive, and *(C)* mixed sleep apneas, Note the large subatmospheric esophageal (pleural) pressures that occur during obstructive and mixed apnea before airflow starts. (Redrawn from Orr, W.C.: Utilization of polysomnography in the assessment of sleep disorders. *Med. Clin. North Am., 69*:1153–1167, 1985.)

women and occurs in light sleep associated with rapid eye movement (REM). The most common patient with sleep apnea is a very sleepy man whose wife complains of excessive snoring and loud sleep sounds.

Two types of central sleep apnea can produce death. *Ondine's curse* is an adult condition named after the fairy whose human lover could not breathe automatically and had to will himself to do so. In this condition, periodic breathing is often reported at night. Patients suffering from Ondine's curse must increase ventilation voluntarily to maintain alveolar P_{CO_2} at a normal level, and some patients require beds that tilt up and down to stimulate the peripheral receptors during sleep. *Sudden infant death syndrome* (SIDS) is a sudden cessation of breathing in newborns occurring during sleep. These conditions may result from either a decreased central sensitivity to P_{CO_2} or a decreased number of chemosensitive cells. It is now common to monitor breathing in infants who are prone to the development of SIDS.

Obstructive sleep apnea occurs during inspiration when the airway is oc-

TABLE 11–1. Characteristics of Patients with Sleep Apnea

Central	Obstructive
Normal body habitus	Commonly obese
Insomnia; hypersomnolence rare	Daytime hypersomnolence
Awaken during sleep	Rarely awaken during sleep
Snoring mild and intermittent	Loud snoring
Depression	Intellectual deterioration
	Morning headache
	Nocturnal enuresis
	Pulmonary hypertension

cluded by the tongue or by closure of the larynx or pharynx. In many cases, apnea is preceded by loud snoring and may be related to excess body fat, which compresses and reduces the diameter of the upper airway. Lack of coordination between laryngeal and diaphragmatic muscle activity can also contribute to the problem. Laryngeal abductor muscles normally maintain the patency of the airway through centrally mediated Pa_{CO_2} receptors. However, the decreased sensitivity of the CO_2 receptors during sleep affects airway muscles to a greater extent than the diaphragm. Most of these subjects respond immediately to the application of continuous positive airway pressure (CPAP) applied throughout the night. This therapy results in a dramatic improvement in the patient's condition.

Irregular Breathing Patterns

Another abnormal breathing pattern associated with periods of apnea is termed *Cheyne-Stokes breathing* (Fig. 11–15). This type of breathing pattern is characterized by a gradual waxing and waning of respiration, i.e., a higher than normal depth and frequency of ventilation for a period of minutes, followed by a cessation of breathing. Periodic ventilation and apnea occur for approximately the same amount of time. Usually, Cheyne-Stokes breathing occurs after head injury or during cardiac failure. This periodic breathing pattern occurs because the central chemoreceptors overdrive ventilation when the circulatory transit time between the lungs and brain increases. The abnormally high alveolar ventilation greatly decreases P_{CO_2} in the blood leaving the lungs, but the time of arrival of the blood to the brain is delayed. Once this hypocapneic blood arrives in the brain, a period of apnea ensues, and the P_{CO_2} increases in the pulmonary capillary blood. When this hypercapneic blood reaches the

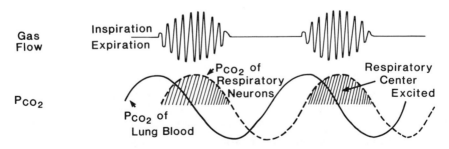

FIGURE 11–15. Pattern of Cheyne-Stokes breathing (top tracing). The changes in P_{CO_2} in pulmonary blood (solid line) and cerebrospinal fluid bathing the central chemoreceptor neurons (dashed line) are shown. Note the time delay between events occurring in pulmonary blood and at the respiratory center. The shaded area represents the activation of the central chemoreceptor by the high P_{CO_2}. (From Guyton, A.C.: *Textbook of Medical Physiology*, 4th ed., Philadelphia: W.B. Saunders, 1971, p. 504.)

brain, another period of hyperventilation is generated and another Cheyne-Stokes cycle begins.

VENTILATORY RESPONSE TO EXERCISE

One of the most obvious and physiologically important responses to sustained exercise is increased ventilation. Oxygen consumption can increase from a normal resting value of 250 ml/min to over 4 l/min in well-trained athletes. Oxygen consumption and delivery are remarkably well matched to workload over a wide range of exercise intensities. As shown in Figure 11–16, there is a linear increase in $\dot{V}_{O_2}$ with increasing work rate in human subjects. $\dot{V}_E$ and $\dot{V}_{CO_2}$ are also linearly matched to work rate at moderate levels of exercise, but, at higher work rates, $\dot{V}_E$ and $\dot{V}_{CO_2}$ increase more rapidly than does $\dot{V}_{O_2}$. The $\dot{V}_{O_2}$ at which this occurs is the *anaerobic threshold* and represents the work rate at which lactic acid production begins to exceed its metabolism. A net increase in blood lactic acid causes acidemia, and excess CO_2 must be eliminated to maintain pH homeostasis. This becomes evident when the ratios of $\dot{V}_E/\dot{V}_{O_2}$ and $\dot{V}_{CO_2}/\dot{V}_{O_2}$ increase. Note that the initial decrease in pH is minimized by body buffer systems. Initially, there is not a significant decrease in $P_{A CO_2}$ because the buffering of lactic acid with bicarbonate produces CO_2. However, at higher workloads, $P_{A CO_2}$ does decrease and $P_{A O_2}$ actually increases owing to hyperventilation. At high work rates, this hyperventilation attenuates the fall in blood pH caused by lactic acid. At high workloads, the maximal $\dot{V}_{O_2}$ is reached when there is no increase in $\dot{V}_{O_2}$ with an increase in workload.

The anaerobic threshold, which indicates the efficiency of O_2 metabolism by the tissues, is increased by endurance training and decreased in the presence of cardiac and pulmonary disease. An increase in anaerobic threshold occurs because hydrogen ions are now more rapidly transported into mitochondria and oxidized. Endurance training increases the number of mitochondria, the number of capillaries, and the myoglobin content of muscle, all of which enhance the oxidative capacity of muscle tissue. In addition, O_2 delivery is enhanced by an increase in the maximal cardiac output due to an increased stroke volume and heart rate. During exercise, an improved O_2 extraction by the tissues can increase the arteriovenous O_2 content difference, and the alveolar-arterial O_2 gradient may increase. The O_2 uptake at the anaerobic threshold can increase by 45 per cent after training in a sedentary individual, and the $\dot{V}_{max O_2}$ can increase by 15 per cent. Improved exercise tolerance can also be realized in persons with chronic disease.

Exercise testing has become a valuable tool for the differential diagnosis of patients with exertional dyspnea as well as for monitoring the progress of exercise training in both cardiac and pulmonary disease patients. Tests can be conducted using incremental exercise on either a treadmill or a bicycle ergometer. Usually maximal exercise is normally limited by the maximal cardiac

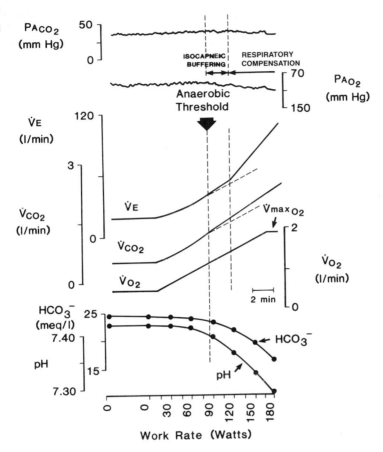

FIGURE 11–16. Measurements of $\dot{V}_E$, $\dot{V}_{CO_2}$, $\dot{V}_{O_2}$, P_{AO_2}, P_{ACO_2}, arterial pH, and bicarbonate ion in a human subject during incremental exercise on a bicycle ergometer. Note the increases in $\dot{V}_E$ and $\dot{V}_{CO_2}$ relative to $\dot{V}_{O_2}$ above a work rate of 90 watts. The $\dot{V}_{O_2}$ at this work rate is the *anaerobic threshold,* and the flat portion of the $\dot{V}_{O_2}$ curve that occurs at a high workload is defined as the $\dot{V}max_{O_2}$. Note that the P_{ACO_2} does not change (isocapneic buffering) until the body buffers allow pH to decrease sufficiently to increase ventilation, which then decreases alveolar P_{CO_2} and buffers the lactic acid (Resp Comp). (Redrawn from Wasserman, K., Whipp, B.J., and Davis, J.A.: Respiratory physiology of exercise: Metabolism gas exchange and ventilatory control. *Int. Rev. Physiol.* 23:149–211, 1981.)

output, but in patients with chronic obstructive or restrictive lung disease, gas exchange capacity of the lungs is limited by the mechanical properties of the respiratory system. Such subjects may not attain their anaerobic threshold or maximal $\dot{V}_{O_2}$ during exercise because a precipitous decrease in Pa_{O_2} and dyspnea often limit maximal exercise. Patients with cardiac disease generally are capable of attaining an anaerobic threshold and a maximal $\dot{V}_{O_2}$ capacity, but these values are usually lower than normal.

Control of ventilation during exercise has been of interest to physiologists because of the ability of the respiratory system to match ventilation to workload and O_2 consumption, even in the absence of sufficient changes in arterial P_{O_2}, P_{CO_2}, and pH to produce the high ventilation. At the onset of exercise, the change in ventilation has a characteristic time course, as shown in Figure 11–17 for four different levels of exercise (0, 300, 600, and 800 Watts). An instantaneous jump in ventilation occurs at the onset of exercise (phase I), followed by a slow transient increase over the next 4 to 5 minutes (phase II) until a plateau level of ventilation is attained (phase III). The increased minute ventilation is due to increases in both rate and depth of respiration. Phase I appears to be neurally mediated by a learned response related to an anticipation of exercise and/or an increased proprioceptor input from muscles and joints at the onset of exercise. Phase I is load independent and accompanied by increases in heart rate and sympathetic activity. The rate of rise in phase II is related to the transit time of gases in the blood. Phase III reaches a steady-state $\dot{V}E$ below anaerobic threshold but may continue to increase during heavy exercise.

The exact mechanism for matching ventilation to workload is unknown, but a possible stimulus for the increased respiratory drive is the slight decrease in pH that occurs at all exercise levels. Very heavy exercise can decrease blood pH by 0.05 to 0.1 units, and this reduction in pH will stimulate carotid body receptors. Wide fluctuations in the alveolar P_{CO_2} have also been implicated as stimuli for the increased ventilation during exercise. These fluctuations in alveolar P_{CO_2} cause oscillations in arterial P_{CO_2} and pH that are sensed by peripheral chemoreceptors. Support for this mechanism to explain the increased ventilation associated with exercise is the observation that subjects

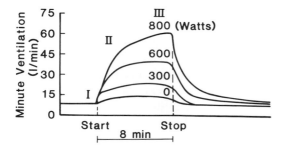

FIGURE 11–17. Ventilatory responses of human subjects at four different workloads, ranging from 0 to 800 Watts. The initial anticipatory neural phase (I), transient humoral phase (II), and plateau level phase (III) are shown for each exercise level. (Redrawn from Pearce, D.H., and Milhorn, H.J. Jr.: Dynamic and steady-state respiratory responses to bicycle exercise. *J. Appl. Physiol.,* 42:959–967, 1977.)

without carotid bodies demonstrate a much slower rise in $\dot{V}E$ during phase II. Another hypothesis is that receptors for O_2 content exist in the pulmonary arteries. These sensors would allow an accurate matching between ventilation and oxygen consumption owing to the larger arteriovenous O_2 difference during exercise.

SUGGESTED READING

Coleridge, H.M., and Coleridge, J.C.G.: Reflexes evoked from tracheobronchial tree and lungs. In Cherniack, N.S., and Widdicombe, J.G. (eds.): *Handbook of Physiology:* Section 3, The Respiratory System, Volume II, Control of Breathing, Part 1. Bethesda: APS, 1986, pp. 395–429.

Euler, C. Von: Brainstem mechanisms for generation and control of breathing pattern. In Cherniack, N.S., and Widdicombe, J.G. (eds.): *Handbook of Physiology:* Section 3, The Respiratory System, Volume II, Control of Breathing, Part 1. Bethesda: APS, 1986, pp. 1–68.

Loeschcke, H.H.: Central chemoreceptors. In Pallot, D.J. (ed.): *Control of Respiration.* New York: Oxford University Press, 1983, pp. 41–77.

Wasserman, K., Whipp, B.J., and Casaburi, R.: Respiratory control during exercise. In Cherniack, N.S., and Widdicombe, J.G. (eds.): *Handbook of Physiology:* Section 3, The Respiratory System, Volume II, Control of Breathing, Part 2. Bethesda: APS, 1986, pp. 594–620.

QUESTIONS

1. What conditions reduce the normal responsiveness of ventilatory control to an increased Pa_{CO_2}?
2. The enhanced sensitivity to Pa_{CO_2} drive induced by simultaneous alveolar hypoxia is mediated by which chemoreceptors?
3. What is the effect of stimulation of the pneumotaxic center nuclei and pulmonary stretch receptors on inspiratory time?
4. Why is Pa_{CO_2} likely to increase in a patient with chronic CO_2 retention who suddenly breathes 100% O_2?
5. What is the anaerobic threshold?

OXYGEN THERAPY
Causes of Hypoxia
Effects of Increased Inspired Oxygen Concentration
O_2 Delivery Systems
Problems Associated with Oxygen Therapy
Oxygen Toxicity

MECHANICAL VENTILATION
Types of Ventilators
Physiologic Effects of Mechanical Ventilation
Positive End-Expiratory Pressure
Continuous Positive Airway Pressure
High-Frequency Ventilation
High-Frequency Positive Pressure Ventilation
High-Frequency Jet Ventilation
High-Frequency Oscillation
Gas Transport During HFO
Indications for Mechanical Ventilation

COMPLICATIONS OF MECHANICAL VENTILATION

12

THERAPEUTIC VENTILATION

OXYGEN THERAPY

Causes of Hypoxia

Tissue hypoxia is caused by inadequate oxygen delivery relative to tissue demand or by toxin-induced interference with mitochondrial oxygen utilization. Hypoxia is classified into four types: (1) hypoxic hypoxemia, (2) anemic hypoxemia, (3) stagnant hypoxia, and (4) histotoxic hypoxia (Table 12–1).

Hypoxic hypoxemia is most commonly caused by ventilation-perfusion abnormalities, increased right-to-left intrapulmonary shunting, inadequate diffusion of oxygen across the alveolar-capillary membrane, or some combination of these. Hypoxic hypoxemia can also occur with hypoventilation or in subjects with normal lung function if the inspired oxygen tension is reduced. Hypoventilation is often due to depression of the respiratory center, upper airway obstruction, respiratory muscle weakness, or flail chest. *Anemic hypoxemia*

217

TABLE 12–1. Hypoxia and Its Effects on Arterial Oxygen Tension, Content, and Saturation

Type of Hypoxia	F_{IO_2}	P_{IO_2}	Pa_{O_2}	Ca_{O_2}	Sa_{O_2}
Hypoxic hypoxemia					
High altitude	N	L	L	L	L
Low insp. O_2 conc.	L	L	L	L	L
Hypoventilation	N	N	L	L	L
$\dot{V}A/\dot{Q}$ abnormality	N	N	L	L	L
Right-to-left shunting	N	N	L	L	L
Diffusion impairment	N	N	L	L	L
Anemic hypoxemia	N	N	N	L	N
Stagnant hypoxia	N	N	N	N	N
Histotoxic hypoxia	N	N	N	N	N

Note: L = low; N = normal. Sa_{O_2} is arterial oxygen saturation.

develops when the oxygen-carrying capacity of arterial blood is insufficient to satisfy the oxygen needs of the tissues. Anemic hypoxemia may be associated with acute or chronic anemia, congenital hemoglobinopathies, methemoglobinemia, or carbon monoxide poisoning. *Stagnant hypoxia* results when the circulation is inadequate to deliver sufficient oxygen for tissue metabolism. An example of stagnant hypoxia occurs in the low cardiac output state seen in hypovolemic or anaphylactic shock. *Histotoxic hypoxia* occurs when the cytochrome oxidative enzymes are poisoned by compounds such as cyanide and can be associated with sepsis or production of toxins in critically ill patients.

Hypoxemia often causes blueness of the skin and mucous membranes, a condition called cyanosis. Cyanosis is an unreliable indicator of hypoxemia, however, since it depends on the type of lighting used during the physical examination, the perception of the examiner, and at least 3 to 5 g of deoxygenated hemoglobin per 100 ml of blood must be present to be detectable. In patients with severe anemic hypoxia, deoxygenated hemoglobin may not be present in sufficient amounts to produce observable cyanosis. For example, if a subject's hemoglobin level was 8 g/dl and the hemoglobin saturation in the capillary was reduced from the normal value of 75 per cent to 50 per cent, only 4 g/dl of hemoglobin would be deoxygenated, and cyanosis might not be present.

In a subject with a healthy cardiovascular system and normal hemoglobin concentration, arterial hypoxemia is well tolerated. A subject can survive for long periods of time with an arterial oxygen tension as low as 50 mmHg but often experiences pulmonary hypertension, polycythemia, and right-sided heart failure. Very low arterial oxygen tensions (20 mmHg or less) can only be tolerated for a few minutes.

Effects of Increased Inspired Oxygen Concentration

Assuming a hemoglobin concentration of 15 g/dl, the oxygen saturation of hemoglobin in arterial blood increases only slightly when normal subjects breathe 100% oxygen, i.e., from 97.5 to 100 per cent. This only increases the amount of oxygen carried by hemoglobin from 20.20 to 20.70 ml/dl of blood. In contrast, the amount of oxygen dissolved in arterial blood increases more than six-fold from 0.30 to 2.00 ml/dl, roughly 10 per cent of the amount combined with hemoglobin. The total increase in the oxygen content of the arterial blood when breathing 100% O_2 is $0.50 + (1.70) = 2.20$ ml/dl of blood. Therefore, breathing 100% oxygen increases oxygen transport capacity to the tissues only slightly.

In contrast to normal subjects, inhalation of 100% oxygen can be life-saving in patients suffering from acute hypoxia. Besides improving blood oxygenation, 100% oxygen in the inspired gas also displaces nitrogen from the ventilated lung regions. This displacement essentially eliminates the effects of ventilation-perfusion abnormalities. Therefore, patients with hypoxemia resulting from ventilation-perfusion abnormalities will benefit significantly from 100% oxygen inhalation. The increased alveolar oxygen tension also elevates the pressure gradient for diffusion of oxygen from the alveoli into the pulmonary capillary blood, which effectively eliminates hypoxemia due to impaired diffusion at the alveolar-capillary membrane. It is important to remember that inhalation of 100% oxygen cannot improve oxygenation of blood that is shunted through the lung, nor can it enhance absorption of oxygen from underperfused lung regions.

To avoid oxygen toxicity, oxygen must never be administered indiscriminately. The goal of oxygen inhalation therapy is to restore arterial oxygen content to an adequate level. Since the slope of the oxyhemoglobin dissociation curve is steep, arterial O_2 content can often be increased considerably using small increases in the inspired oxygen concentration. However, this effect will only be seen in the presence of ventilation-perfusion abnormalities, as seen in patients with chronic obstructive pulmonary disease. It is not seen in the presence of right-to-left intrapulmonary shunting, a condition found frequently in patients with *adult respiratory distress syndrome.*

The effects of various arterial oxygen tensions on oxygen delivery to the tissues are shown in Table 12–2. Pa_{O_2} values of 25, 40, and 100 mmHg (normal)

TABLE 12–2. Relationship Between Oxygen Partial Pressure and O_2 Available to the Tissue

Variable	Life-threatening Hypoxia	Hypoxia	Normoxia
Pa_{O_2} (mmHg)	25	40	100
Sa_{O_2} (%)	50	75	97.5
Ca_{O_2} (ml/dl)	8.0	14.0	20.0
$C\bar{v}_{O_2}$ (ml/dl)	4.0	4.0	4.0
$\dot{Q}$ (l/min)	5	5	5
Oyxgen available to tissue* (ml/min)	200	500	800

*$\dot{Q}(Ca_{O_2} - C\bar{v}_{O_2})$
For definition of abbreviations, see text.

are shown in the upper row. The O_2 available to the tissues was calculated assuming a cardiac output ($\dot{Q}$) of 5 l/min, an oxygen uptake ($\dot{V}_{O_2}$) of 200 ml/min, a hemoglobin concentration of 15 g/dl, a mixed venous O_2 content ($C\bar{v}_{O_2}$) of 4.0 ml/dl, and a normal oxyhemoglobin dissociation curve. A modest increase in Pa_{O_2} from 25 to 40 mmHg increases the available oxygen from 200 to 500 ml/min. Such an increase in Pa_{O_2} could be accomplished by increasing inspired oxygen concentration by only 2 per cent in normal subjects, and the increase in inspired oxygen would only need to be slightly larger to achieve the same effect in patients with ventilation-perfusion abnormalities.

O_2 Delivery Systems

Several ventilation systems are used to deliver oxygen. The low-flow oxygen delivery systems supply oxygen to the lungs at flows less than the patient's inspiratory flow. Since these systems only enrich the subject's inspired gas with O_2, they provide only modest, unpredictable increases in the inspired oxygen concentration. The increase in the inspired concentration of oxygen depends on the flow of oxygen into the system and the subject's inspiratory flow. These systems are only used when modest impairment of oxygenation is present. Nasal catheters and simple oxygen masks are examples of low-flow oxygen delivery systems. In contrast, high-flow gas supply systems provide O_2 flows that exceed the patient's maximal inspiratory flow. These devices permit accurate control of the patient's inspired concentration of oxygen and can be used to deliver a high $F_{I_{O_2}}$. But these systems are wasteful in terms of gas used, and if a subject's lungs are to be ventilated with an $F_{I_{O_2}}$ of 1.0 for any prolonged period, the high-flow devices require a closed gas system and an intubated airway. The Venturi mask is an example of this type of ventilator. In this system, the inspired O_2 concentration is independent of the patient's minute ventilation.

Problems Associated with Oxygen Therapy

Inhalation of high concentrations of oxygen is associated with a number of dangers (including fire and explosion hazards as well as drying of mucous membranes from inadequate humidification), all of which are easily avoided by taking appropriate precautions. In addition, the reduction or absence of nitrogen in the alveoli during inhalation of 100% oxygen may lead to a condition called *absorption atelectasis*. This condition develops when the diffusion of alveolar oxygen into the pulmonary capillaries exceeds the replenishment of alveolar oxygen by ventilation, allowing alveolar collapse. Finally, the administration of oxygen may lead to ventilatory failure in patients with chronic carbon dioxide retention, presumably owing to a reduction in ventilatory drive. This occurs because the peripheral chemoreceptors are no longer stimulated by hypoxia, whereas the central chemoreceptors do not respond to hypercarbia.

Oxygen Toxicity

Morphologic alterations in lungs subjected to high levels of O_2 for a few days include excessive damage to pulmonary capillary endothelium, injury to alveolar epithelium with destruction of alveolar type I cells, development of interstitial edema, and proliferation of alveolar type II cells. The earliest manifestations of pulmonary oxygen toxicity appear to be tracheobronchitis (with cough), substernal discomfort, reduced vital capacity, diminished clearance of secretions, reduced lung compliance, and reduced diffusing capacity. Chronic pulmonary oxygen toxicity causes pulmonary emphysema and fibrosis and, in children, bronchopulmonary dysplasia. Premature infants may develop retrolental fibroplasia.

According to current research, oxygen toxicity is caused by partially reduced oxygen products. These partially reduced oxygen products, called oxygen free radicals, have an unpaired electron, which makes them chemically unstable and highly reactive. Figure 12–1 shows how these free radicals are generated. Molecular oxygen is reduced to superoxide anion (O_2^-) and hydrogen peroxide (H_2O_2). O_2^- can combine with H_2O_2 in the presence of Fe^{+++} (Haber-Weiss reaction) to produce the very toxic hydroxyl radical ($OH^\bullet$).

When the rate of oxygen radical formation exceeds the body's capacity to defend against these very powerful oxidants, oxygen toxicity occurs. Oxygen free radicals act on unsaturated lipids (causing lipid peroxidation), and they also degrade proteins, inactivate enzymes, alter nucleic acid bases, and oxidize

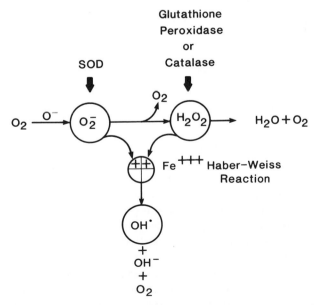

FIGURE 12–1. Schematic representation of pathways for oxygen radical production and the enzymes responsible for their detoxification. SOD = superoxide dismutase.

carbohydrates. These chemical changes lead to cell death. All body cells are susceptible to oxygen toxicity, but cells of the lung are particularly vulnerable because they are exposed to higher oxygen tensions. In fact, after 70 hours of breathing 100% O_2, one-half of the lung's capillaries are destroyed in some animal models.

The lung's defenses against oxygen toxicity include superoxide dismutase, catalase, and glutathione peroxidase, which are enzymatic detoxifiers of these reactive products of oxygen. Superoxide dismutase (SOD) reduces superoxide to hydrogen peroxide, which is then reduced to H_2O by catalase or glutathione peroxidase. In addition, the body uses nonenzymatic antioxidant systems, such as hemoglobin, reduced glutathione, and α-tocopherol (vitamin E), to defend against the reactive products of oxygen. Recent studies have shown that if SOD is given in such a way that it enters the cells of the lung, the cellular damage seen with 100% O_2 is inhibited. This allows for an extended period of 100% O_2 ventilation.

The threshold for oxygen toxicity is not known, since the sensitivity of cells to oxygen injury varies between individuals. Tolerance may develop and is a function of age, nutrition, hormones, drugs, and the subject's ability to detoxify oxygen radicals. It is becoming increasingly clear that enzymatic detoxifiers, iron chelators, or nonenzymatic scavengers may be useful in preventing the O_2 toxicity if they can be modified to enter the lung's cells.

Although pulmonary oxygen toxicity is related to the partial pressure of oxygen and the duration of exposure, oxygen should never be withheld from a patient because of fear of toxicity. Instead, the rule of thumb is to give O_2 at the lowest possible level for the shortest possible period.

MECHANICAL VENTILATION

Types of Ventilators

Ventilators are classified as *flow* or *pressure* generators, depending on their mode of operation. Flow generators deliver a preset flow of gas, regardless of the opposing forces. Any change in impedance of the total respiratory system (combined forces opposing lung inflation, i.e., elastic, resistive, and inertial forces) will be reflected by a change in airway pressure. Flow generators are designed to deliver either a constant or a sinusoidal flow. Pressure generators, on the other hand, deliver a preset pressure, and gas flow is a result of the applied pressure. Since pressure is constant, increased impedance results in decreased gas flow.

The cycling between inspiration and expiration can be controlled by time or volume for flow generators or by pressure for pressure generators. For time-limited ventilators, inspiration is terminated after a given period of time, and cycling occurs regardless of the developed pressure or delivered volume. Volume-limited ventilators cycle when a predetermined volume has been delivered, regardless of the time required or the pressure developed. Volume-limited ventilators compensate for changes in the impedance of the respiratory system but not for gas leaks. Pressure-limited ventilators develop a predetermined pressure and then begin the expiratory cycle. The advantage of pressure-limited as compared with time- or volume-limited ventilators is that they can compensate for small gas leaks between ventilator and patient. The disadvantage of pressure-limited ventilators is that the gas volume delivered to the lungs varies with changes in the impedance of the respiratory system. For pressure generators, an increase in impedance will reduce the delivered volume, whereas a decrease in impedance will increase the delivered volume. Volume-limited ventilators are commonly used in intensive care of adults, whereas pressure-limited ventilators are more often used with neonates.

Most ventilators can operate in several modes. In the *control(ler) mode*, the ventilator controls the volume and the timing of ventilation. In the *assist(or) mode*, the patient's inspiratory efforts trigger the start of inflation. *Intermittent mandatory ventilation* (IMV) allows the patient to assume most of the work of breathing but provides mechanical inflation of the lungs at predetermined intervals during spontaneous breathing. If inappropriately applied, IMV may cause severe respiratory muscle fatigue. When using *synchronous intermittent mandatory ventilation* (SIMV), the lung inflations during IMV are synchronized to coincide with the patient's own inspiratory efforts. Both IMV and SIMV are frequently used to help facilitate weaning of a patient from a ventilator, which is a major problem in patients whose lungs have been ventilated for long periods of time. Some ventilators have incorporated a "sigh," i.e., an intermittent deep breath used to periodically hyperinflate the lungs, which helps to prevent or reverse the tendency for some portions of the lung to collapse. Patients are very likely to experience this collapse when their lungs are ventilated with a constant, low tidal volume.

Physiologic Effects of Mechanical Ventilation

Mechanical ventilation of the lungs affects both the respiratory and cardiac systems. The increased airway pressure is accompanied by an increase in alveolar gas and pleural pressures during the inspiratory phase of mechanical ventilation (Fig. 12–2). During the expiratory phase, airway and alveolar gas pressures decrease to normal levels.

Any rise in intrathoracic pressure during mechanical ventilation increases right atrial pressure and reduces the pressure gradient between peripheral veins and right atrium, tending to impede venous return of blood to the heart. Subjects with normal blood volumes and nervous systems re-establish the necessary pressure gradient by increasing the peripheral venous pressure. However, patients with low blood volumes cannot employ this type of compensatory mechanism to increase their peripheral venous pressures, since their veins are

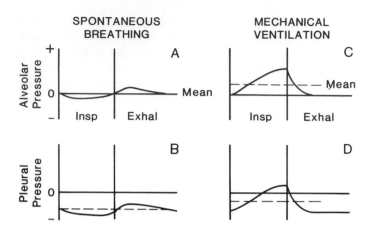

FIGURE 12–2. Both alveolar and pleural pressures increase during the inspiratory phase of mechanical ventilation *(C and D)*. This is shown in contrast to the subatmospheric pressures generated during spontaneous inspiration *(A and B)*.

already constricted; therefore, in these patients mechanical ventilation decreases cardiac output.

In healthy persons, gas distribution remains nonuniform when the lungs are passively inflated. In these subjects, however, intrapulmonary distribution of inspired gas is different during mechanical ventilation than during spontaneous breathing. During spontaneous breathing, ventilation of dependent lung regions is greater than that of nondependent regions when the inspiration is initiated from a lung volume equal to or greater than the functional residual capacity (FRC). During mechanical ventilation under general anesthesia, the respiratory muscles are usually paralyzed, and the pattern of gas distribution is altered in all but the prone position (Fig. 12–3). In both the lateral decubitus and supine positions, gas distribution is more uniform (as measured by the ventilation index; see Fig. 12–3 legend) during mechanical ventilation than during spontaneous breathing, whereas in the sitting position the opposite is true.

This alteration in gas distribution seen during mechanical ventilation is associated with a different pattern of diaphragmatic motion. The motion of the dependent portion of the diaphragm is greater than that of the nondependent portion during spontaneous breathing, as seen in Figure 12–4A for a supine subject (hatched area). Conversely, the nondependent portions of the diaphragm move more than the dependent portions during mechanical ventilation in a paralyzed subject, as shown in Figure 12–4B. The relative contribution of the rib cage to the tidal volume is also altered during mechanical ventilation. In recumbent persons, the relative contribution of the rib cage is greater during mechanical ventilation than during spontaneous breathing.

During spontaneous breathing, the pattern of chest wall motion is deter-

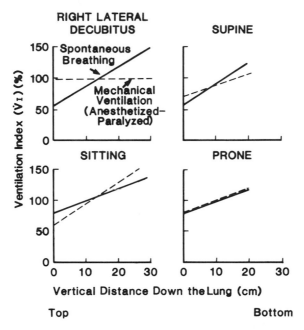

FIGURE 12–3. Intrapulmonary inspired gas distribution is different during mechanical ventilation in anesthetized-paralyzed subjects (dashed lines) from spontaneous breathing in normal subjects (solid lines). The ventilation index is the ratio of measured regional ventilation to that predicted if inspired gas distribution had been uniform. A ventilation index of 100 per cent indicates uniform ventilation; a larger index indicates regional hyperventilation, and a lower index indicates regional hypoventilation. Inspiration was initiated from functional residual capacity, and the tidal volume was equal to 10 per cent of total lung capacity. During spontaneous breathing, gas distribution is nonuniform in all four positions. Compared with that in spontaneous breathing, gas distribution during mechanical ventilation is virtually uniform in the right lateral decubitus position, becomes more uniform in the supine position and becomes less uniform in the seated position. Only in the prone position is there virtually no difference in gas distribution between spontaneous breathing and mechanical ventilation. (Modified from Rehder, K., Knopp, T.J., and Sessler, A.D.: Regional intrapulmonary gas distribution in awake and anesthetized-paralyzed prone man. *J. Appl. Physiol., 45*:528–535, 1978.)

mined by the balance between the regional muscular expanding forces and the regional impeding forces. During mechanical ventilation, the regional expanding forces are no longer dependent on muscle contraction but are provided by the relatively uniform increase in alveolar gas pressure. Thus, the pattern of motion during mechanical ventilation at conventionally used respiratory frequencies is determined by the distribution of regional elastances (reciprocal of compliance) within the lung and chest wall. Therefore, nonuniform lung disease may alter gas distribution during mechanical ventilation. The alteration in gas distribution during mechanical ventilation suggests that the action of the respiratory muscles is an important determinant of inspired gas distribution during spontaneous breathing. Consider the gas distribution in the prone and supine

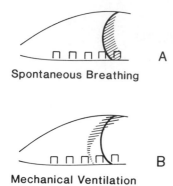

Spontaneous Breathing

A

Mechanical Ventilation

B

FIGURE 12–4. Diagrammatic representation of the pattern of motion of the diaphragm in a supine subject. The hatched area depicts the motion of the diaphragm during spontaneous breathing *(A)* and mechanical ventilation *(B)*. The solid line represents the position of the diaphragm in the awake subject lying supine at end-expiration. Note different movements of the diaphragm between spontaneous breathing and mechanical ventilation. (Modified from Froese, A.B., and Bryan, A.C.: Effects of anesthesia and paralysis on diaphragmatic mechanics in man. *Anesthesiology, 41:*242–255, 1974.)

positions during spontaneous breathing (see Fig. 12–3). The respiratory muscles cause the different gas distribution, since gas distribution in these two positions is similar when the muscles are not functioning during mechanical ventilation. Gas distribution is also different during mechanical ventilation in various body positions (see Fig. 12–3), suggesting that the direction in which gravity acts on the respiratory system is a major determinant of gas distribution.

Positive End-Expiratory Pressure

Positive end-expiratory pressure (PEEP) is used in conjunction with mechanical ventilation (Fig. 12–5). Interestingly, certain subjects maintain an increased end-expiratory pressure (*physiologic PEEP*) and lung volume spontaneously through activation of inspiratory muscles or through adduction of the vocal cords (called glottic throttling). Endotracheal intubation of such patients leads to a loss of the "physiologic PEEP" and a reduction in end-expiratory lung volume.

PEEP is used clinically to improve arterial oxygenation. The rationale for the use of PEEP is that end-expiratory lung volume is low in patients with

FIGURE 12–5. Diagrammatic representation of airway pressure during mechanical ventilation with 0 end-expiratory pressure *(A)* and with positive end-expiratory pressure (PEEP) *(B)*.

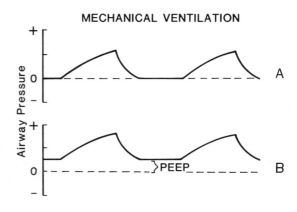

MECHANICAL VENTILATION

acute respiratory failure. The low lung volume is often associated with closure of small airways, particularly in the dependent lung regions. Lung regions that have closed airways are not ventilated, and perfusion of these regions results in arterial hypoxemia. PEEP can hold the airways open throughout the entire respiratory cycle and may restore ventilation to previously perfused but unventilated regions, improving oxygenation.

PEEP has many disadvantages, however. Hyperinflation of previously expanded alveoli can impair their perfusion (producing zone I conditions), resulting in an increase in physiologic dead space. Increased perfusion to lung regions with low ventilation-to-perfusion ratios results in a lower arterial P_{O_2} because PEEP causes blood flow to shift from the well-ventilated nondependent lung regions to the poorly ventilated dependent regions, resulting in a further reduction of their $\dot{V}_A/\dot{Q}$. PEEP can also decrease tissue oxygenation by decreasing cardiac output; this reduction in cardiac output is primarily caused by a decrease in venous return. High levels of PEEP (greater than 15 cmH$_2$O) may also impair left ventricular function by causing a shift in the interventricular septum. Normally, the interventricular septum bulges into the right ventricle (Fig. 12–6). With high levels of PEEP, however, the septum becomes flat, reducing left ventricular size. A larger pressure is now necessary to fill the left ventricle to a given volume (decreased left ventricular compliance). This decrease in left ventricular compliance is amplified by an intact, nondistensible pericardium.

On the other hand, cardiac output occasionally increases during the application of PEEP because a severe systemic hypoxemia has been corrected. The carotid and aortic chemoreceptors cause an increased peripheral vascular resistance during hypoxia; when hypoxia is corrected, vascular resistance falls. As a result, left ventricular afterload is reduced, and cardiac output may increase. The ultimate effect of PEEP on the cardiovascular system depends on the interrelationships among lung mechanics, intravascular blood volume, and effects on cardiac function.

The magnitude of the increase in lung volume caused by PEEP is determined by the slope and position of the pressure-volume curve as well as by the pressure applied to the airway, as seen in Figure 12–7. Point A refers to the change in lung volume during mechanical ventilation with an increase in airway pressure of 10 cmH$_2$O without PEEP. With 20 cmH$_2$O of PEEP, an increase in airway pressure of 10 cmH$_2$O results in a larger increase in lung volume (point B). In patients with acute respiratory failure, airways that have

FIGURE 12–6. Short-axis view of right (RV) and left (LV) ventricles. *A,* The normal ventricular septum (convex to the right ventricle). *B,* The flattening of the ventricular septum with PEEP. This flattening reduces the size of the left ventricle and therefore reduces cardiac output.

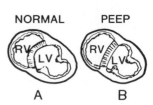

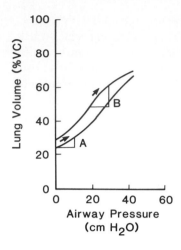

FIGURE 12–7. Pressure-volume curve of a subject with respiratory failure and a low lung volume without PEEP (lower curve). Inflation of the lungs with a peak pressure of 10 cmH_2O airway pressure results in only a small increase in lung volume (A). Application of 20 cmH_2O PEEP causes a shift of the pressure-volume curve upward and an increased end-expiratory lung volume as shown by the zero pressure intercept. Now inflation of the lungs from an airway pressure of 20 to 30 cmH_2O results in a larger increase in lung volume (B).

closed may be reopened by PEEP. Recruitment of these regions reduces the elastic forces opposing the inflation of the lung. This recruitment also reduces the resistive forces opposing lung inflation since airway diameters increase as lung volume increases. Because of this combined effect, less pressure is required to inflate the lungs using a set volume with PEEP than without PEEP.

Originally, it was believed that PEEP reduced extravascular water in normal or edematous lungs. However, this is not true. PEEP can actually increase fluid accumulation in the lung by increasing filtration of fluid out of the extraalveolar vessels when the perivascular pressure becomes more subatmospheric owing to lung distension. Interstitial or alveolar water is still removed by the pulmonary lymphatics, but this removal is slightly decreased with PEEP. Although PEEP does not reduce fluid accumulation, it does improve pulmonary gas exchange by increasing the surface area of the alveoli, which spreads the accumulated fluid out into a thin layer.

Continuous Positive Airway Pressure

Continuous positive airway pressure (CPAP) is defined as positive end-expiratory pressure administered during *spontaneous* breathing (Fig. 12–8). CPAP is usually applied via an endotracheal tube or with an appropriate face mask. When CPAP is used, resistance to gas flow in the inspiratory limb of the CPAP circuit should be sufficiently low to ensure that the inspiratory effort of the patient does not lower the airway pressure. Also, gas flow into the system should always be in excess of the patient's need. In general, the physiologic effects of CPAP are similar to those of PEEP.

High-Frequency Ventilation

High-frequency ventilation is accomplished by ventilating with small tidal volumes at high frequencies. High-frequency ventilation is categorized into

SPONTANEOUS BREATHING

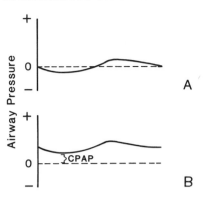

FIGURE 12–8. Diagrammatic representation of airway pressure during spontaneous breathing (A) and during spontaneous breathing with CPAP (B).

three major groups (Fig. 12–9): high-frequency positive pressure ventilation (HFPPV), high-frequency jet ventilation (HFJV), and high-frequency oscillation (HFO) (sometimes also referred to as high-frequency ventilation, HFV). With HFPPV, tidal volumes larger than the anatomic dead space are delivered at frequencies ranging between 60 and 120 breaths/min. With HFJV, a jet of gas is introduced into the airway at frequencies ranging between 100 and 300 breaths/min. HFO uses frequencies as great as 3000 or more per minute.

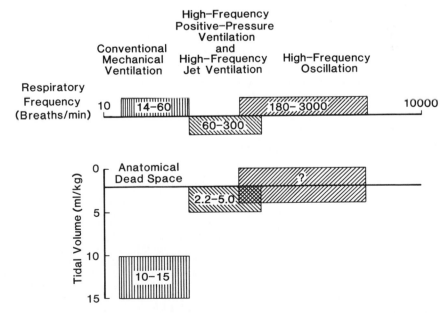

FIGURE 12–9. Tidal volume and breathing frequency (logarithmic scale) during four different modes of mechanical ventilation.

Oscillatory pressure swings are delivered to either the airway or the chest wall to produce HFO.

HIGH-FREQUENCY POSITIVE PRESSURE VENTILATION

HFPPV was developed to study the control of blood pressure by the carotid sinus baroreceptors. These studies required a means to attenuate the fluctuations in blood pressure caused by mechanical ventilation. To reduce these thoracic pressure swings, the lungs were ventilated with small tidal volumes at rates of 60 to 100 breaths/min, which provided adequate alveolar ventilation. For clinical applications, the technique has been modified. Compressed gas is insufflated through the side arm of the system, which functions as a pneumatic valve (Fig. 12–10). At a certain angle between the side arm and the straight tube of the pneumatic valve, the exhalation port is functionally occluded by the streaming gas during insufflation. At end-insufflation, pressure in the side arm approaches 0, allowing the patient to exhale through the straight tube by virtue of the elastic recoil of the respiratory system.

Clinically, HFPPV is used for endoscopic procedures and during general anesthesia. Experience with this technique in patients with respiratory failure is still limited.

HIGH-FREQUENCY JET VENTILATION

HFJV combines the principle of transtracheal jet ventilation with that of high-frequency ventilation. Intermittent jets of gas are delivered into the airways at high frequencies through a small-bore catheter or needle ("jet" in Fig. 12–11). The timing of gas delivery by the jet is controlled by either a rotary valve or an electronic solenoid valve. Gas leaves the small-bore catheter at an extremely high velocity. This high gas velocity lowers the lateral pressure surrounding the jet (Bernoulli principle or Venturi effect), and thus gas is suctioned from the outside, augmenting the gas volume delivered per cycle.

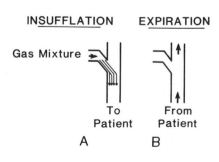

INSUFFLATION   **EXPIRATION**

Gas Mixture

To Patient   From Patient

A   B

FIGURE 12–10. A, The system used for high-frequency positive pressure ventilation (HFPPV). Using a cannula with a correct angle between the side arm and the straight tube, the exhalation port is functionally occluded by the gas flow during insufflation. B, During expiration the pressure in the side arm becomes 0 and the subject exhales, by virtue of the elastic recoil pressure of the respiratory system, through the straight tube. (From Sjöstrand, U.: Review of the physiological rationale for and development of high-frequency positive-pressure ventilation—HFPPV. Acta Anaesthesiol. Scand., Suppl. 64:7–27, 1977.)

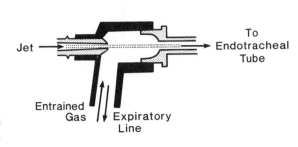

FIGURE 12–11. With high-frequency jet ventilation (HFJV), intermittent jets of gas (dots) are delivered through the cannula inserted into the lumen of the airway. When the jet is stopped, the subject exhales using the elastic recoil pressure of the respiratory system. (Modified from Carlon, G.C., Miodownik, S., Ray, C. Jr., and Kahn, R.C.: Technical aspects and clinical implications of high frequency jet ventilation with a solenoid valve. *Crit. Care Med.* 9:47–50, 1981.)

The delivered gas volume is a function of the diameter of the catheter, the velocity of the gas, and the alveolar gas pressure.

HFJV provides adequate pulmonary gas exchange, but CO_2 is retained at rates higher than 300 breaths/min. HFJV has been advocated for certain surgical operations and for treatment of bronchopleural fistulas, but more information is needed to judge the efficacy of its usage in these conditions. It is not known whether the stress on the bronchial wall during HFJV is less than, equal to, or greater than that associated with conventional mechanical ventilation.

When the upper airway is partially obstructed, transtracheal HFJV can have lethal consequences. This occurs because gas continues to enter the lungs owing to the high inflation pressure generated by the ventilator, but the respiratory system's recoil is insufficient to properly empty the lung. Therefore, gas volume continues to accumulate in the lung during ventilation. The lungs rapidly become overdistended and rupture. Recently, ventilators have been modified with built-in safeguards to prevent overdistension.

HIGH-FREQUENCY OSCILLATION

With HFO, displacement of gas volume is generated by the movement of a piston pump or some other type of oscillator. The output from the oscillator is directed to a manifold (Fig. 12–12) to which several other tubes are connected. Gas flows through the manifold into the endotracheal tube, and excess gas plus expired gas exit via the manifold through a bias tube. The diameter and length of the bias tube are such that the tube offers a high impedance to high frequencies and a low impedance to low frequencies. Therefore, the bias tube directs most of the high-frequency oscillations to the lungs. The gas volume delivered to the lungs depends on the relative impedances of the bias tube and the respiratory system. Impedance of the respiratory system increases if the lungs become stiff and/or airway resistance increases. With HFO, this increase in impedance results in more gas leaving through the bias tube and less gas being delivered to the lungs.

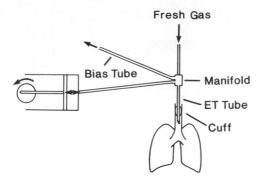

FIGURE 12–12. The output from an oscillation generator (in this example, a piston pump) is directed into a manifold. The bias tube has a high impedance to the high frequencies generated by the pump but a low impedance to low frequencies. ET = cuffed endotracheal tube.

It has been assumed, but not necessarily validated, that the gas volume delivered by HFO is less than the stroke volume of the ventilator (the volume of gas moved per oscillation). But the delivered gas volume can actually exceed the stroke volume of the oscillation generator. This amplification is due to resonance. When the ventilator produces oscillations at the resonant frequency of the entire circuit, the volume of gas delivered will be enhanced. Because of resonant amplification of the delivered gas volume, lung volume must be carefully controlled during HFO to prevent overinflation.

CO_2 elimination during HFO can be adjusted by changing the combination of stroke volume and oscillatory frequency. The optimal combinations of stroke volume and oscillatory frequency for CO_2 elimination have not been defined. Oxygenation during HFO is regulated by adjusting the inspired oxygen concentration and the lung volume.

The magnitude of cyclic airway pressure swings associated with HFO is different from that during conventional mechanical ventilation. With HFO, the amplitude of airway pressure swings is small and is symmetrically distributed about the mean airway pressure (Fig. 12–13). Compared with conventional mechanical ventilation, the minimal airway pressure is higher and the maximal pressure is lower with HFO. As a result, more alveoli remain open during expiration, but fewer are recruited during inspiration. Intermittent sustained hyperinflations of 15 to 30 seconds' duration have been recommended to promote and maintain recruitment of closed lung units.

Earlier reports suggested that pulmonary gas exchange was improved with HFO. It now appears that pulmonary gas exchange during HFO is no better than that obtained using conventional mechanical ventilation in adult patients with acute respiratory failure. In our opinion, no clear indication for the clinical use of HFO in adults has been established. Whether HFO will be more useful in neonates with infant respiratory distress syndrome is questionable.

GAS TRANSPORT DURING HFO

During spontaneous breathing and conventional mechanical ventilation, gas is moved to the respiratory zone by convection. Once gas arrives in the

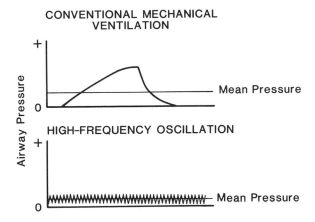

FIGURE 12–13. Diagrammatic representation of airway pressure during conventional mechanical ventilation without PEEP and during high-frequency oscillation. The maximal pressure is less and the minimal pressure is larger with high-frequency oscillation than with conventional mechanical ventilation. Mean airway pressure is also lower during high-frequency oscillation than during conventional mechanical ventilation.

respiratory zone, molecular diffusion is the predominant means of gas movement. With HFO, the gas volume delivered to the lungs with each respiratory cycle is often less than the volume of the anatomic dead space. According to conventional thinking, pulmonary gas exchange should not occur under this condition. How then can pulmonary gas exchange occur when the tidal volume is less than the anatomic dead space?

Several mechanisms have been suggested to explain this phenomenon. First, some airways are shorter than others. Thus, bulk convection may supply fresh gas to the respiratory zone of these lung regions, even when the total gas volume delivered per cycle is less than the anatomic dead space volume. Second, velocity profiles in the airways are different during inspiration from those during expiration. This difference in velocity profiles may increase the net transport of gas. To understand this phenomenon, it is useful to consider a model with a tracer placed into a straight tube to which an oscillatory flow with equal displacements to the left and right is imposed (Fig. 12–14). Assume that a parabolic velocity profile develops during the movement of the plug of tracer to the right, and that a flat velocity profile exists as the tracer moves to the left. As a consequence, a net movement of the tracer to the right occurs in the center of the tube, whereas the tracer close to the wall moves to the left (Fig. 12–14C). This would cause a to-and-fro motion of gas. Finally, a combination of axial convection and radial mixing may be the most important mechanism for gas transport. During HFO, molecular diffusion contributes to gas transport in the respiratory zone, but convection is the predominant means of gas transport.

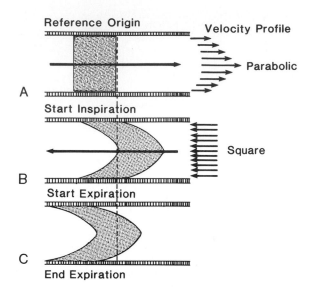

FIGURE 12–14. Diagrammatic representation of gas transport during high-frequency oscillation (HFO) due to the different velocity profiles during inspiration and expiration. A parabolic velocity profile develops during inspiration *(A)*, whereas a flat velocity profile exists during expiration *(B)*. This results in net movement of the tracer to the right (toward the lung) in the center of the tube, whereas a net movement to the left occurs close to the wall at end-expiration *(C)*. (From Haselton, F.R., and Scherer, P.W.: Bronchial bifurcations and respiratory mass transport. *Science, 208*:69–71, 1980.)

Indications for Mechanical Ventilation

Mechanical ventilation for short periods is widely used in surgical anesthesia. Curare-like drugs are used to induce muscle paralysis, allowing anesthesiologists to maintain patients at light planes of anesthesia while providing excellent surgical conditions. The resulting respiratory muscle paralysis makes mechanical ventilation necessary. Even when curare-like drugs are not administered, mechanical ventilation is often used during general anesthesia, since many anesthetics and narcotics depress ventilatory drive and limit the efficacy of spontaneous breathing.

Long-term mechanical ventilation is necessary to treat patients with respiratory failure. Mechanical ventilation is also indicated in patients with primary ventilatory failure, i.e., when disturbances of the nervous, muscular, or skeletal apparatus (such as myasthenia gravis, poliomyelitis, polyneuritis, tetanus, chest wall trauma, or chronic hypoventilation syndrome) exist. Patients with bronchial asthma are candidates for mechanical ventilation when hypercapnia and respiratory muscle failure develop.

Mechanical ventilation is also used prophylactically in patients with impending respiratory failure. Respiratory muscles, including the diaphragm, will fatigue when their rate of energy consumption is greater than the energy supplied to them. Reduced cardiac output and/or hypoxemia favor the development of muscle fatigue, since they reduce energy supply. Subjects breathing at high lung volume are particularly susceptible to muscle fatigue because respiratory muscles can develop only small pressures, yet their energy consumption is high. Muscular atrophy or neuromuscular disease also predisposes the respiratory muscles to fatigue. Hypophosphatemia has been associated with respiratory muscle fatigue owing to depletion of ATP stores.

Even though general guidelines are available to indicate when mechanical ventilation should be used (Table 12–3), good clinical judgment is also required to assess the trend of the disease.

COMPLICATIONS OF MECHANICAL VENTILATION

Mechanical ventilation usually requires endotracheal intubation or a tracheostomy to ensure a patent airway. The trachea can be intubated via the mouth (orotracheal intubation) or the nares (nasotracheal intubation). The latter should probably be avoided in subjects who have a tendency for nose bleeding. Excessive movement of the tube against the vocal cords may lead to ulcers of the vocal cords, with subsequent development of granulomas. Edema of the larynx and trachea also occurs, but tracheal stenosis, tracheomalacia, and tracheal perforation at the site of the endotracheal tube cuff or the tracheostomy stoma are rare. The incidence of serious complications has declined with the widespread use of plastic nontoxic endotracheal tubes equipped with low-pressure, high-volume cuffs. Sinusitis, otitis media, and nosocomial infections of the respiratory system are complications associated with nasotracheal intubation.

TABLE 12–3. General Indications for Tracheal Intubation and Conventional Mechanical Ventilation in Adults

Variable	Range of Normal Values	Tracheal Intubation and Mechanical Ventilation Indicated
Mechanics		
Respiratory rate (breaths/min)	12–20	>35
Vital capacity (ml/kg*)	65–75	<15
FEV$_1$ (ml/kg)	50–60	<10
Maximal inspiratory force at FRC (cmH$_2$O)	90–130	<25
Oxygenation		
Pa$_{O_2}$ (mmHg)	75–100	<70 (on mask O$_2$)
(A − a)D$_{O_2}$ (mmHg)	25–65	>450 (on mask O$_2$)
Ventilation		
Pa$_{CO_2}$ (mmHg)	35–45	>55†
V$_D$/V$_T$	0.25–0.40	>0.60

*Ideal rather than real weight is used if patient is grossly overweight or underweight.
†Except in patients with chronic hypercapnia.

A frequent complication associated with tracheal intubation is intubation of a mainstem bronchus, which prevents proper ventilation of the opposite lung. In the adult, right-sided endobronchial intubation is more common than left-sided, but in the infant or small child there is an equal disposition to intubate either main bronchus. In the adult, the right mainstem bronchus is more likely to be intubated because it branches at a less acute angle than the left. Intubation of the mainstem bronchus is diagnosed on the basis of absent breath sounds over the nonventilated lung, the roentgenogram of the chest, asymmetric chest wall motion, and/or hypoxemia. Occasionally, the cuff at the distal end of the endotracheal tube "herniates" over the distal tip of the endotracheal tube, causing a ball-valve-type obstruction of the airway. When this herniation occurs, the lungs can be inflated, but the patient cannot exhale. This is a serious complication resulting in cardiovascular insufficiency, which must be corrected immediately by deflating the cuff.

Mechanical ventilation is not a totally innocuous intervention, particularly when used on a long-term basis. Inadequate humidification of the inspired gas mixture may lead to retention of secretions, resulting in airway obstruction. Constant volume ventilation with low or normal tidal volumes is often associated with the development of atelectasis, which is suspected when the compliance of the respiratory system decreases and when hypoxemia develops. In the past, a high incidence of bleeding from stress ulcers of the gastric mucosa has been associated with long-term mechanical ventilation, but this problem has been almost eliminated by routinely using an antacid combined with a histamine H-2 receptor blocker.

Barotrauma of the lungs may occur, particularly when high airway pressures are necessary to adequately oxygenate the blood. Emphysematous blebs or injured lung regions are the predominant sites for lung rupture. A tension pneumothorax, which is usually associated with hypoxia and progressive increases in peak inflation pressure, may develop. With barotrauma, gas usually follows the perivascular and peribronchial spaces, moving into the mediastinum and subcutaneous tissue (subcutaneous emphysema). In rare instances, gas enters the vascular system, resulting in air emboli.

Hepatic dysfunction and reduction in urine output with salt and water retention are other complications sometimes associated with mechanical ventilation in patients with acute respiratory failure. The underlying mechanisms for the hepatic dysfunction are complex and are probably related to a reduction in splanchnic blood flow. The release of antidiuretic hormone, lowered renal perfusion, and enhanced angiotensin-aldosterone secretion are probably responsible for the observed salt and water retention.

SUGGESTED READING

Fisher, A.B., and Forman, H.J.: Oxygen utilization and toxicity in the lungs. In Fishman, A.P., and Fisher, A.B. (eds.): *Handbook of Physiology.* The Respiratory System, Volume I: Circulation and nonrespiratory functions. Bethesda: APS, 1985, pp. 231–254.

Froese, A.B., and Bryan, A.C.: High frequency ventilation. *Am. Rev. Respir. Dis.*, *135*:1363–1374, 1987.

Rehder, K., and Marsh, H.M.: Respiratory mechanics during anesthesia and mechanical ventilation. In Macklem, P.T., and Mead, J. (eds): *Handbook of Physiology:* Section 3, The Respiratory System, Volume III. Bethesda: APS, 1986, pp. 737–752.

QUESTIONS

1. List the types of hypoxemia and their most common causes.
2. What is the underlying mechanism for oxygen toxicity?
3. Name the mechanisms that can contribute to low cardiac output with PEEP.
4. Describe the effect of PEEP on extravascular lung water.
5. What are the three types of high-frequency ventilation?

ACID-BASE BUFFER SYSTEMS
Henderson-Hasselbalch Equation
Physiologic Buffers
The Carbonic Acid, HCO_3^- Buffer System

RENAL H^+ and HCO_3^- REGULATION
HCO_3^- Salvage
Formation of Titratable Acid
Ammonia/Ammonium System

TYPES OF ACIDOSIS AND ALKALOSIS
Davenport pH-HCO_3^- Diagram
Respiratory Acidosis
Respiratory Alkalosis
Metabolic Acidosis
Metabolic Alkalosis
Siggaard-Andersen Nomogram
Anion Gap
Other Measurements

13

REGULATION OF ACID-BASE BALANCE

Before describing the body's response to changes in hydrogen ion concentration ($[H^+]$) in the body fluids, a brief review of acid-base theory is necessary. An acid is a substance that can donate a proton (H^+), whereas a base is a substance that can accept a proton. Although most protons in the body react with water to form hydronium ions (H_3O^+, $H_5O_2^+$, $H_7O_3^+$, and $H_9O_4^+$), assume, for the sake of simplicity, that only hydrogen ion is formed. The $[H^+]$ in plasma is extremely low (40 nmoles/l) as compared with the concentrations of sodium and potassium ions (140 $\times$ 10^6 and 4 $\times$ 10^6 nmoles/l, respectively). The $[H^+]$ of the interstitial fluid is slightly lower than that of plasma because of the Donnan effect related to plasma proteins, whereas the $[H^+]$ within the cell is higher (about 160 nmoles/l).

The $[H^+]$ is expressed in terms of pH, which is a measure of the acidity or alkalinity of a solution. pH is defined as the negative logarithm of the $[H^+]$:

$$pH = -\log[H^+]$$

A solution with a pH greater than 7 is basic, whereas one with a pH of less than 7 is acidic. Extracellular body fluids have an average pH of 7.4, i.e., they are slightly basic.

Expressing $[H^+]$ in terms of pH has two main advantages. First, it is convenient for expressing a wide range of hydrogen ion concentrations. Second, it is useful when evaluating different buffer systems, as will be discussed later. Use of the pH scale, however, may cause problems in conceptualizing the amount of acid in solution. For instance, a relatively small change in pH from 7.7 (20 nmoles/l) to 7.4 (40 nmoles/l) corresponds to a doubling of H^+ concentration.

Acids are defined as weak or strong according to how well they dissociate in H_2O. HCl is a very strong acid since it almost completely dissociates into H^+ and Cl^-, but most other biologic acids (such as carbonic acid, H_2CO_3) are weak acids and dissociate to a much smaller extent.

Hydrogen ions are very reactive, and their small size allows them to diffuse rather easily in biologic fluids. Hydrogen ions interact readily with negatively charged ions. Binding of hydrogen ions to negatively charged sites on an enzyme can alter the enzyme's specificity and activity by causing conformational changes in protein structure. Similarly, structural proteins can be damaged in the presence of excessive hydrogen ions. To prevent excessive changes in pH, several systems are present in the body in which the addition of acid or alkali causes far smaller changes in pH than would occur in water alone. The simplest of these systems, which are called buffer systems, is a combination of a weak acid (HA) and its conjugate base (A-).

ACID-BASE BUFFER SYSTEMS

Henderson-Hasselbalch Equation

Acids (HA) dissociate in water:

$$[HA] + [H_2O] \underset{k_2}{\overset{k_1}{\rightleftarrows}} [H_3O^+] + [A^-] \tag{13-1}$$

where k_1 and k_2 are reaction constants. The rate of the reaction from left to right (v_1) is proportional to the undissociated acid and water concentrations:

$$v_1 = k_1 [HA] [H_2O] \tag{13-2}$$

and from right to left (v_2) is proportional to the hydronium and conjugate base concentrations:

$$v_2 = k_2 [H_3O^+] [A^-] \tag{13-3}$$

In a steady state, $v_1 = v_2$. Therefore,

$$k_1 [HA] [H_2O] = k_2 [H_3O^+] [A^-]$$

and

$$\frac{k_1}{k_2} = \frac{[H_3O^+] [A^-]}{[HA] [H_2O]} \tag{13-4}$$

where k_1/k_2 is defined as the equilibrium constant (K). Equation 13-4 can be rewritten as:

$$K = \frac{[H_3O^+] [A^-]}{[HA] [H_2O]} \tag{13-5}$$

or, more simply

$$K' = \frac{[H^+] [A^-]}{[HA]} \tag{13-6}$$

where K' is the dissociation constant. The larger the K', the stronger the acid, since K' is a ratio of the concentration of dissociated acid ($[H^+] [A^-]$) to the concentration of undissociated acid (HA).

To obtain the Henderson-Hasselbalch equation, Equation 13-6 is rewritten as:

$$[H^+] = K' \frac{[HA]}{[A^-]}$$

or

$$\log [H^+] = \log K' + \log \frac{[HA]}{[A^-]}$$

Since pH $= -\log[H^+]$, $-\log K' = pK$, and $-\log [HA]/[A^-] = \log [A^-]/[HA]$ then

$$pH = pK + \log \frac{[A^-]}{[HA]} \tag{13-7}$$

The ability of a buffer system to minimize fluctuations in pH is dependent on two factors. The first of these factors is the pH of the buffer relative to the pH of the body fluids. When pH equals pK, the amount of the dissociated acid equals the concentration of undissociated acid, and their ratio is 1. Since log 1 = 0, the buffer is at its maximum buffering capacity because it can accept acid or alkali equally well. The second factor is the concentration of the buffer. If more buffer is available to act with the acid or alkali, the system is more effective. For instance, the phosphate buffer has an ideal pK (6.8) for buffering changes in pH since its pK is near body pH, but its concentration is so low that it is not an effective plasma buffer.

The *isohydric principle* states that all buffer systems contribute to buffering changes in body fluid pH and are in dynamic equilibrium:

$$pH = pK_1 + \log \frac{[A_1^-]}{[HA_1]} = pK_2 + \log \frac{[A_2^-]}{[HA_2]} = pK_n + \log \frac{[A_n^-]}{[HA_n]} \quad (13\text{--}8)$$

Although all buffers must finally reach an equilibrium with respect to pH in plasma, it should be understood that plasma and red blood cells cannot be considered to be in the same isohydric system, since their pHs are different.

Physiologic Buffers

Table 13–1 shows the various components of the major buffer systems in body fluids and their efficiencies in buffering changes in fixed acid concentrations. In plasma, phosphate ions contribute 2 per cent, plasma proteins contribute 23 per cent, and bicarbonate ions contribute 75 per cent to the buffering of fixed acids. Similar buffers are present in the interstitial fluids, but the lower protein concentration limits their buffering capacity. Red cells contain large amounts of hemoglobin, which contributes 60 per cent of the buffering capacity of this cell. In addition, red cells also contain organic phosphates and HCO_3^-, which are responsible for the remaining buffering capacity. Within other cells of the body, such as muscle, the cellular proteins provide about one-half of the buffering capacity, whereas organic phosphates provide most of the remaining buffering capacity.

TABLE 13–1. Buffering Components of Body Fluids Compartments

Buffer	pK	Relative or Actual Concentrations	Fixed Acid Buffering (%)
Plasma			
Phosphate buffer	6.8	Low	2
Plasma proteins (histidine)	5.5–8.5	7 gm%	23
HCO_3^-	6.1	24 meq/l	75
Red Cells			
Proteins (Hb, histidine, N-terminal valine)	5.5–8.5	High	60
HCO_3^-	6.1	10 meq/l	30
Phosphate buffer	6.8	Low	10
Interstitial Fluid			
HCO_3^-	6.1	26 meq/l	90
Phosphate buffer	6.8	Low	1
Proteins	5.5–8.5	2 gm%	9
Other Cells			
HCO_3^-	6.1	10 meq/l	2
Proteins (histidine)	5.5–8.5	High	50
Phosphate buffer	6.8	High	48

The Carbonic Acid, HCO_3^- Buffer System

Figure 13–1 is a graphic representation of the Henderson-Hasselbalch equation for the bicarbonate buffer system. Note that the change in pH is the smallest for added acid or added base (i.e., the buffering capacity is maximal) on either side of the pK. At a normal plasma pH of 7.4 (which is more than one pH unit above the pK of the bicarbonate buffer system), pH changes greatly with only small additions in acid or base. For instance, the addition of base at a pH equal to the pK causes an increase in pH from point A to point B (0.4 unit). Addition of another equal amount of base causes the pH to change from point B to point C (1.5 units). This example illustrates that the buffer capacity of the bicarbonate system is relatively poor at normal plasma pH (7.4).

Why then is the bicarbonate system such an important buffer? The answer to this question can be seen from the basic Henderson-Hasselbalch equation:

$$pH = pK + \log [(HCO_3^-)/(H_2CO_3)]$$

for the reaction

$$CO_2 + H_2O \rightarrow H_2CO_3 \rightarrow H^+ + HCO_3^- \qquad (13\text{–}9)$$

Since CO_2 has a concentration 400 times greater than that of H_2CO_3, the Henderson-Hasselbalch equation can be rewritten with only $[CO_2]$ to represent the total carbonic acid pool ($[CO_2] + [H_2CO_3]$). Therefore,

$$pH = pK + \log \frac{[HCO_3^-]}{[CO_2]} \qquad (13\text{–}10)$$

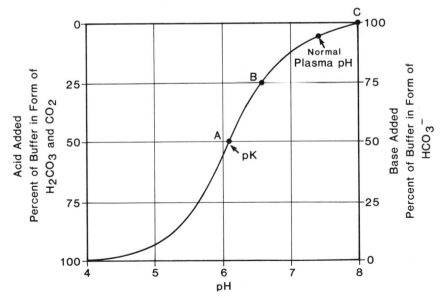

FIGURE 13–1. Titration curve for the bicarbonate buffer system (pH = 6.1 + log $[HCO_3^-]$/$[CO_2]$).

The concentration of CO_2 is directly proportional to its partial pressure (P_{CO_2}) and its solubility coefficient in plasma, which is equal to 0.03 meq/l/mmHg. Therefore,

$$pH = 6.1 + \log \frac{[HCO_3^-]}{0.03\ P_{CO_2}} \qquad (13–11)$$

where P_{CO_2} is in mmHg and $[HCO_3^-]$ is in meq/l. When acid is added to the body fluids, H^+ combines with HCO_3^-, producing H_2CO_3. H_2CO_3 then dissociates to H_2O and CO_2. The CO_2 is then eliminated by the lungs, which decreases P_{CO_2} and lessens the fall in pH that would otherwise occur. Bicarbonate is such an important buffer system because P_{CO_2}, and consequently H_2CO_3 concentration, can be controlled by respiration. Changes in the numerator of Equation 13–11 are almost perfectly balanced with changes in the denominator by the lung's elimination of CO_2, so that the pH change is minimized.

From Equation 13–11, it can be seen that pH is inversely related to P_{CO_2}:

$$pH \propto \frac{1}{P_{CO_2}}$$

and CO_2 is inversely related to alveolar ventilation ($\dot{V}_A$) (as derived in Equation 2–11):

$$P_{CO_2} \propto 1/\dot{V}_A$$

So,

$$pH \propto \dot{V}_A \qquad (13–12)$$

Therefore, when alveolar ventilation is increased, pH increases because CO_2 is eliminated and vice versa. Once body pH is changed, the respiratory system rapidly responds to return the pH toward normal. Figure 13–2 shows the relationship between pH and alveolar ventilation. When alveolar ventilation doubles, pH changes from 7.4 (point A) to 7.63 (point B), showing how effectively changes in ventilation can alter pH. The ability of the lungs to quickly eliminate CO_2 provides a buffering capacity two times greater than that of all other buffering components in the body. The final pH value is then fine tuned by the kidney's ability to regulate hydrogen and bicarbonate ion concentrations in the plasma as well as by elimination of organic acids, which occurs more slowly.

RENAL H^+ AND HCO_3^- REGULATION

In addition to eliminating organic acids, the kidney uses three basic mechanisms to regulate the acid-base balance of body fluids: (1) the salvage of bi-

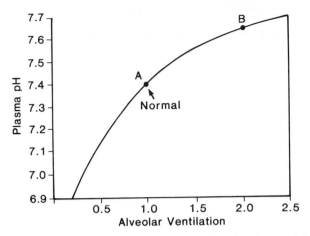

FIGURE 13–2. Change in plasma pH associated with relative alveolar ventilation. Normal alveolar ventilation = 1. Point A is normal pH, and point B represents the change in pH associated with a two-fold increase in alveolar ventilation.

carbonate from tubular fluids in exchange for CO_2, (2) the formation of titratable acid, which represents an actual loss of body H^+ into the urine, and (3) hydrogen removal from the body as ammonium ions.

HCO_3^- Salvage

Figure 13–3 is a schematic of a renal epithelial cell showing the pathways involved in the salvage of HCO_3^-. This involves the hydration of CO_2 to H_2CO_3 in the presence of carbonic anhydrase (CA) within the cell. The H_2CO_3 then dissociates into H^+ and HCO_3^-. Hydrogen ions move into the lumen of the renal tubules via a countertransport system with Na^+. The H^+ combines with filtered HCO_3^- to form H_2CO_3, which then forms H_2O and CO_2. CO_2 then diffuses back into the cell to again combine with water, and the cycle starts again. The HCO_3^- generated in the cell enters the interstitium in combination with the Na^+, which is actively transported across the basal epithelial membrane, and enters the peritubular fluid. The overall effect is that H^+ is recycled; no net H^+ is added to the tubular fluids, but 90 per cent of the total filtered load of HCO_3^- is salvaged in this fashion, and the water moves into the tissues to maintain isotonic transport. The amount of HCO_3^- removed from the filtrate is directly related to body P_{CO_2}. When P_{CO_2} is low, less CO_2 enters the tubular cells and less HCO_3^- can be recovered. Conversely, when P_{CO_2} is high in body fluids, more HCO_3^- is removed from the filtrate in an attempt to buffer the changes in plasma pH. When plasma K^+ levels are high, H^+ may not be adequately secreted into the lumen of the renal tubules, since K^+ and H^+ compete for the same active transport system.

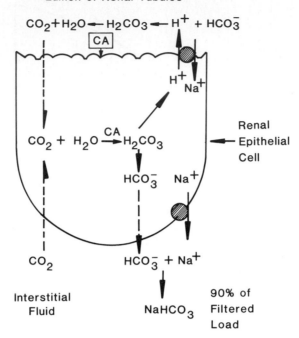

FIGURE 13–3. Bicarbonate salvage from renal tubular fluid. ↑ refers to an active transport process, and the dashed arrows refer to passive diffusion.

Formation of Titratable Acid

The H^+ actively secreted into the renal tubular fluids can combine with $H_2PO_4^-$ to form a titratable acid (TA), which enters the urine (Fig. 13–4). In the tubular epithelium, CO_2 is rapidly hydrated to form H_2CO_3 in the presence of carbonic anhydrase. The H_2CO_3 then dissociates into HCO_3^- and H^+. The intracellular H^+ is secreted by the Na^+ countertransport system into the tubule, where it combines with HPO_4^- to form $H_2PO_4^-$, which is then excreted into the urine as NaH_2PO_4. The HCO_3^- formed within the epithelial cells does not come from an exchange process with the tubular fluids; it is a new HCO_3^-. The newly formed HCO_3^- then moves down its concentration gradient into the interstitial fluids. The net effect is to rid the body fluids of excess H^+ as well as form new HCO_3^-. Since phosphate is concentrated in luminal fluid, and the pH of this fluid is near the pK of the phosphate buffer system (6.8), its buffer capacity is great. The more serious the acidosis, the greater the H^+ elimination and new HCO_3^- formation.

Ammonia/Ammonium System

Figure 13–5 shows how ammonia (NH_3) formed by the renal tubular cells causes H^+ excretion and HCO_3^- conservation. In the presence of carbonic

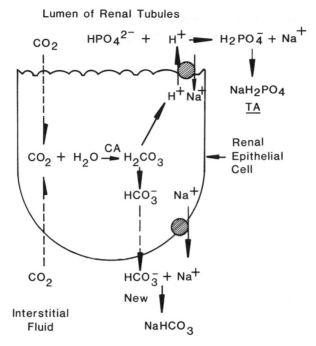

FIGURE 13–4. Renal phosphate buffer system showing tubular excretion of H^+ and conservation of HCO_3^-. TA refers to titratable acid, ↑ signifies an active transport process, and the dashed arrows refer to passive diffusion.

anhydrase, the CO_2 entering the cell is rapidly converted to H_2CO_3, which dissociates into H^+ and HCO_3^-. The HCO_3^- diffuses from the cell down its electrochemical gradient to combine with the actively transported Na^+ in the interstitial fluid. The H^+ is actively secreted into the lumen via sodium countertransport. Ammonia, which is produced in the cell from glutamine, diffuses into the lumen of the tubule down its concentration gradient. Once in the lumen, ammonia combines with H^+ and forms ammonium ion (NH_4^+), which cannot diffuse back into the tubular cells and is therefore trapped in the lumen. The NH_4^+ combines with either chloride or sulfate ions to form weak bases. This process reduces the formation of strong acids (such as HCl) in the tubules. Formation of ammonia increases in acidosis, and this increases renal buffering capacity. Table 13–2 shows the amount of titratable acid (TA) and ammonium ion in urine of normal individuals and those with two conditions that alter acid-base balance. Note the large amount of ammonium ion (NH_4^+) and titratable acid (TA) excreted in the patient with diabetic acidosis and the small amount excreted in renal disease. Note that the kidney, even in diabetic acidosis, cannot eliminate over 750 meq/day of acid. Contrast this to the 12,000 meq/day of acid removed by CO_2 elimination in the lungs.

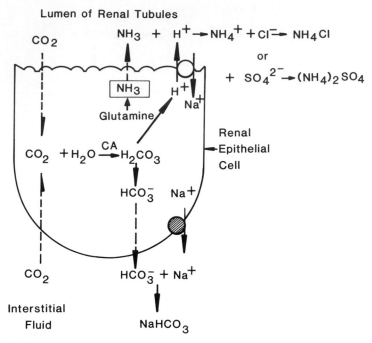

FIGURE 13–5. Tubular H^+ excretion and HCO_3^- conservation related to the ammonium ion. ↑ signifies active transport systems, and dashed arrows refer to passive diffusion.

TYPES OF ACIDOSIS AND ALKALOSIS

Table 13–3 lists several causes of disturbances in acid-base balance and categorizes them in terms of origin (metabolic or respiratory). Respiratory acid-base changes are related to CO_2 elimination. By contrast, metabolic distur-bances in acid-base balance involve either a gain or loss of a fixed acid or bicarbonate in the extracellular fluid. Metabolic acid-base imbalances are op-posed by (1) rapidly altering the amount of CO_2 eliminated by ventilation and (2) renal excretion of excess base or acid into the urine, which requires a longer period of time. A single type of acid-base disturbance is rarely seen; instead, disturbances are usually of mixed origin. Acid-base imbalances are defined as respiratory alkalosis, respiratory acidosis, metabolic acidosis, and metabolic

TABLE 13–2.   Urinary Excretion of H^+ as Ammonium Ion (NH_4^+) and Titratable Acid (TA) in Humans

Condition	Ammonium	Titratable Acid
	(meq of Urinary H^+/day)	
Normal	30–50	10–30
Diabetic acidosis	300–500	75–250
Chronic renal disease	0.5–15	2–20

TABLE 13–3. Causes of Acid-Base Disturbances*

METABOLIC

Acidosis
 Hyperchloremic
  Diarrhea
  Acetazolamide
  IV hyperalimentation
  Interstitial renal disease
  Renal tubular acidosis
 Increased Undetermined Anion
  Generalized renal failure
  Diabetic ketoacidosis
  Alcoholic ketoacidosis
  Lactic acidosis

Alkalosis
  Vomiting
  Nasogastric suction
  Diuretics
  Alkali treatment
  Corticoid treatment
  Severe K^+ depletion
  Cl^- restriction

RESPIRATORY

Acidosis
  Respiratory failure
   Obstructive lung disease
   Chest wall disease
   Mechanical hypoventilation
  CNS depression
  Severe pulmonary edema
  Status asthmaticus
  Primary hypoventilation
  Pneumothorax
  Abdominal distension

Alkalosis
  Hyperventilation
  Gram-negative sepsis
  Pulmonary emboli
  Pneumonia
  Hepatic failure
  High altitude
  Severe anemia

*Revised from Masoro, E.J., and Siegel, P.D.: *Acid-Base Regulation: Its Physiology, Pathophysiology, and the Interpretation of Blood-Gas Analysis,* 2nd ed. Philadelphia: W.B. Saunders, 1977.

alkalosis. Usually, changes in pH tend to be compensated for by either metabolic or respiratory mechanisms. By convention, when the pH of blood is less than 7.4, the condition is referred to as acidemia, and when pH is greater than 7.4, it is called alkalemia.

Davenport pH-HCO$_3^-$ Diagram

The body's response to acidosis or alkalosis can be illustrated using a Davenport diagram, which relates $[HCO_3^-]$ to pH (see Fig. 13–6). Three different buffer lines were drawn by measuring the $[HCO_3^-]$ and pH in response to infusing a fixed acid or base into plasma. In addition, the $[HCO_3^-]$ values are plotted as a function of pH for three different plasma P_{CO_2} values. Point A represents a normal pH (7.4), normal bicarbonate concentration (24 meq/l), and a normal P_{CO_2} of 40 mmHg.

Respiratory Acidosis

Point B in Figure 13–6 defines respiratory acidosis, which is caused by alveolar hypoventilation. Plasma P_{CO_2} increases to 60 mmHg and plasma pH falls below 7.4. In response to acidosis, the kidney conserves HCO_3^- and increases its secretion of H^+. These renal effects cause the plasma pH to approach normal (along the line B $\rightarrow$ D). This condition is *respiratory acidosis* with *renal compensation*.

Respiratory Alkalosis

Point C defines respiratory alkalosis and is due to alveolar hyperventilation. Plasma P_{CO_2} decreases to 20 mmHg, and plasma pH is above 7.4. In response, the kidney secretes less H^+ into the urine and reduces its HCO_3^- absorption, both of which cause the pH of plasma to become more acidic (line C $\rightarrow$ F). This condition defines *respiratory alkalosis* with *renal compensation*.

Metabolic Acidosis

Point G defines metabolic acidosis associated with an abnormal accumulation of fixed acids in plasma. Note that plasma P_{CO_2} is 40 mmHg, plasma pH is below 7.4, and plasma $[HCO_3^-]$ is below normal. The central chemoreceptors are activated, and alveolar ventilation increases (line G $\rightarrow$ F), increasing CO_2 elimination and decreasing pH. This type of acid-base derangement is defined as *metabolic acidosis* with *respiratory compensation*. Strangely, this compensation results in a further reduction in plasma $[HCO_3^-]$. This occurs because the lowered plasma P_{CO_2} decreases renal hydrogen ion secretion and bicarbonate ion absorption. In this case, the renal response to the respiratory compensation associated with the metabolic acidosis is in the wrong direction. However, the respiratory response to acidosis is so strong that the pH returns almost to normal.

Metabolic Alkalosis

Point E defines metabolic alkalosis resulting from loss of H^+ due to nasogastric suction. Plasma P_{CO_2} is 40 mmHg, plasma pH is greater than 7.4, and plasma $[HCO_3^-]$ is above normal. Because of the high plasma pH, the central chemoreceptors are depressed and alveolar ventilation decreases, causing pH to fall as P_{CO_2} builds up in the plasma (line E $\rightarrow$ D). This acid-base derangement is defined as *metabolic alkalosis* with *respiratory compensation*. Again, note that the renal response to the respiratory compensation results in a paradoxic change in plasma $[HCO_3^-]$, i.e., an increase.

In most instances, the patient will not totally compensate for the acid-base imbalance, and the plasma pH will not be normal. Such a patient could have either alkalemia or acidemia.

Siggaard-Andersen Nomogram

There are many ways to plot the variables appearing in the Henderson-Hasselbalch equation, such as that shown in the Davenport diagram (Fig. 13–6), which describes the relationship between plasma pH, $[HCO_3^-]$, and P_{CO_2}.

DAVENPORT DIAGRAM

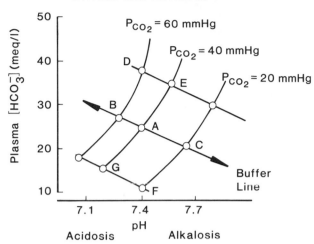

FIGURE 13-6. A Davenport diagram showing [HCO$_3^-$] as a function of pH and P$_{CO_2}$.

Unfortunately, one important component of acid-base balance cannot be obtained from the Davenport plot: *base excess* (BE). Base excess is defined as the amount of acid or base that will restore 1 liter of blood to a normal pH and [HCO$_3^-$] at a P$_{CO_2}$ of 40 mmHg. Base excess can be better understood by using a Siggaard-Andersen nomogram (Fig. 13-7). The log of plasma P$_{CO_2}$ forms the vertical axis, whereas the plasma pH is the horizontal axis. The plasma [HCO$_3^-$] is shown as a series of parallel straight lines (plasma isobicarbonate lines). A base excess curve is shown in the lower quadrants. Positive base excess values indicate alkalosis, whereas negative values indicate acidosis.

Point 0 on the figure represents normal plasma P$_{CO_2}$, pH, and [HCO$_3^-$] of 40 mmHg, 7.4, and 24 meq/l, respectively. When plasma P$_{CO_2}$ is increased to 80 mmHg, plasma pH decreases to 7.08 (point A). Point B is a plasma P$_{CO_2}$ of 20 mmHg, a plasma [HCO$_3^-$] of 24 meq/l, and a plasma pH of 7.71. All possible P$_{CO_2}$ and pH values for a plasma [HCO$_3^-$] of 24 meq/l are on the isobicarbonate line limited by line A → B. Also, note that the isobicarbonate line crosses the base excess curve at 0. The values on line A → 0 define respiratory acidosis, whereas those on line 0 → B define respiratory alkalosis.

If another buffer, in this case hemoglobin, is added to the H$_2$CO$_3$ in plasma, the resulting curve (line C → D) will not lie on a plasma isobicarbonate line. Instead, the curve will be rotated in a clockwise direction, since hemoglobin provides a greater buffering capacity and decreases the net effect of changes in plasma P$_{CO_2}$ on pH as compared with plasma without hemoglobin.

With pure respiratory acidosis or alkalosis, as shown by lines AB and CD, respectively, there is *no* base excess regardless of the buffer present, and plasma pH can be corrected simply by returning ventilation to normal values. Note that in respiratory acidosis all plasma P$_{CO_2}$ and pH values will always be in the

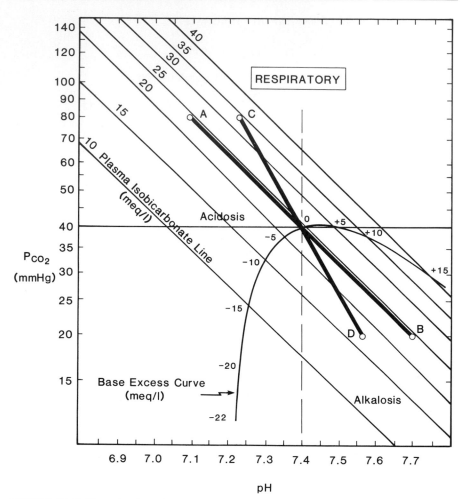

FIGURE 13–7. Normal values for plasma P_{CO_2}, pH, and $[HCO_3^-]$ are shown on a Siggaard-Andersen nomogram at point 0. Also shown are parallel plasma isobicarbonate lines. The base excess curve is shown in the lower quadrants. Line A → B is a normal isobicarbonate line for a plasma $[HCO_3^-]$ of 24 meq/l. Line C → D is constructed by adding hemoglobin to plasma containing a normal $[HCO_3^-]$. Note that lines A → B and C → D intercept the base excess line at 0.

upper left quadrant, whereas all plasma values for P_{CO_2} and pH in respiratory alkalosis are confined to the lower right quadrant.

Figure 13–8 shows plots of metabolic alkalosis and acidosis on a Siggaard-Andersen nomogram for plasma. The metabolic alkalosis point was obtained by increasing plasma $[HCO_3^-]$ to 35 meq/l while holding plasma P_{CO_2} constant at 40 mmHg, which increases plasma pH to 7.55 (point A). The metabolic acidosis point was generated by decreasing plasma $[HCO_3^-]$ to 12 meq/l while holding plasma P_{CO_2} at 40 mmHg, producing a pH of 7.11 (point B). In alkalosis,

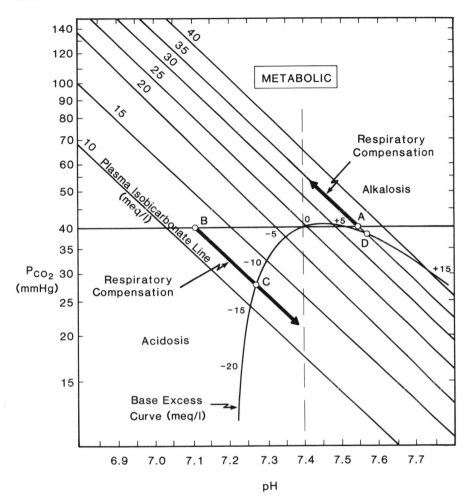

FIGURE 13–8. Metabolic acidosis and alkalosis with respiratory compensation are shown on a Siggaard-Andersen nomogram for plasma P_{CO_2} and pH value. Acidosis is compensated by increasing CO_2 elimination, which returns plasma pH toward normal. Note for metabolic acidosis that the respiratory compensation line crosses the base excess curve at − 13 meq/l (point C). In metabolic alkalosis, CO_2 elimination is decreased, causing plasma pH to return toward normal. In this case the respiratory compensation line crosses the base excess curve at + 11 meq/l (point D).

ventilation rate will decrease, increasing P_{CO_2} along the heavy line in the upper right quadrant, and pH will approach normal. Note that the heavy line intersects the base excess curve at + 11 meq/l (point D), indicating an excess of base. In metabolic acidosis, ventilation rate increases and plasma P_{CO_2} decreases along the heavy line in the lower left quadrant. Note the base excess is now − 13 meq/l (point C), indicating a deficit of 13 meq/l of plasma [HCO_3^-]. This information can be used to calculate the amount of $NaHCO_3$ needed to correct the base deficit and the accompanying acidosis. Assuming that extracellular fluid volume is 30 per cent of body weight, the amount of base that must be added for a 70-kg man equals:

$$NaHCO_3 \text{ added} = 0.3 \times 70 \times BE = 0.3 \times 70 \times 13 \text{ meq/l} = 273 \text{ meq}$$

In practice, one should give one-half this amount and then reassess the acid-base balance before giving more sodium bicarbonate. Note that metabolic acidosis plasma values for P_{CO_2} and pH are confined to the lower left quadrant, whereas all plasma values for metabolic alkalosis are confined to the upper right quadrant.

Anion Gap

Another quick way to estimate the acid-base balance of body fluids is to calculate the anion gap (or undetermined anion concentration). The anion gap, [A-], is defined as the difference between the plasma concentrations of the major cations ($[Na^+] + [K^+]$) and anions ($[Cl^-] + [HCO_3^-]$), i.e.,

$$[A^-] = ([Na^+] + [K^+]) - ([Cl^-] + HCO_3^-]) \qquad (13-13)$$

Figure 13–9 shows the normal concentration of these anions and cations and a normal anion gap of 16 meq/l (A). For metabolic acidosis (B), the excess fixed acids will decrease $[HCO_3^-]$ and cause an increased anion gap (28 meq/l). However, in hyperchloremic acidosis (C), the anion gap may be normal (16 meq/l), showing the potential problem associated with measuring only the anion

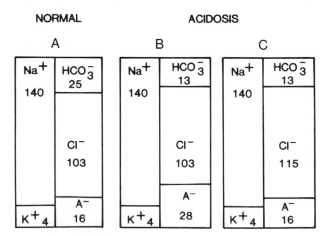

$$\frac{\text{Anion}}{\text{Gap}} = [A^-] = ([Na^+] + [K^+]) - ([Cl^-] + [HCO_3^-]) \text{ (meq/l)}$$

FIGURE 13–9. [Na+], [K+], [HCO₃⁻], [Cl-], and a normal anion gap (A). Metabolic acidosis with increased anion gap (B), and hyperchloremic metabolic acidosis with normal anion gap and increased [Cl-] (C) are also shown.

gap to assess acid-base status. But the anion gap is useful for determining base excess as the difference between the anion gap of the acidosis case and normal values (e.g., $28 - 16 = 12$ meq/l).

Other Measurements

Other measurements related to acid-base include the *standard bicarbonate*, which is measured by equilibrating blood to a P_{CO_2} of 40 mmHg. This will yield a normal plasma $[HCO_3^-]$ if the acid-base imbalance is only due to ventilatory abnormalities (see Fig. 13–7); any change in standard bicarbonate is due to metabolic acidosis or alkalosis. The *actual bicarbonate* is the $[HCO_3^-]$ measured in anaerobically drawn blood plasma.

SUGGESTED READING

Davenport, H.W.: *The ABC of Acid-Base Chemistry*, 6th ed. Chicago: University of Chicago Press, 1974.
Guyton, A.C.: *Textbook of Medical Physiology*, 7th ed. Philadelphia: W.B. Saunders, 1986, Chap. 37.
Masoro, E.J., and Siegel, P.D.: *Acid-Base Regulation: Its Physiology, Pathophysiology, and the Interpretation of Blood-Gas Analysis*, 2nd ed. Philadelphia: W.B. Saunders, 1977.
Mines, A.H.: *Respiratory Physiology.* New York: Raven Press, 1981.
Siggaard-Andersen, O., and Engle, K.: A new acid-base nomogram. An improvised method for the calculation of the relevant blood acid-base data. *Scand. J. Clin. Lab. Invest.*, 12:177–186, 1960.

QUESTIONS

1. If plasma bicarbonate concentration is 23 meq/l and plasma Pa_{CO_2} is 50 mmHg, calculate arterial pH using the Henderson-Hasselbalch equation.
2. Name the three mechanisms the kidney uses to maintain acid-base balance.
3. For each of the conditions below, indicate whether pH, P_{CO_2}, and $[HCO_3^-]$ are increased or decreased.
   a. Respiratory acidosis with renal compensation
   b. Respiratory alkalosis with renal compensation
   c. Metabolic acidosis with respiratory compensation
   d. Metabolic alkalosis with respiratory compensation
4. Given a plasma bicarbonate concentration of 15 meq/l and P_{CO_2} of 50 mmHg, determine the arterial pH and base excess using the Siggaard-Andersen nomogram (see Fig. 13–8) and calculate the amount of sodium bicarbonate required to correct this abnormality in a 70-kg man.

ALTITUDE ADAPTION
  Ventilatory Adjustments to Altitude
  Circulatory Adjustments to Altitude
  Medical Problems at Altitude
    Acute Mountain Sickness
    Chronic Mountain Sickness

DIVING PHYSIOLOGY
  Effect of Depth on Gas Volume and Density
  Gas Partial Pressures at Depth
  Diving Reflex
  Medical Problems Associated with Diving
    Decompression Sickness
    Nitrogen Narcosis
    Oxygen Toxicity

14

ALTITUDE
ADAPTION AND
DIVING
PHYSIOLOGY

Humans can ascend to high altitudes or descend underwater to great depths. In these environments, the body is subjected to conditions that result in hypoxia, hypothermia, and radiation exposure at high altitude; and asphyxia, decompression problems, oxygen toxicity, and high pressure effects during underwater diving. Therefore, it is important to understand the physiologic adaptions that maintain homeostasis under these extreme conditions.

ALTITUDE ADAPTION

The major environmental change associated with living at altitudes much above sea level is a low ambient P_{O_2}. The ambient barometric pressure (P_B) at sea level is 760 mmHg. P_B decreases progressively by approximately one-half for each 5,500 m (18,000 ft) above sea level. The highest continuously inhabited city in the world is Morococha, Peru, located at an altitude of approximately 4,575 m (15,000 ft) above sea level. Leadville, Colorado, the highest city in the United States, is approximately 3,660 m (12,000 ft) above sea level. Figure 14–1 shows the inspired P_{O_2}, alveolar P_{O_2}, and blood P_{O_2} of subjects living either at sea level or at Morococha. At high altitudes, the partial pressures of CO_2 and water vapor in the alveoli are independent of the ambient pressure. Alveolar P_{O_2} (P_{AO_2}) is approximately:

$$P_{AO_2} = P_{IO_2} - 1.2 \ P_{ACO_2}$$

P_{IO_2} equals barometric pressure (P_B) minus partial pressure of water (P_{H_2O}) times the fractional concentration of O_2 ($F_{IO_2} = 0.21$, see Chap. 8). P_B decreases with increasing altitude, whereas P_{ACO_2} can only decrease by about 25 mmHg owing to hyperventilation. P_{AH_2O} remains constant (47 mmHg) because P_{H_2O} is determined only by body temperature. Thus, water vapor and CO_2 in the alveoli decrease P_{AO_2} to a relatively greater extent at high altitude than at sea

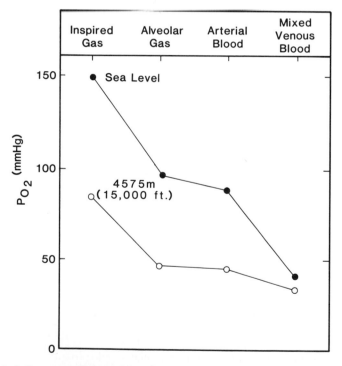

FIGURE 14–1. Oxygen partial pressures of inspired gas, alveolar gas, arterial blood, and mixed venous blood at sea level and in residents at an altitude of 4,575 m (15,000 ft). (Redrawn from Hurtado, A.: Animals in high altitudes: resident man. In: Dill, D.B., Adolph, E.F. (eds): *Handbook of Physiology. Adaptation to the Environment,* Washington, D.C., American Physiological Society, 1964, pp. 843–860.)

level. Fortunately, the P_{O_2} drop from alveolar gas to mixed venous blood is also reduced in subjects adapted to high altitudes. This is due to physiologic changes that enhance O_2 transport so that, even with the diminished inspired P_{O_2}, sufficient oxygen is maintained in the tissues to sustain proper oxidative metabolism.

Ventilatory Adjustments to Altitude

As shown in Figure 14–2, when a subject ascends from sea level to 4,575 m (15,000 ft) the $P_{I_{O_2}}$ decreases from 150 to 83 mmHg. Resting alveolar ventilation increases acutely at high altitudes from 4 to 7 l/min (as shown by the first two dashed vertical lines), and $P_{A_{O_2}}$ decreases from 100 mmHg at sea level (point A) to about 46 mmHg at an altitude of 4575 m (point C). The increased alveolar ventilation decreases $P_{A_{CO_2}}$ from 40 mmHg (point B) to about 28 mmHg (point D). This decreased $P_{A_{CO_2}}$ allows $P_{A_{O_2}}$ to be higher (point C) than it would have been without the hyperventilation (point G). Within several days to weeks (shown as chronic adaption in Fig. 14–2), alveolar ventilation increases further, to 10 l/min in this example, and this allows $P_{A_{O_2}}$ to rise from point C to point E and $P_{A_{CO_2}}$ to decrease from point D to point F. This new resting alveolar ventilation occurs because HCO_3^- ions are transported out of the cer-

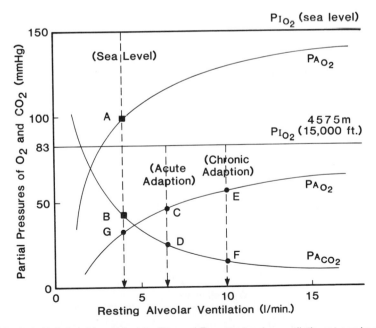

FIGURE 14–2. Relationship of alveolar P_{O_2} and P_{CO_2} to alveolar ventilation at sea level and at 4,575 m (15,000 ft) altitude. Dashed lines intercept $P_{A_{O_2}}$ and $P_{A_{CO_2}}$ curves at sea level and high altitude for different ventilations seen at different stages of high altitude adaption.

ebrospinal fluid into blood, thereby removing the braking effect of the high brain tissue $[HCO_3^-]$ on the central chemoreceptors.

In a high altitude native, vital capacity, functional residual capacity, and total lung capacity are all increased. Resting alveolar ventilation is approximately 20 per cent higher than in an altitude-adapted non-native. This increased ventilation is caused by an increased tidal volume, with no significant increase in respiratory frequency. Another aspect of chronic adaption to altitude is an increased pulmonary diffusing capacity of about 30 per cent, which is due to an increased surface area for gas exchange associated with the increased lung volume.

Circulatory Adjustments to Altitude

Individuals adapted to high altitude living have an increased hematocrit and blood volume. Hematocrit can increase from a normal value of 40% to as much as 60%. This increased hematocrit is associated with a normal or slightly elevated cardiac output, a 10 to 20 per cent increase in blood volume, and a decreased plasma volume. Within only a few hours after exposure to hypoxia, the kidney releases erythropoietin, a 40,000 molecular weight glycoprotein, which stimulates red blood cell production by the bone marrow (Fig. 14–3). The increased hematocrit increases the oxygen-carrying capacity of the blood, providing more oxygen to the tissues. Renal hypoxia is then reduced by the increased O_2 delivery (dashed arrow), and the erythropoietin production decreases. Thus, a negative feedback system operates between tissue hypoxia and oxygen delivery to control erythropoietin production and the subsequent increase in red blood cell production leading to an increased O_2 delivery to the

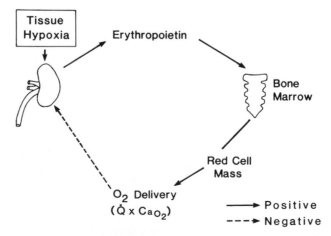

FIGURE 14–3. Diagram showing how erythropoietin production increases red cell mass, increasing O_2 delivery and relieving tissue hypoxia.

tissues. Hematocrit usually reaches a plateau level after about 2 months of living at high altitude.

Figure 14–4 summarizes the physiologic basis for the increased O_2 delivery to the tissues that occurs in high altitude adaption. The figure shows an idealized curve that relates cardiac output ($\dot{Q}$) and arterial O_2 content (CaO_2) to O_2 delivery ($\dot{Q} \times CaO_2$). The figure illustrates the inverse relationship between cardiac output and hematocrit and the direct relationship between arterial O_2 content and hematocrit. The product of blood flow and O_2 content (solid curved line for an individual living at sea level, $\dot{Q} \times CaO_2$) determines oxygen delivery. The oxygen delivery curve is bell shaped and attains a maximal value at a hematocrit of 45% for this particular sea level resident (vertical dotted line). After acclimatization (dashed lines for $\dot{Q} \times CaO_2$), the optimal hematocrit increases in this example to 50% (vertical dashed line). This increased hematocrit, combined with the increased cardiac output, causes O_2 delivery to approximately double. An increased red cell mass (polycythemia) facilitates oxygen delivery even in the presence of smaller arterial-to-venous PO_2 differences.

Figure 14–5 shows oxyhemoglobin dissociation curves for an individual living at sea level and a chronically altitude-adapted individual. In subjects chronically adapted to high altitude, both arterial (a) and mixed venous ($\bar{v}$) PO_2's fall on the steep portion of the oxyhemoglobin dissociation curve. Therefore, oxygen extraction is maintained at a level approximately equal to that seen in

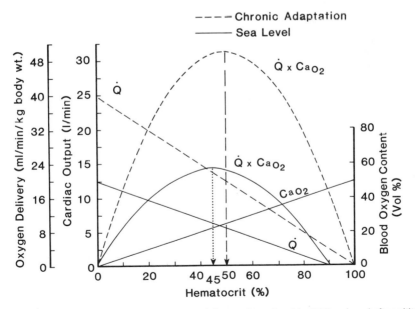

FIGURE 14–4. Optimal hematocrit for oxygen delivery at sea level (solid lines) and after altitude adaption (dashed lines). Relationships of cardiac output ($\dot{Q}$), arterial oxygen content (CaO_2), and oxygen delivery ($\dot{Q} \times CaO_2$) to hematocrit are shown. Arrows refer to sea level hematocrit (dotted) and chronic adaptation hematocrit (dashed).

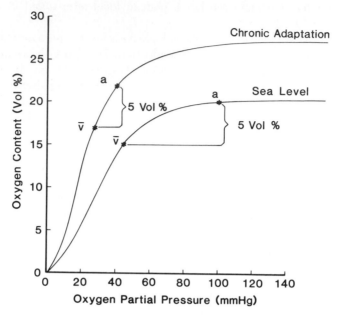

FIGURE 14–5. Oxyhemoglobin dissociation curves at sea level and during chronic altitude adaptation. The increased oxygen content for the chronic adaptation is due to an increased hemoglobin content. Note the same oxygen extractions for the two conditions.

a subject at sea level even though a smaller mixed arterial-to-venous P_{O_2} difference exists. In this example, no change in cardiac output is necessary because the arterial-to-venous difference in O_2 content is identical for both examples (5 vol %). The increased hemoglobin results in a larger O_2 content for the same oxygen partial pressure.

At high altitude, the oxyhemoglobin dissociation curve is affected by the

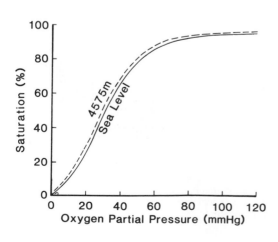

FIGURE 14–6. Oxyhemoglobin dissociation curves at sea level and after ascent to 4,575 m.

increased red cell 2,3-diphosphoglycerate (2,3-DPG) content (see Chap. 4), which should produce a right shift in the dissociation curve. Figure 14–6 shows the oxygen dissociation curve in terms of per cent saturation, which normalizes for the differences in hemoglobin content between sea level and altitude-adapted individuals as shown in Figure 14–5. In reality, the oxyhemoglobin curve is not shifted to the right at high altitudes but is actually slightly shifted to the left because the respiratory alkalosis overrides the 2,3-DPG effect (see Fig. 14–6).

Because of the low Pao_2 present at high altitudes, the pressure gradient for O_2 diffusion between capillaries and the tissues is also significantly lowered. To compensate for this reduced gradient for oxygen transfer into cells, new capillaries grow in the tissues. This decreases the distance for O_2 transfer from blood to tissues and slightly reduces the total vascular resistance (5 per cent). In addition, muscle myoglobin content increases, and this facilitates oxygen diffusion through the tissue.

Prolonged hypoxia at high altitude also has a striking effect on body fluid volume and blood pressure. The plasma volume decreases about 12 per cent owing to the water loss associated with hyperventilation and reduced water intake associated with loss of appetite. This decrease in plasma volume, and the existing tissue hypoxia, stimulate the secretion of renin by the kidney. Renin converts angiotensinogen to angiotensin I, which is then converted by the angiotensin converting enzyme (ACE) to angiotensin II. The increased angiotensin II level stimulates the release of aldosterone from the adrenal glands with subsequent sodium and fluid retention (Fig. 14–7). However, this response does not totally restore the plasma volume to normal, because the aldosterone release associated with angiotensin is reduced after high altitude adaption.

Medical Problems at Altitude

Central sleep apnea (see Chap. 11) can occur in normal sea level residents after they ascend to high altitudes. This breathing pattern is most likely to occur during rapid eye movement sleep and consists of periods of hyperventilation followed by apnea. The hyperventilation induced by the low arterial Po_2 in unacclimatized subjects reduces arterial Pco_2 and $[H^+]$ to levels approaching the apnea threshold. During sleep, the central chemoreceptor sensitivity to Pco_2 is reduced. This increased apnea threshold, in conjunction with the reduced respiratory drive, results in periods of apnea. The hypoxemia resulting from apnea excites the peripheral chemoreceptors, and the $Paco_2$ increases to levels that now excite the central chemoreceptors. The resulting hyperventilation decreases the $Paco_2$ to levels below the apnea threshold at the central chemoreceptor, and the increased Po_2 decreases the stimulation of the peripheral chemoreceptors so that another apneic period begins. Usually

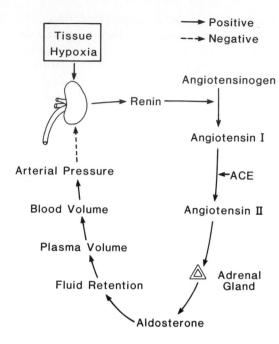

FIGURE 14–7. Diagram showing the acute effects of renal hypoxia and low plasma volume on fluid balance.

sleep apnea does not occur, but most subjects do experience some changes in their sleeping patterns at high altitudes.

ACUTE MOUNTAIN SICKNESS

Some individuals experience a physical and mental incapacity, called *acute mountain sickness*, 5 to 100 hours after ascending to high altitudes. The symptoms include headache, lightheadedness, irritability, dyspnea, weakness, lassitude, insomnia, and nausea. These symptoms usually subside over several days without any treatment and appear to be related to acute fluid retention (see Fig. 14–7). When severe, this problem can be treated with a diuretic.

A more serious problem that can occur at altitudes above 3000 m is pulmonary edema (high altitude pulmonary edema, HAPE). This condition sometimes occurs in unacclimatized subjects who rapidly ascend to high altitude. The condition is more often seen when a healthy, athletic person vigorously exercises at high altitudes. Surprisingly, mountain dwellers who return to high altitude after a period at sea level are particularly susceptible to the development of HAPE. Also, persons who develop edema are very prone to developing HAPE with each ascent to high altitude. The edema is thought to be due to pulmonary hypertension, which results from increased vascular volume, high cardiac output, and pulmonary hypoxic vasoconstriction. However, the exact mechanisms are not known, and very few unacclimatized individuals actually develop HAPE. The edema associated with high altitude occurs in the upper and middle lobes of the lung rather than the expected dependent portions of lungs. The high cardiac output and the pulmonary hypoxic vasoconstriction may produce sufficiently high pressures in large and small pulmonary arteries to damage the pulmonary vessels, causing them to more easily form edema. The pulmonary edema can be treated by having the subject inhale gas containing high oxygen concentrations and return to low altitudes.

Chronic Mountain Sickness

Chronic mountain sickness (Monge's disease) is seen in young or middle-aged men but rarely in women. Headache, dizziness, insomnia, and exercise intolerance are the usual symptoms. Cyanosis, clubbing of the fingers, congestive heart failure, and right heart hypertrophy are the most common findings. An essential component of this disease is a sustained secretion of erythropoietin and renin, which produces an abnormal hematocrit as high as 80% and can double the blood volume. Mean pulmonary artery pressure may increase to values exceeding 50 mmHg. Peripheral vascular resistance increases, owing to the increased blood viscosity, to such an extent that tissue perfusion is often inadequate, and the left heart may become overloaded and fail. Patients suffering from chronic mountain sickness should be moved to lower altitudes as soon as possible.

DIVING PHYSIOLOGY

Men working in deep underground mines or at depths beneath the ocean surface are exposed to very high ambient pressures. Tissue damage can occur as a result of changing gas volumes in enclosed spaces within the body, such as the thoracic cavity. In addition, the high partial pressures of respiratory gases can produce other serious pathophysiologic effects, such as N_2 narcosis, O_2 toxicity, and CO_2 toxicity.

Effect of Depth on Gas Volume and Density

Boyle's law dictates that a gas volume decreases in direct proportion to the applied pressure when temperature remains constant. Conversely, the volume of gas increases in proportion to a decrease in ambient pressure. This effect of pressure on gas volume is illustrated by the diving bell shown in Figure 14–8. The pressure surrounding the bell increases by 1 atm for every 10 m (33 ft) below sea level. Since ambient pressure is 1 atm at sea level, the gas volume will be decreased by one-half at a depth of 10 m (2 atm) and halved again at 30 m (4 atm). When a volume of gas expands or contracts within a rigid body space, severe stresses can be generated across its walls. If the pressure is not

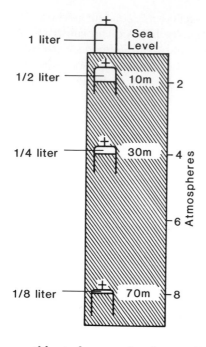

FIGURE 14–8. Effect of depth below sea level on gas volumes and ambient pressures.

equilibrated across the chest wall and lungs, paranasal sinuses, middle ear, and portions of the gastrointestinal tract, catastrophic tissue damage can occur.

During a breath-holding dive the ambient water pressure will compress the volume of gas in the lungs to one-fourth its original volume at a depth of 30 m. Since residual volume in the lung averages one-fourth of total lung capacity (TLC), the lung volume will be equal to residual volume if the lungs were filled to TLC at sea level. In some individuals, the residual volume may be as low as 16 per cent of TLC, such that a limiting depth of 50 m can be attained; at that depth, gas volume will equal residual volume. When lung volume becomes smaller than residual volume, alveolar pressure becomes sub-ambient, causing a condition referred to as *lung squeeze*. This condition results from reaching the limit of chest wall compressibility. This leads to pulmonary vascular engorgement, edema formation, and lung hemorrhage. As much as 1 liter of blood can enter the pulmonary vasculature to replace the lost gas volume. This allows some trained divers to descend to depths below 80 m.

When a scuba diver, breathing compressed air, ascends from a depth of 10 m (2 atm) while holding a breath of 50 per cent TLC, his lung volume expands to TLC at the water's surface. If this diver were to hold a breath equal to 75 per cent TLC at 10 m's depth, then his lungs would not be able to expand to 150 per cent of TLC at the water's surface and lung rupture would occur. In fact, ascent from only 1 m may damage the lungs when holding a breath equal to TLC while surfacing. Lung rupture produces pneumothorax, gas dissection along the mediastinum into the neck, and gas emboli in the blood vessels. Severe lung damage is accompanied by cough, chest pain, and dyspnea ("the chokes") and is best diagnosed using a chest roentgenogram. Treatment is immediate recompression to a similar pressure, followed by slow decompression.

Other gas-filled body spaces can be damaged during descent and subsequent ascent if significant transmural pressure gradients are allowed to develop across these boundaries. In particular, the middle ear may be damaged when middle ear pressure does not equilibrate with pressures in the outer ear canal and inner ear (Fig. 14–9). If the eustachian tube is blocked during a dive, a pressure gradient develops across the tympanic membrane, causing a sensation known as *ear squeeze*. This same phenomenon occurs when an airplane descends, a condition most readers should be able to appreciate. When the pressure difference between the outer and middle ear exceeds 60 mmHg, the pain of ear squeeze develops, and the tympanic membrane usually ruptures when the pressure difference is 100 to 150 mmHg. Although the round window is more resistant to rupture than the tympanic membrane, it can also rupture. If a diver attempts to clear a blocked eustachian tube by increasing his oral pressure when a large pressure gradient already exists across the round window, the round window can rupture, resulting in loss of fluid from the inner ear into the middle ear space. Damage to either membrane produces severe pain and a hearing impairment.

Paranasal sinuses are also susceptible to barotrauma during dives when sinus openings are blocked by swollen mucosa or polyps. Local sinus pain and mucosal contusions can occur on ascent or descent if the sinus block is not relieved. Expansion of trapped gas in dental caries and the gastrointestinal tract can also produce pain when ascending from depths. A common type of compressive "squeeze" occurs when one dives without equilibrating face mask pressure with ambient pressure. Facial edema, conjunctival hemorrhage, and

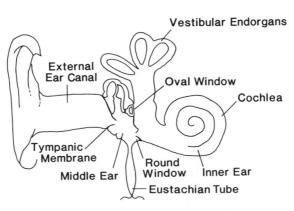

FIGURE 14–9. Diagram of outer, middle, and inner ear structures showing the location of possible rupture points at the tympanic membrane and round window.

pain can result. A severe form of "squeeze" can occur in helmet diving if a diver suddenly loses helmet pressure at a great depth. In some instances the diver has been squeezed into the diving helmet, experiencing total "body squeeze."

In addition to reducing the volume of a gas, high ambient pressures also increase the density of the gas in proportion to the reduction of gas volume. Because gas flow velocity is inversely proportional to the square root of gas density, the flow velocity of compressed air breathed at 30 m below sea level will be one-half that at sea level for the same muscular effort. At 15 atm (150 m) the density effect will reduce gas velocity to one-fourth of that occurring at sea level for the same pressure gradient. For practical purposes, however, density effects do not markedly limit work performance at depth, since breathing during work is still significantly lower than the maximal breathing capacity. Only at depths below 30 m does the density effect on gas velocity begin to limit the work capacity of a diver. Above this depth, the resistance of the external breathing circuit limits the ventilation to a greater extent. Below 30 m, the problem of nitrogen narcosis places practical limits on compressed air breathing. At greater depths, helium is substituted for nitrogen in the breathing mixture since helium is less dense than air and greatly reduces the work of breathing at great depths.

Gas Partial Pressures at Depth

High ambient pressures, encountered in undersea diving, also modify alveolar gas partial pressures. As a person holds his breath and dives, the alveolar gases are compressed and their partial pressures increase. During descent to 10 m (Fig. 14–10), O_2 consumption remains constant. The removal of O_2 from the alveoli into the blood tends to reduce alveolar P_{O_2}, but this effect is almost exactly offset by the increase in $P_{A_{O_2}}$ with depth. The alveolar P_{CO_2} increases during descent, and an alveolar-to-arterial P_{CO_2} gradient is established that actually causes CO_2 uptake into the blood. Obviously, the body CO_2 stores are increased during descent. On ascent, the alveolar P_{O_2} and P_{CO_2} decrease precipitously so that $P_{A_{O_2}}$ decreases to levels equal to venous blood and no exchange of oxygen occurs at the end of the dive, whereas the elimination of CO_2 returns toward normal. Note that N_2 is absorbed from the lung during descent and is not released during ascent, resulting in a net increase in body N_2 during the dive.

This effect of diving on gas exchange has been implicated in many of the over 7000 drownings that occur each year in the United States. Breath-hold dive time is limited by the build-up of Pa_{CO_2} because the central chemoreceptors sense a change in CO_2, whereas the peripheral carotid body inputs only sense a normal Pa_{O_2}. Longer breath-holding times can be attained by hyperventilating prior to diving, which reduces Pa_{CO_2} and delays the onset of

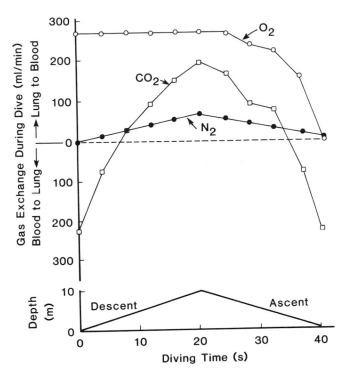

FIGURE 14–10. Effects of a 10-m breath-hold dive and subsequent ascent on O_2, CO_2, and N_2 exchange across the alveolar capillary membrane. (Redrawn from Hong, S.K., Lin, Y.C., Lally, D.A., Yim, B.J.B., Kominami, N., Hong, P.W. and Moore, J.O.: Alveolar gas exchanges and cardiovascular functions during breath holding with air. *J. Appl. Physiol., 30*:540–547, 1971.)

the urge to breathe. If the dive is extended for too long, P_{AO_2} falls, resulting in unconsciousness, which may lead to drowning.

Diving Reflex

The cardiovascular changes that occur during diving are described as the *diving reflex*. Hemodynamic variables measured in a human during a 60-sec breath-hold dive are shown in Figure 14–11. Bradycardia, decreased forearm blood flow, and increased mean systemic arterial pressure associated with increased peripheral resistance are seen in the diving reflex. These responses serve to maintain a supply of oxygenated blood to the heart and brain at the expense of skeletal muscle. The heart and brain cannot tolerate ischemia for more than 3 min, whereas skeletal muscle can tolerate over 12 hr of ischemia. The muscular energy used during the dive is supplied by anaerobic glycolysis, and the lactate is metabolized after completion of the dive. The diving reflex is developed to a remarkable degree in diving marine mammals. Weddell seals and sperm whales can dive to depths of 600 and 1000 m, respectively. Such

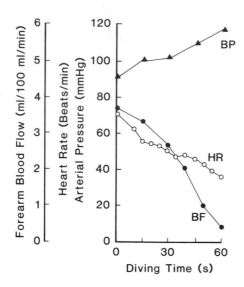

FIGURE 14–11. Effect of diving on mean arterial blood pressure (BP), heart rate (HR), and forearm blood flow (BF) in a human subject. (Redrawn from Campbell, L.B., Gooden, B.A., Horowitz, J.D.: Cardiovascular responses to partial and total immersion in man. *J. Physiol. [London]* 202:239–250, 1969.)

mammals have an enlarged compliant aortic root that can store the cardiac stroke volume and maintain a constant arterial pressure during intense vasoconstriction in peripheral muscles and visceral organs. Large quantities of blood hemoglobin and muscle myoglobin increase body oxygen stores and can extend breath-hold dives of these animals to over 1 hr.

Medical Problems Associated with Diving

DECOMPRESSION SICKNESS

The high partial pressures encountered when diving can cause respiratory gases to produce life-threatening effects. The most common complication seen in diving is decompression sickness, also called the "bends" or "caisson disease," which is due to ascending too rapidly. Since nitrogen obeys Henry's Law, large quantities can dissolve in body fluids because of the high pressure associated with deep diving. When a diver ascends rapidly to the surface, the ambient pressure decreases well below the partial pressure of the nitrogen dissolved in the tissues. Because of the high N_2 partial pressure, bubbles form in body fluids, much like the bubbles in champagne that form when the high bottle pressure is released by removing the cork. Tissues with the highest blood flow equilibrate more rapidly with the ambient N_2 partial pressures on ascents and descents. The brain, spinal cord, and adipose tissue can absorb large quantities of N_2 because of their high lipid content. Brain and spinal cord equilibrate rapidly with N_2, whereas adipose tissue equilibrates very slowly because of its low blood flow.

The probability of decompression sickness increases in proportion to the depth and length of time of the dive and the rapidity of ascent. Decompression tables are available that describe the amount of time required for a safe decompression for dives of various depths and durations. If nitrogen bubbles form within the thoracic and lumbar cord, paresthesias and hyperesthesias ("pins and needles") in the lower trunk and extremities may result. If gas bubbles form in the cerebral vessels, hemiplegia and permanent paralysis may result. Gas emboli to the coronary arteries can produce angina and arrhythmias. Pain is often present around joints. Aseptic necrosis of the articular portions of the proximal upper and lower extremity long bones can occur after multiple cycles of compression and decompression.

The best treatment for severe decompression sickness is immediate recompression followed by slow decompression. Mild cases are often treated by simply breathing 100% oxygen, which creates a large partial pressure gradient of N_2 between tissue and blood and facilitates N_2 clearances.

NITROGEN NARCOSIS

At high partial pressures, additional N_2 dissolves in the lipid of CNS tissue and acts as an anesthetic gas. Nitrogen narcosis or "the rapture of the deep" refers to the euphoria, lightheadedness, and drunken-like state that occurs in divers breathing compressed air at depths below 30 m. Below a depth of 50 m, symptoms become severe and a diver may become mentally impaired. Divers at that depth have mistakenly thought that an assigned task was completed and have even been known to offer a mouthpiece to a passing fish. At 100 m, unconsciousness can occur. These problems can be prevented by substituting helium in the gas mixture for N_2. Helium is much less soluble and does not have the anesthetic properties of N_2 at these depths.

OXYGEN TOXICITY

An additional hazard associated with deep dives is related to the high partial pressure of oxygen. Breathing 100% oxygen for extended periods damages the alveolar epithelial and endothelial membranes. When breathing compressed air, the alveolar P_{O_2} would be approximately 800 mmHg at a depth of 40 m and increase to approximately 3,360 mmHg at 200 m. These higher P_{O_2}s can produce oxidative damage to tissues in short periods of time. Superoxide anion, hydrogen peroxide, and hydroxyl radicals produce lipid peroxidation of cell membranes, inhibit enzyme function, and interrupt nerve conduction. Neurologic damage usually precedes pulmonary damage, but both can be prevented by using the proper helium and oxygen mixtures. Oxygen concentration is progressively reduced with depth. Only a low O_2 concentration is required to maintain alveolar oxygen partial pressures near normal, e.g., only 1% O_2 is needed, at a depth of 200 m, to produce a $P_{A_{O_2}}$ of 150 mmHg.

SUGGESTED READING

Elsner, R., and Gooden, B.: *Diving and Asphyxia*. London: Cambridge University Press, 1983.
Guyton, A.C.: *Textbook of Medical Physiology.* 7th ed., Philadelphia: W.B. Saunders, 1986, Chapters 44 and 45.
Heath, D., and Williams, D.R.: *Men at High Altitude*. Edinburgh: Churchill Livingstone, 1977.
Strauss, R.H.: *Diving Medicine*. New York: Grune and Stratton, 1976.
Weil, J.V.: Ventilatory control at high altitude. In Cherniack, N.S., and Widdicombe, J.G. (eds.): *Handbook of Physiology:* Section 3, The Respiratory System, Volume 2, Control of Breathing. Part 2. Bethesda: APS, 1986.
West, J.B., and Lahiri, S. (eds.): *High Altitude and Man*. Bethesda: APS, 1984.

QUESTIONS

1. A diver at 600 ft below sea level must breathe an oxygen-helium mixture with approximately what per cent O_2 to attain a normal inspired air P_{O_2} of 150 mmHg?

2. If 2 l of compressed air were inspired at 300 ft below the ocean surface, calculate the volume of the air at sea level.

3. Given that barometric pressure is 500 mmHg and $P_{A_{CO_2}}$ is 30 mmHg, calculate $P_{A_{O_2}}$.

4. Describe what happens to the following parameters during chronic altitude acclimatization:

   a. Bicarbonate ion concentration in the cerebrospinal fluid and $P_{A_{CO_2}}$ and $P_{A_{CO_2}}$

   b. Resting ventilation

   c. Blood volume and hematocrit

   d. Vital capacity

APPENDIX A
DERIVATION OF
ALVEOLAR GAS
EQUATION

At end-inspiration, some of the inhaled gas remains in the dead space, whereas the major portion reaches the respiratory zone of the lung. The latter is referred to as the inspiratory alveolar ventilation ($\dot{V}_{AI}$). By convention, the expired (not the inspired) alveolar gas volume per unit time is defined as alveolar ventilation ($\dot{V}_{A}$). Differentiating the inspired from the expired alveolar ventilation may seem superfluous, but it is important because in a steady state O_2 uptake exceeds CO_2 elimination; thus, the inspired alveolar ventilation is somewhat larger than the expired alveolar ventilation.

To derive the alveolar gas equation, two assumptions are made: (1) inspired volume of nitrogen per unit time ($\dot{V}_I \times F_{IN_2}$) equals expired volume of nitrogen per unit time ($\dot{V}_E \times F_{EN_2}$) (see Chap. 4), and (2) gas exchange does not occur in the dead space. $\dot{V}_{N_2}$ being the nitrogen exchange, the two assumptions can be stated in mathematical terms:

$$\dot{V}_{N_2} = (\dot{V}_I \times F_{IN_2}) - (\dot{V}_E \times F_{EN_2}) = 0$$

or

$$\dot{V}_{N_2} = (\dot{V}_{AI} \times F_{IN_2}) - (\dot{V}_A \times F_{AN_2}) = 0$$

Solving for $\dot{V}_{AI}$ in the latter equation:

$$\dot{V}_{AI} = \dot{V}_A (F_{AN_2}/F_{IN_2})$$

273

From Equation 4–7:

$$\dot{V}_{CO_2} = (\dot{V}_E \times F_{ECO_2}) - (\dot{V}_I \times F_{ICO_2})$$

which can be rewritten as:

$$\dot{V}_{CO_2} = (\dot{V}_A \times F_{ACO_2}) - (\dot{V}_{AI} \times F_{ICO_2})$$

Inserting $\dot{V}_{AI}$ yields:

$$\dot{V}_{CO_2} = \dot{V}_A (F_{ACO_2} - F_{ICO_2} \times F_{AN_2}/F_{IN_2})$$

A similar equation can be derived for the oxygen consumption:

$$\dot{V}_{O_2} = \dot{V}_A (F_{IO_2} \times F_{AN_2}/F_{IN_2} - F_{AO_2})$$

Dividing $\dot{V}_{CO_2}$ by $\dot{V}_{O_2}$ and substituting partial pressures for fractional gas concentrations yields the important alveolar gas equation:

$$P_{AO_2} = P_{IO_2} + \left[F_{IO_2} \frac{(1 - R)}{R} - \frac{(1)}{R} \right] P_{ACO_2} \qquad (8\text{--}10)$$

in which R is the respiratory exchange ratio, that is, $\dot{V}_{CO_2}/\dot{V}_{O_2}$.

APPENDIX B
ANSWERS TO
CHAPTER QUESTIONS

CHAPTER 1:

1. True. Increases from 2 to approximately 1000 cm^2 (Fig. 1–6).
2. False. Produced by type II cells.
3. True.
4. False. The postganglionic parasympathetic system is excitatory; the non-cholinergic-nonadrenergic system is the inhibitory system in man.

CHAPTER 2:

1. a and d *cannot* be measured by simple spirometry.
2. $FRC = \dfrac{V_1(C_1 - C_2)}{C_2} = \dfrac{4(10 - 5)}{5} - 4\,l.$
3. $\dot{V}_A = 863$ mmHg (400 ml/min)/(40 mmHg)
   $= 8.63$ l/min.

CHAPTER 3:

1. The diffusion of CO_2 across the alveolar-capillary membrane is 20 times faster for CO_2 than for O_2, but the rate of chemical reactions involving CO_2 in the blood is much slower than for O_2.
2. Hemoglobin has an extremely high affinity for CO, that is, large amounts of CO can combine with hemoglobin without appreciably raising the partial

pressure of CO in blood. Hence, the amount of CO that is transferred is not limited by the uptake in blood, but rather by the properties of the alveolar-capillary membrane.

3. The most common cause for a reduction in the CO diffusing capacity of the lung is a reduction in the surface area for diffusion, not an increase in the thickness of the alveolar-capillary membrane.

CHAPTER 4:

1. The oxygen content is the total amount of oxygen carried in blood, that is, the oxygen in solution in plasma plus that combined with hemoglobin. Oxygen capacity is the maximal volume of oxygen that can be bound by hemoglobin. Oxygen saturation is the amount of oxygen chemically combined, with hemoglobin expressed as a percentage of the oxygen capacity.

2. The oxygen hemoglobin dissociation curve is flat at high oxygen tensions. It thus provides a protective effect against fluctuations in oxygen content when alveolar oxygen tension is lowered. The steepness of the oxyhemoglobin dissociation curve at low oxygen tensions facilitates the unloading of oxygen from hemoglobin, because small changes in oxygen tension greatly reduce the oxygen content of the blood.

3. The position of the CO_2 dissociation curve is affected by the degree of hemoglobin oxygenation. When oxygen is released from the hemoglobin into the tissue, the capacity of the blood to carry CO_2 increases. In the absence of the Haldane effect, the P_{CO_2} in the blood, and therefore the tissue, would need to increase more than it does in the presence of the Haldane effect.

4. Most carbon dioxide in the body is stored as bicarbonate in bone. Approximately 850 ml of oxygen can be stored by hemoglobin in a subject with a blood volume of 5 l. If the hemoglobin concentration is 16 g/dl and if the hemoglobin is completely saturated with oxygen in the arterial blood, then 1 l of arterial blood can store 220.8 ml. If the venous blood volume is 4 l and if its hemoglobin is saturated to 75% with oxygen, then it can store 662.4 ml.

5. $\dot{V}_{O_2} = \{[(F_{E_{N_2}}/F_{I_{N_2}}) \times F_{I_{O_2}}] - F_{E_{O_2}}\} \times \dot{V}_E$
   $= \{[(0.85/0.80) \times 0.20] - 0.15\} \times 7,500$ ml/min
   $= 468.8$ ml/min.

6. a. $P_{O_2}/760 \times \alpha_{O_2} = 85/760 \times 2.3 = 0.26$ ml/100 ml. The subject, therefore, has $22 - 0.26 = 21.74$ ml O_2 combined with hemoglobin in 100 ml of blood.

   b. The maximum O_2 that can combine with 16 g of hemoglobin is 22.1 ml. The O_2 saturation of hemoglobin is, therefore, 21.74/22.1, or 98.4%.

7. $\dot{V}_{O_2} = \dot{Q}(Ca_{O_2} - C\bar{v}_{O_2})$

$$\dot{Q} = \frac{\dot{V}_{O_2}}{(Ca_{O_2} - C\bar{v}_{O_2})}$$

$$= \frac{400 \text{ ml/min}}{19 \text{ ml/100 ml} - 16 \text{ ml/100 ml}}$$

$$= \frac{400 \text{ ml/min}}{3 \text{ ml/100 ml}}$$

$$= 13333 \text{ ml/min}$$

$$= 13.33 \text{ l/min}.$$

8. $\dot{V}_{CO_2} = F_{ECO_2} \times \dot{V}_E$
   $$= (0.05) \times (7,500 \text{ ml/min})$$
   $$= 375 \text{ ml/min}.$$

CHAPTER 5:

1. 2.5 cmH$_2$O/l/min.
2. 33 ml/min.
3. 12 times.
4. Distension and recruitment decrease regional vascular resistance down zone III, but a reduced lung recoil narrows extra-alveolar vessels down zone IV.

CHAPTER 6:

1. a. 0.8 l ÷ 4 cmH$_2$O.
2. a. The dependent right lung is ventilated better than the nondependent lung.
3. True. The time constant of region A has been increased three-fold.

CHAPTER 7:

1. At the increased atmospheric pressure gas density is increased tenfold. This increases the Reynolds number, resulting in turbulent flow and increased airway resistance, which leads to dyspnea. Resistance, and hence effort, during turbulent flow can be decreased by administering a gas with a lower density than air. The density of the He:O$_2$ mixture is about one-third that of air.

2. False. Resistance is decreased, but conductance is increased near TLC.
3. See Fig. 7–16B. Once dynamic compression has occurred you are on the plateau of the IVPF curve and increased effort does not increase flow (effort independent).

CHAPTER 8:

1. The V_D/V_T for this patient is 0.67, that is, 67% of the tidal volume is wasted in terms of carbon dioxide exchange (Eq. 8–4).
2. The arteriovenous oxygen content difference can be calculated from the rearranged Fick equation:

a. $(Ca_{O_2} - C\bar{v}_{O_2}) = \dfrac{\dot{V}_{O_2}}{\dot{Q}} \times 100 = \dfrac{0.240}{6.0} \times 100 = 4.0$ vol %.

b. $\dot{Q}s/\dot{Q} = \dfrac{(P_{A_{O_2}} - Pa_{O_2}) \times 0.0031}{(P_{A_{O_2}} - Pa_{O_2}) \times 0.0031 + 4} = \dfrac{0.558}{4.558} \times 100$

$= 12.2\%$ of the cardiac output.

3. The perfusion of region 1 is $[\dot{V}_A/(\dot{V}_A/\dot{Q})] = 0.5/0.2$ or 2.5 l/min, and the perfusion of region 2 is (3.9/2.0) or 1.95 l/min, i.e., overall $\dot{Q}$ is (2.5 + 1.95), or 4.45 l/min. Therefore, the fractional perfusion of region 1 is (2.5/4.45) or 56%, and that of region 2 is (1.95/4.45) or 44%. The overall alveolar ventilation is 4.4 l/min. The fractional ventilation of region 1 is (0.5/4.4) or 0.11, and that of region 2 is (3.9/4.44) or 0.89.

The overall $P_{A_{CO_2}}$ calculated from the weighted average of the $P_{A_{CO_2}}$ in the two regions is $[(0.11 \times 46) + (0.89 \times 35)] = 36.2$ mmHg, and the overall $P_{A_{O_2}}$ is $[(0.11 \times 53) + (0.89 \times 129)] = 120.6$ mmHg.

The overall Pa_{O_2} and Pa_{CO_2} *cannot* be calculated from the weighted average of the regional gas tension. One must first determine the weighted average of the overall O_2 and CO_2 contents in blood and then determine the appropriate overall Pa_{O_2} and Pa_{CO_2} from the oxyhemoglobin and CO_2 dissociation curve, respectively. The carbon dioxide content of region 1 is 51.2 vol %, and that of region 2 is 46 vol %, that is, the overall carbon dioxide content is $[(0.56 \times 51.2) + (0.44 \times 46)] = 48.9$ vol %. This is equivalent to a Pa_{CO_2} of 41 mmHg. The oxygen content of region 1 is 17.4 vol %, and that of region 2 is 19.8 vol %, that is, the overall oxygen content is $[(0.56 \times 17.4) + (0.44 \times 19.8)] = 18.45$ vol %. This is equivalent to an overall Pa_{O_2} of 78.0 mmHg. Therefore, the $(A - a)D_{O_2} = (120.6 - 78.0) = 42.6$ mmHg, and the $(a - A)D_{CO_2} = (41.0 - 36.2) = 4.8$ mmHg.

	Region 1	Region 2	Overall
$\dot{V}_A/\dot{Q}$	0.20	2.0	0.99
Gas phase:			
$\dot{V}_A$, l/min	0.5	3.9	4.4
$\dot{V}_A\%$ of overall	(11%)	(89%)	(100%)
P_{ACO_2}, mmHg	46	35	36.2
P_{AO_2}, mmHg	53	129	120.6
Blood phase:			
$\dot{Q}$, l/min	2.5	1.95	4.45
$\dot{Q}\%$ of overall	(56%)	(44%)	(100%)
Pa_{CO_2}, mmHg	46	35	41
Ca_{CO_2}, vol %	51.2	46	48.9
Pa_{O_2}, mmHg	53	129	78.0
Ca_{O_2}, vol %	17.4	19.8	18.45

$(A - a)D_{O_2} = 120.6 - 78 = 42.6$ mmHg

$(a - A)D_{CO_2} = 41 - 36.2 = 4.8$ mmHg

4. $P_{AO_2} = (760 - 47) - 30 = 713 - 30 = 683$ mmHg.
$(A - a)D_{O_2} = 683 - 100 = 583$ mmHg.

$(Ca - C\bar{v})_{CO_2} = \dfrac{0.250}{3.0} \times 100 = 8.33$ vol %.

$\dot{Q}s/\dot{Q} = \dfrac{583 \times 0.0031}{(583 \times 0.0031) + 8.33} = \dfrac{1.81}{10.14} = 0.179.$

$\dot{Q}s = 0.179 \times 3.0 = 0.535$ l/min.

5. $(Ca - C\bar{v})_{O_2} = \dfrac{0.25}{6.0} \times 100 = 4.17$ vol %.

$\dot{Q}s/\dot{Q} = \dfrac{583 \times 0.0031}{(583 \times 0.0031) + 4.17} = \dfrac{1.81}{5.98} = 0.303.$

$\dot{Q}s = 0.303 \times 6.00 = 1.82$ l/min.

CHAPTER 9:

1. a. Obstructive.
   b. Increased TLC (hyperinflation), reduced FEV_1 (severe obstruction).
   c. Yes. Suggests emphysema based on low D_{LCO}.
   d. A significant reduction in lung recoil at TLC (Pst,L_{TLC}) would be very suggestive of pure emphysema. Indeed, this patient proved to have alpha 1–antitrypsin deficiency. Pure emphysema was proven at post mortem 5 years later. The family history is very consistent with this diagnosis.
2. a. Mild obstructive.

    b. The reduction in the FEV_1 to 63% predicted but especially the FEV_1% of 3/5, or 60%.

    c. The marked improvement to essentially normal following bronchodilator administration indicates hyperreactive airways, most likely asthma. In addition, the supranormal D_{LCO} is seen in asthma.

    d. No further testing is warranted at this time. The patient was placed on regular bronchodilator therapy and the cough subsided. Cough is frequently the first symptom of bronchospasm even before the patient notes wheezing.

3. a. Restrictive.

    b. Reduced TLC and FVC in face of a normal FEV_1% (2.0/2.2 = 91%). Most important is the associated marked reduction in D_{LCO}.

    c. In view of the very low D_{LCO}, this is most likely due to parenchymal lung disease, such as idiopathic pulmonary fibrosis (IPF).

    d. A crucial bit of evidence is the chest roentgenogram, which showed a diffuse interstitial pattern consistent with IPF. In this case, a lung biopsy confirmed the diagnosis. Pst,L_{TLC} was increased to -50 cmH_2O, and both static and dynamic compliance were markedly reduced. Pa_{CO_2} was 32 mmHg, and Pa_{O_2} was only 50 mmHg at rest. Cough is often a complaint in these patients, and clubbing of the fingers may occur, as in this woman.

4. a. Obstructive.

    b. Severely reduced FEV_1 and FEV_1% and increased RV/TLC ratio.

    c. Yes. Suggests chronic bronchitis based on smoking history and symptoms and the near normal D_{LCO}; also, there is no response to bronchodilator therapy, in contrast to what you would expect in asthma.

    d. Finding a normal Pst,L_{TLC} would make this case very consistent with chronic bronchitis secondary to tobacco abuse. Additional supportive data were a Pa_{O_2} of 55 mmHg and a Pa_{CO_2} of 45 mmHg measured at rest.

5. a. Restrictive.

    b. Reduced TLC and FVC with a normal FEV_1% (90%).

    c. A restrictive pattern with a normal D_{LCO} suggests an extraparenchymal problem.

    d. There is no obvious skeletal deformity, so the next step is to measure the strength of the respiratory muscles. This man had marked weakness with a maximal expiratory pressure of $+120$ cmH_2O and maximal inspiratory pressure of -60 cmH_2O. Normal predicted values were $+220$ and -160 cmH_2O, respectively. Pst,L_{TLC} was normal at -20 cmH_2O. The ineffective cough reflected the expiratory muscle weakness. Careful neurologic exam revealed early stages of amyotrophic lateral sclerosis.

6. a. Obstructive.

    b. The reduced FEV_1 and FEV_1% of 60. The fact that the RV/TLC ratio is normal is puzzling.

c. It is difficult to subclassify further on the basis of Table 9–1. The normal RV/TLC and DL_{CO} speak against emphysema. The lack of a history of smoking or of repeated respiratory infections speaks against chronic bronchitis, as does the normal RV/TLC ratio. Against asthma is the lack of improvement following bronchodilator therapy. We need more information.

d. On physical examination, inspiratory stridor was noted during rapid breathing. The MVV test was markedly reduced. Respiratory muscle strength was measured and was normal. Flow-volume loops (inspiratory and expiratory) were obtained and were markedly abnormal. The pattern was that of a fixed lesion (see Fig. 9–5). Peak expiratory flow was reduced to 1.5 l/s and peak inspiratory flow to 2 l/s. On bronchoscopy a stricture at the site of the tracheostomy was seen to narrow the airway to 4 mm in diameter. The stricture was resected and the trachea reanastomosed. The patient became symptom-free, and all tests returned to normal.

CHAPTER 10:

1. $Jv = 1$ ml/min/mmHg $\{[7-(-7)] - 0.9(28 - 13)\}$
   $= 1$ ml/min/mmHg $[14 - 0.9 (15)]$
   $= 1$ ml/min/mmHg $(14 - 13.5) = 0.5$ ml/min.
2. $Jv = 3$ ml/min/mmHg $[(7 - 0) - 0.5 (28 - 20)]$
   $= 3$ ml/min/mmHg $[7 - 0.5 (8)]$
   $= 3$ ml/min/mmHg $(7 - 4) = 9$ ml/min.
3. The tissue fluid pressure increases to 0 mmHg, lymph flow provides a safety factor equal to about 7 mmHg, and the tissue colloid osmotic pressure decreases to 7 mmHg.

Change in Starling forces
$Jv = 1$ ml/min/mmHg $[(20 - 0) - 0.9 (28 - 7)]$
$= 1$ ml/min/mmHg $[20 - 0.9 (21)]$
$= 1$ ml/min/mmHg $(20 - 19.8)$
$= 0.2$ ml/min.

No change in Starling forces
$Jv = 1$ ml/min/mmHg $[20 - (-7) - 0.9 (28 - 13)]$
$= 1$ ml/min/mmHg $(27 - 13.5)$
$= 13.5$ ml/min.

Since lymph flow can only carry away a fluid volume of about 7 ml/min (7 mmHg safety factor $\times$ Kfc) and the capillaries are filtering 13.5 ml/min, fluid will accumulate in the tissues, resulting in edema.

CHAPTER 11:

1. Sleep, depressant drugs, and adaption of central chemoreceptors to a sustained increase in Pa_{CO_2}.
2. Peripheral chemoreceptors.
3. Inspiratory time is shortened.
4. An acute loss of hypoxic peripheral chemoreceptor drive after adaption of the central chemoreceptors to a sustained elevation of Pa_{CO_2}.
5. The $\dot{V}_{O_2}$ at which $\dot{V}_E$ begins to exceed the rate required to meet metabolic O_2 demands. Carbon dioxide in excess of that produced by oxidative metabolism must be expired to compensate for metabolic acidosis.

CHAPTER 12:

1. a. Hypoxic hypoxemia: increased $\dot{V}_A/\dot{Q}$ mismatching, increased right-to-left shunting, inadequate diffusion, reduced inspired oxygen tension.
   b. Anemic hypoxemia: chronic anemia, methemoglobinemia, carbon monoxide poisoning.
   c. Stagnant hypoxia: inadequate circulation with low cardiac output or anaphylactic shock.
   d. Histotoxic hypoxia: cyanide poisoning.
2. According to current thinking, oxygen toxicity is caused by partially reduced oxygen products (oxygen-free radicals). Molecular oxygen is reduced to superoxide anion (O_2^-) and hydrogen peroxide (H_2O_2). These two combine (Haber-Weiss reaction) to form the very toxic hydroxyl radical ($OH\cdot$).
3. Decreased venous return is the primary cause. Reduced left ventricular function due to the shift of the ventricular septum also contributes to the decrease in cardiac output.
4. PEEP may increase fluid accumulation in the lung. This is caused by the lung distension associated with PEEP, which results in a more subatmospheric perivascular pressure, causing increased filtration of fluid from extra-alveolar vessels.
5. High-frequency ventilation is categorized into three major groups. (1) High-frequency positive pressure ventilation (HFPPV), which is sometimes used for endoscopic procedures. (2) High-frequency jet ventilation (HFJV) has been advocated for treatment of bronchopleural fistulas and certain surgical operations. (3) High-frequency oscillation has not found a clear indication in clinical practice.

CHAPTER 13:

1. The Henderson-Hasselbalch equation can be written as:

$$pH = 6.1 + \log \frac{[HCO_3^-]}{(0.03)P_{CO_2}}$$

So, $$pH = 6.1 + \log \frac{23 \text{ meq/l}}{(0.03) \, 50}$$

$$= 6.1 + \log (15.3)$$
$$= 6.1 + 1.19$$
$$= 7.29.$$

2. a. Bicarbonate salvage.
   b. Formation of titratable acids.
   c. Formation of ammonium ions.

3.

	pH	$P_{CO_2^-}$	$[HCO_3^-]$
Respiratory acidosis with renal compensation	Decreased	Increased	Increased
Respiratory alkalosis with renal compensation	Increased	Decreased	Decreased
Metabolic acidosis with respiratory compensation	Decreased	Decreased	Decreased
Metabolic alkalosis with respiratory compensation	Increased	Increased	Increased

4. Base excess = −10 meq/l.
   Arterial pH = 7.1.
   $NaHCO_3$ required = (0.30) (70 kg) (base excess)
   $$= 21(10 \text{ meq/l})$$
   $$= 210 \text{ meq/l.}$$
   (Note: Sodium bicarbonate must be *added*, since negative base excess represents a base deficit. Hence, the negative sign used in calculation of $NaHCO_3$ required has been dropped.)

CHAPTER 14:

1. Recall that the pressure of a gas increases by 1 atmosphere for each 33 ft a diver descends.
   $$\frac{600 \text{ ft}}{33 \text{ ft}} = 18.2 \text{ atm}$$
   Total pressure at 600 ft = 18.2 atm + 1 atm = 19.2 atm (at sea level).

Since $P_{O_2} = F_{I_{O_2}} (P_{Ambient} - 47 \text{ mmHg})$, solve for $F_{I_{O_2}}$.

$$F_{I_{O_2}} = \frac{P_{O_2}}{(P_{Ambient} - 47)}$$

$$F_{I_{O_2}} = \frac{150}{[19.2(760) - 47]}$$

$$F_{I_{O_2}} = 0.01$$

or about 1% of the mixture breathed at 600 ft.
2. At 300 ft below sea level, total pressure is:

$$\frac{300 \text{ ft}}{33 \text{ ft}} + 1 \text{ atm (at sea level)} =$$

9.1 atm + 1 atm = 10.1 atm.

Since the volume of a gas is inversely proportional to its pressure, it is possible to solve for the volume at sea level using Henry's Law.

(Pressure at 300 ft below sea level) (2 l) = (pressure at sea level) ($\times$ l)

$$(10.1 \text{ atm}) (2 \text{ l}) = (1 \text{ atm}) (\times 1 \text{ l}) \times = 20.2 \text{ l}$$

3. Recall that:
   (1) $P_{A_{O_2}} = P_{I_{O_2}} - 1.2 \, P_{A_{CO_2}}$
   (2) $P_{I_{O_2}} = F_{I_{O_2}} \times (P_B - P_{H_2O})$
   $\qquad = 0.21 \times (500 \text{ mmHg} - 47 \text{ mmHg})$
   $\qquad = 95.1 \text{ mmHg}.$

   Therefore,
   $\qquad P_{A_{O_2}} = 95.1 \text{ mmHg} - (1.2) (30 \text{ mmHg})$
   $\qquad\qquad = 95.1 \text{ mmHg} - 36 \text{ mmHg}$
   $\qquad\qquad = 59.1 \text{ mmHg}.$

4. During chronic altitude adaptation:
   a. Bicarbonate ion in the cerebrospinal fluid decreases, and $P_{A_{CO_2}}$ and $P_{A_{CO_2}}$ both decrease.
   b. Resting ventilation increases.
   c. Blood volume and hematocrit increase.
   d. Vital capacity increases.

APPENDIX C
INDICATOR DILUTION
MEASUREMENTS OF
PULMONARY BLOOD
FLOW AND VOLUME

Pulmonary blood flow can be measured by injecting an intravascular indicator into the right atrium and sampling at the pulmonary artery. Cardiogreen dye is a commonly used indicator because it binds to plasma proteins and is confined to the circulation. The rate of appearance of the injected dye is directly proportional to the flow and inversely proportional to the volume of distribution. Pulmonary blood flow ($\dot{Q}$) can be calculated by integrating the area under the outflow time-concentration (Ct) curve when the quantity of dye injected (Qd) is known.

$$\dot{Q} = Qd / \int_{o}^{t} Ct \, dt. \tag{C–1}$$

The mean transit time ($\bar{t}$) of the dye can be calculated by:

$$\bar{t} = \int_{o}^{t} t \cdot Ct \cdot dt / \int_{o}^{t} Ct \cdot dt. \tag{C–2}$$

The pulmonary blood volume (V_B) is calculated using the calculated mean transit time of the vascular marker between pulmonary artery and left atrium and pulmonary blood flow by:

$$V_B = \dot{Q} \cdot \bar{t}. \tag{C–3}$$

A bolus of cold saline is also used to measure blood flow when the volume

285

(Vi) and temperature (Ti) of injectate, the blood temperature (TB), and the specific gravity (SB, Si) and densities (DB, Di) of blood and injectate, respectively, are known using the following equation:

$$\dot{Q} = K \cdot Vi \cdot \left(\frac{Si\ Di}{SB\ DB}\right) \left(\frac{TB - Ti}{\int_o^t TB(t)\ dt}\right) \qquad (C–4)$$

Using a thermal indicator the distribution volume measures both the lung tissue fluid volume and blood volume when measured at the left atrium. Using this information, the differences in thermal and dye distribution volumes are used to evaluate extravascular lung water.

APPENDIX D
TABLE OF SYMBOLS

V_T	tidal volume
FRC	functional residual capacity
ERV	expiratory reserve volume
RV	residual volume
IC	inspiratory capacity
IRV	inspiratory reserve volume
TLC	total lung capacity
VC	vital capacity
V_D	dead space volume
V_A	alveolar gas volume
V_I	inspired volume
V_E	expired volume
V_D/V_T	ratio of dead space volume to tidal volume (fractional dead space)
$\dot{V}$	volume of ventilation per minute
$\dot{V}_I$	inspired volume of ventilation per minute
$\dot{V}_E$	expired volume of ventilation per minute
$\dot{V}_A$	alveolar ventilation per minute
$\dot{V}_{O_2}$	rate of oxygen uptake per minute (oxygen consumption)
$\dot{V}_{CO_2}$	rate of carbon dioxide elimination per minute
$\dot{V}max_{O_2}$	maximal oxygen consumption at high work loads
$\dot{V}max_{CO_2}$	maximal rate of carbon dioxide production at high work loads
R	respiratory exchange ratio

$\dot{V}_{N_2}$	rate of nitrogen uptake per minute
$\dot{V}_{CO}$	rate of carbon monoxide uptake per minute
DL_{O_2}	diffusing capacity of the lung for oxygen
DL_{CO}	diffusing capacity of the lung for carbon monoxide
DM_{CO}	diffusing capacity of the total alveolar membrane for carbon monoxide
Raw	airway resistance to air flow into the lung
RL	lung tissue resistance
$Cdyn,L$	dynamic compliance of the lung
Cst,L	static compliance of the lung
Pst,L	static recoil pressure of lung tissue
Pst,L_{TLC}	static recoil pressure of the lung tissue at TLC
FVC	forced expired vital capacity
FEV_1	volume of gas expired in the first second of forced expiration
FEF_{25-75}	average expiratory flow rate over the middle 50% of forced vital capacity
MEFV	maximal expiratory flow volume
$\dot{V}max_{50}$	maximal expiratory flow rate at 50% of vital capacity
$\dot{V}max_{50,He}$	$\dot{V}max_{50}$ measured when breathing a helium gas mixture
$\dot{V}max_{50,air}$	$\dot{V}max_{50}$ measured when breathing air
$\Delta\dot{V}max_{50}$	the change in $\dot{V}max_{50}$ measured when breathing a helium-oxygen mixture compared with that measured when breathing air
FI_{O_2}	fractional concentration of oxygen in inspired gas
FI_{CO_2}	fractional concentration of carbon dioxide in inspired gas
FI_{N_2}	fractional concentration of nitrogen in inspired gas
FI_{CO}	fractional concentration of carbon monoxide in inspired gas
FA_{CO_2}	fractional concentration of carbon dioxide in alveolar gas
FA_{N_2}	fractional concentration of nitrogen in alveolar gas
FA_{CO}	fractional concentration of carbon monoxide in alveolar gas
FE_{O_2}	fractional concentration of oxygen in expired gas
FE_{CO_2}	fractional concentration of carbon dioxide in expired gas
FE_{N_2}	fractional concentration of nitrogen in expired gas
FE_{CO}	fractional concentration of carbon monoxide in expired gas

$F\bar{E}_{CO_2}$	fractional concentration of carbon dioxide in mixed expired gas
P_B	atmospheric pressure
P_A or Palv	alveolar pressure
Ppl	pleural pressure
P_{O_2}	partial pressure of oxygen
P_{CO_2}	partial pressure of carbon dioxide
P_{N_2}	partial pressure of nitrogen
Pa_{O_2}	partial pressure of oxygen in arterial blood
Pa_{CO_2}	partial pressure of carbon dioxide in arterial blood
$P\bar{v}_{O_2}$	partial pressure of oxygen in mixed venous blood
$P\bar{v}_{CO_2}$	partial pressure of carbon dioxide in mixed venous blood
$P_{A_{O_2}}$	partial pressure of oxygen in alveolar gas
$P_{A_{CO_2}}$	partial pressure of carbon dioxide in alveolar gas
$P\bar{E}_{CO_2}$	partial pressure of carbon dioxide in mixed expired gas
$(A-a)D_{O_2}$	alveolar to arterial gradient for the partial pressure of oxygen
$(a-A)D_{CO_2}$	arterial to alveolar gradient for partial pressure of carbon dioxide
P_{H_2O}	partial pressure of water
$P_{A_{CO}}$	partial pressure of carbon monoxide in alveolar gas
$P_{A_{He}}$	partial pressure of helium in alveolar gas
$P_{I_{He}}$	partial pressure of helium in inspired gas
V_B	blood volume
$\dot{Q}$	blood flow
$\dot{Q}s$	shunt blood flow
$\dot{V}_A/\dot{Q}$	alveolar ventilation perfusion ratio
$\dot{Q}s/\dot{Q}t$	fractional shunt blood flow
C_{O_2}	concentration of oxygen
C_{CO_2}	concentration of carbon dioxide
Ca_{O_2}	concentration of oxgyen in arterial blood
$C\bar{v}_{O_2}$	concentration of oxygen in mixed venous blood
Ca_{CO_2}	concentration of carbon dioxide in arterial blood
$C\bar{v}_{CO_2}$	concentration of carbon dioxide in mixed venous blood
Cc'_{O_2}	concentration of oxygen in pulmonary end capillary blood

$(Ca-C\bar{v})_{O_2}$	arterial to mixed venous difference in blood oxygen concentration
$(C\bar{v}-Ca)_{CO_2}$	mixed venous to arterial difference in blood carbon dioxide concentration
S_{O_2}	percent saturation of hemoglobin with oxygen
Sa_{O_2}	percent saturation of hemoglobin with oxygen in arterial blood
$S\bar{v}_{O_2}$	percent saturation of hemoglobin with oxygen in mixed venous blood
Ppc	pulmonary capillary hydrostatic pressure
Ppa	pulmonary arterial hydrostatic pressure
Pla	left atrial hydrostatic pressure
P$_T$	interstitial hydrostatic pressure
P$_{LYM}$	lymphatic hydrostatic pressure
Ppl,f	pleural fluid hydrostatic pressure
πP	plasma colloid osmotic pressure for total proteins
πT	tissue fluid colloid osmotic pressure for total proteins
C$_P$	concentration of protein in plasma
C$_T$	concentration of protein in tissue fluid
Kfc	pulmonary capillary filtration coefficient
JV	rate of transcapillary fluid movement
σd	osmotic reflection coefficient for total proteins
ΔLF	change in lymph flow
ΔP$_T$	change in tissue hydrostatic pressure

The authors wish to thank Dr. Mary I. Townsley for compiling this table of symbols.

INDEX

Note: Numbers in *italic* refer to illustrations; numbers followed by t indicate tables.

291